WITHDRAWN
WRIGHT STATE UNIVERSITY LIBRARIES

ADVANCES IN NEUROLOGY

Volume 62

Advances in Neurology

INTERNATIONAL ADVISORY BOARD

Julius Axelrod, *Bethesda*
H. J. M. Barnett, *London, Canada*
Thomas Brandt, *Munich*
Donald B. Calne, *Vancouver*
Macdonald Critchley, *Somerset*
Roger C. Duvoisin, *New Brunswick*
Stanley Fahn, *New York*
Robert A. Fishman, *San Francisco*
Sid Gilman, *Ann Arbor*
Gilbert H. Glaser, *New Haven*
Gary W. Goldstein, *Baltimore*
Herbert H. Jasper, *Montreal*
Bryan Jennett, *Glasgow*
Richard T. Johnson, *Baltimore*
Harold L. Klawans, *Chicago*
Donlin M. Long, *Baltimore*
C. David Marsden, *London, UK*
Joseph B. Martin, *Boston*
W. Ian McDonald, *London, UK*
J. Kiffin Penry, *Winston-Salem*
Alfred Pope, *Belmont*
Dominick P. Purpura, *Bronx*
Pasko Rakic, *New Haven*
Roger N. Rosenberg, *Dallas*
Lewis P. Rowland, *New York*
Arnold B. Scheibel, *Los Angeles*
Peritz Scheinberg, *Miami*
Richard P. Schmidt, *Gainesville*
Donald B. Tower, *Chevy Chase*
John N. Walton, *Oxford*
Arthur A. Ward, Jr., *Seattle*
Stephen G. Waxman, *New Haven*
Melvin D. Yahr, *New York*
Anne B. Young, *Boston*

Advances in Neurology
Volume 62

Cerebral Small Artery Disease

Editors

Patrick M. Pullicino, M.D., Ph.D.
*Assistant Professor
Department of Neurology
State University of New York at Buffalo
Buffalo, New York*

Louis R. Caplan, M.D.
*Professor and Chairman
Department of Neurology
Tufts New England Medical Center
Boston, Massachusetts*

Marc Hommel, M.D.
*Neurologist
Department of Clinical and Biological Sciences
Stroke Unit
Centre Hospitalier Universitaire Régional de Grenoble
Grenoble, France*

RAVEN PRESS ● NEW YORK

Raven Press, Ltd., 1185 Avenue of the Americas, New York, New York 10036

© 1993 by Raven Press, Ltd. All rights reserved. This book is protected by copyright. No part of it may be reproduced, stored in a retrieval system, or transmitted, in any form or by any means, electronic, mechanical, photocopying, recording, or otherwise, without prior written permission of the publisher.

Made in the United States of America

Library of Congress Cataloging-in-Publication Data

Cerebral small artery disease / edited by Patrick M. Pullicino, Louis R. Caplan, Marc Hommel.
    p. cm.
  Includes bibliographical references and index.
  ISBN 0-7817-0051-5
  1. Cerebral infarction. 2. Cerebrovascular disease.
I. Pullicino, Patrick M. II. Caplan, Louis R. III. Hommel, Marc.
  [DNLM: 1. Cerebral Artery Diseases. WL 355 C4125 1993]
RC394.I5C47 1993
616.8'1—dc20
DNLM/DLC
for Library of Congress   92-48462
                                                                    CIP

The material contained in this volume was submitted as previously unpublished material, except in the instances in which credit has been given to the source from which some of the illustrative material was derived.

Great care has been taken to maintain the accuracy of the information contained in the volume. However, neither Raven Press nor the editors can be held responsible for errors or for any consequences arising from the use of the information contained herein.

Materials appearing in this book prepared by individuals as part of their official duties as U.S. Government employees are not covered by the above-mentioned copyright.

9 8 7 6 5 4 3 2 1

Advances in Neurology Series

Vol. 62: Cerebral Small Artery Disease: *P. M. Pullicino, L. R. Caplan, and M. Hommel*, editors. 256 pp., 1993.
Vol. 61: Inherited Ataxias: *A. Harding and T. Deufel*, editors. 240 pp., 1993.
Vol. 60: Parkinson's Disease: From Basic Research to Treatment: *H. Narabayashi, T. Nagatsu, N. Yanagisawa, and Y. Mizuno*, editors. 800 pp., 1993.
Vol. 59: Neural Injury and Regeneration: *F. J. Seil*, editor. 384 pp., 1993.
Vol. 58: Tourette Syndrome: Genetics, Neurobiology, and Treatment: *T. N. Chase, A. J. Friedhoff, and D. J. Cohen*, editors. 400 pp., 1992.
Vol. 57: Frontal Lobe Seizures and Epilepsies: *P. Chauvel, A. V. Delgado-Escueta, E. Halgren, and J. Bancaud*, editors. 752 pp., 1992.
Vol. 56: Amyotrophic Lateral Sclerosis and Other Motor Neuron Diseases: *L. P. Rowland*, editor. 592 pp., 1991.
Vol. 55: Neurobehavioral Problems in Epilepsy: *D. B. Smith, D. Treiman, and M. Trimble*, editors. 512 pp., 1990.
Vol. 54: Magnetoencephalography: *S. Sato*, editor. 284 pp., 1990.
Vol. 53: Parkinson's Disease: Anatomy, Pathology, and Therapy: *M. B. Streifler, A. D. Korczyn, E. Melamed, and M. B. H. Youdim*, editors. 640 pp., 1990.
Vol. 52: Brain Edema: Pathogenesis, Imaging, and Therapy: *D. Long*, editor. 640 pp., 1990.
Vol. 51: Alzheimer's Disease: *R. J. Wurtman, S. Corkin, J. H. Growdon, and E. Ritter-Walker*, editors. 308 pp., 1990.
*Vol. 50: Dystonia 2: *S. Fahn, C. D. Marsden, and D. B. Calne*, editors. 688 pp., 1988.
*Vol. 49: Facial Dyskinesias: *J. Jankovic and E. Tolosa*, editors. 560 pp., 1988.
Vol. 48: Molecular Genetics of Neurological and Neuromuscular Disease: *S. DiDonato, S. DiMauro, A. Mamoli, and L. P. Rowland*, editors. 288 pp., 1987.
Vol. 47: Functional Recovery in Neurological Disease: *S. G. Waxman*, editor. 640 pp., 1987.
Vol. 46: Intensive Neurodiagnostic Monitoring: *R. J. Gumnit*, editor. 336 pp., 1987.
Vol. 45: Parkinson's Disease: *M. D. Yahr and K. J. Bergmann*, editors. 640 pp., 1986.
*Vol. 44: Basic Mechanisms of the Epilepsies: Molecular and Cellular Approaches: *A. V. Delgado-Escueta, A. A. Ward, Jr., D. M. Woodbury, and R. J. Porter*, editors. 1,120 pp., 1986.
Vol. 43: Myoclonus: *S. Fahn, C. D. Marsden, and M. H. Van Woert*, editors. 752 pp., 1986.
Vol. 42: Progress in Aphasiology: *F. Clifford Rose*, editor. 384 pp., 1984.
Vol. 41: The Olivopontocerebellar Atrophies: *R. C. Duvoisin and A. Plaitakis*, editors. 304 pp., 1984.
Vol. 40: Parkinson-Specific Motor and Mental Disorders, Role of Pallidum: Pathophysiological, Biochemical, and Therapeutic Aspects: *R. G. Hassler and J. F. Christ*, editors. 601 pp., 1984.
*Vol. 39: Motor Control Mechanisms in Health and Disease: *J. E. Desmedt*, editor. 1,224 pp., 1983.
Vol. 38: The Dementias: *R. Mayeux and W. G. Rosen*, editors. 288 pp., 1983.
Vol. 37: Experimental Therapeutics of Movement Disorders: *S. Fahn, D. B. Calne, and I. Shoulson*, editors. 339 pp., 1983.
Vol. 36: Human Motor Neuron Diseases: *L. P. Rowland*, editor. 592 pp., 1982.
Vol. 35: Gilles de la Tourette Syndrome: *A. J. Friedhoff and T. N. Chase*, editors. 476 pp., 1982.
*Vol. 34: Status Epilepticus: Mechanisms of Brain Damage and Treatment: *A. V. Delgado-Escueta, C. G. Wasterlain, D M. Treiman, and R. J. Porter*, editors. 579 pp., 1983.
*Vol. 33: Headache: Physiopathological and Clinical Concepts: *M. Critchley, A. Friedman, S. Gorini, and F. Sicuteri*, editors. 417 pp., 1982.
*Vol. 32: Clinical Applications of Evoked Potentials in Neurology: *J. Courjon, F. Mauguiere, and M. Revol*, editors. 592 pp., 1982.
Vol. 31: Demyelinating Diseases: Basic and Clinical Electrophysiology: *S. Waxman and J. Murdoch Ritchie*, editors. 544 pp., 1981.
Vol. 30: Diagnosis and Treatment of Brain Ischemia: *A. L. Carney and E. M. Anderson*, editors. 424 pp., 1981.

*Vol. 29: Neurofibromatosis: *V. M. Riccardi and J. J. Mulvihill, editors*. 288 pp., 1981.
Vol. 28: Brain Edema: *J. Cervós-Navarro and R. Ferszt, editors*. 539 pp., 1980.
Vol. 27: Antiepileptic Drugs: Mechanisms of Action: *G. H. Glaser, J. K. Penry, and D. M. Woodbury, editors*. 728 pp., 1980.
Vol. 26: Cerebral Hypoxia and Its Consequences: *S. Fahn, J. N. Davis, and L. P. Rowland, editors*. 454 pp., 1979.
*Vol. 25: Cerebrovascular Disorders and Stroke: *M. Goldstein, L. Bolis, C. Fieschi, S. Gorini, and C. H. Millikan, editors*. 412 pp., 1979.
*Vol. 24: The Extrapyramidal System and Its Disorders: *L. J. Poirier, T. L. Sourkes, and P. Bédard, editors*. 552 pp., 1979.
*Vol. 23: Huntington's Chorea: *T. N. Chase, N. S. Wexler, and A. Barbeau, editors*. 864 pp., 1979.
Vol. 22: Complications of Nervous System Trauma: *R. A. Thompson and J. R. Green, editors*. 454 pp., 1979.
*Vol. 21: The Inherited Ataxia: Biochemical, Viral, and Pathological Studies: *R. A. Kark, R. Rosenberg, and L. Schut, editors*. 450 pp., 1978.
Vol. 20: Pathology of Cerebrospinal Microcirculation: *J. Cervós-Navarro, E. Betz, G. Ebhardt, R. Ferszt, and R. Wüllenweber, editors*. 636 pp., 1978.
*Vol. 19: Neurological Epidemiology: Principles and Clinical Applications: *B. S. Schoenberg, editor*. 672 pp., 1978.
*Vol. 18: Hemi-Inattention and Hemisphere Specialization: *E. A. Weinstein and R. P. Friedland, editors*. 176 pp., 1977.
*Vol. 17: Treatment of Neuromuscular Diseases: *R. C. Griggs and R. T. Moxley, editors*. 370 pp., 1977.
Vol. 16: Stroke: *R. A. Thompson and J. R. Green, editors*. 250 pp., 1977.
*Vol. 15: Neoplasia in the Central Nervous System: *R. A. Thompson and J. R. Green, editors*. 394 pp., 1976.
*Vol. 14: Dystonia: *R. Eldridge and S. Fahn, editors*. 510 pp., 1976.
Vol. 13: Current Reviews: *W. J. Friedlander, editor*. 400 pp., 1975.
Vol. 12: Physiology and Pathology of Dendrites: *G. W. Kreutzberg, editor*. 524 pp., 1975.
*Vol. 11: Complex Partial Seizures and Their Treatment: *J. K. Penry and D. D. Daly, editors*. 486 pp., 1975.
*Vol. 10: Private Models of Neurological Disorders: *B. S. Meldrum and C. D. Marsden, editors*. 270 pp., 1975.
*Vol. 9: Dopaminergic Mechanisms: *D. B. Calne, T. N. Chase, and A. Barbeau, editors*. 452 pp., 1975.
*Vol. 8: Neurosurgical Management of Epilepsies: *D. P. Purpura, J. K. Penry, and R. D. Walter, editors*. 370 pp., 1975.
Vol. 7: Current Reviews of Higher Nervous System Dysfunction: *W. J. Friedlander, editor*. 202 pp., 1975.
Vol. 6: Infectious Diseases of the Central Nervous System: *R. A. Thompson and J. R. Green, editors*. 402 pp., 1974.
*Vol. 5: Second Canadian-American Conference on Parkinson's Disease: *F. McDowell and A. Barbeau, editors*. 526 pp., 1974.
*Vol. 4: International Symposium on Pain: *J. J. Bonica, editor*. 858 pp., 1974.
*Vol. 3: Progress in the Treatment of Parkinsonism: *D. B. Calne, editor*. 402 pp., 1973.
*Vol. 2: The Treatment of Parkinsonism—The Role of DOPA Decarboxylase Inhibitors: *M. D. Yahr, editor*. 304 pp., 1973.
Vol. 1: Huntington's Chorea: 1872–1972: *A. Barbeau, T. N. Chase, and G. W. Paulson, editors*. 902 pp., 1973.

---

*Out of print.

Contents

Contributing Authors		ix
Preface		xi
Acknowledgments		xiii
1.	Historical Aspects of Lacunes and the "Lacunar Controversy" *Gérard Besson and Marc Hommel*	1
2.	The Course and Territories of Cerebral Small Arteries *Patrick M. Pullicino*	11
3.	Diagrams of Perforating Artery Territories in Axial, Coronal and Sagittal Planes *Patrick M. Pullicino*	41
4.	Computed Tomography and Magnetic Resonance of Subcortical Ischemic Lesions *Patrick M. Pullicino and Reza Pordell*	73
5.	Pathology of Small Artery Disease *Peter T. Ostrow and Lucia L. Miller*	93
6.	Pathogenesis of Lacunar Infarcts and Small Deep Infarcts *Patrick M. Pullicino*	125
7.	Lacunar Syndromes *Gérard Besson and Marc Hommel*	141
8.	Clinical Features of Lacunar and Small Deep Infarcts at Specific Anatomical Sites *Marc Hommel and Gérard Besson*	161
9.	Clinical Features of Multiple Lacunar and Small Deep Infarcts *Marc Hommel and Gérard Besson*	181
10.	Lacunar Syndromes Due to Non-Ischemic Small Deep Lesions *Gérard Besson and Marc Hommel*	187
11.	Binswanger's Disease *John C. van Swieten and Louis R. Caplan*	193
12.	Incidence, Natural History, and Risk Factors in Lacunar Infarction *Jan Lodder and Jelis Boiten*	213
Index		229

Contributing Authors

Gérard Besson, M.D. *Neurologist, Department of Clinical and Biological Neurosciences, Stroke Unit, Centre Hospitalier, Universitaire Régional de Grenoble, BP 217, 38043 Grenoble CEDEX 9, France*

Jelis Boiten, M.D., Ph.D. *Neurologist, Department of Neurology, University Hospital Maastricht, State University of Limburg, P. Debyelaan 25, P.O. Box 5800, NL-6202 AZ Maastricht, The Netherlands*

Louis R. Caplan, M.D. *Professor and Chairman, Department of Neurology, Tufts University of Medicine, Neurologist-in-Chief, New England Medical Center, 171 Harrison Avenue, Boston, Massachusetts 02111*

Marc Hommel, M.D. *Neurologist, Department of Clinical and Biological Neurosciences, Stroke Unit, Centre Hospitalier Universitaire Régional de Grenoble, BP 217, 38043 Grenoble CEDEX 9, France*

Jan Lodder, M.D., Ph.D. *Neurologist, Department of Neurology, University Hospital Maastricht, State University of Limburg, P. Debyelaan 25, P.O. Box 5800, NL-6202 AZ Maastricht, The Netherlands*

Lucia L. Miller, M.D. *Fellow in Neuropathology, Department of Pathology, State University of New York at Buffalo, Buffalo General Hospital, 100 High Street, Buffalo, New York 14203*

Peter T. Ostrow, M.D., Ph.D. *Associate Professor, Department of Pathology, State University of New York at Buffalo, Director of Neuropathology, Buffalo General Hospital, 100 High Street, Buffalo, New York 14203*

Reza Pordell, M.D. *Chief, Division of Neuroradiology; Clinical Assistant Professor, Department of Radiology, State University of New York at Buffalo, Buffalo General Hospital, 100 High Street, Buffalo, New York 14203*

Patrick M. Pullicino, M.D. Ph.D. *Assistant Professor, Department of Neurology, State University of New York at Buffalo, Buffalo General Hospital, 100 High Street, Buffalo, New York 14203*

John C. van Swieten, M.D. *Neurologist, Department of Neurology, University Hospital Dykzigt, Dr. Molewaterplein 40, 3015 GD Rotterdam, The Netherlands*

Preface

Stroke is a major public health problem. It is the third most common cause of death in the United States and in many other countries, and an even more important cause of morbidity, long-term disability, and the need for chronic care. Small deep infarcts, customarily called *lacunes*, are the most common abnormality found in human brains at post-mortem examination. Lacunes represent one of the most frequent subtypes of stroke diagnosed clinically and/or by neuroimaging.

Although lacunes were first recognized nearly a century ago, the recent introduction and wide dissemination of high quality CT and MRI scanners now makes it possible to confirm the presence of a small deep infarct during life and even very soon after it first gives rise to symptoms. The findings of neuroimaging have, however, raised many questions and controversies. Both the wealth of data now available, as well as controversies that have been recently raised, prompted us to develop this book.

The history of stroke can be conveniently divided into four distinct but overlapping epochs. During the first, rather long era (Cheyne, 1808 to Foix, circa 1927), interest in stroke centered mostly on the correlation of the anatomy of the brain lesions with the associated clinical symptoms and signs found during life. Physicians were interested in how the brain worked and how small focal brain lesions affected normal function. Since stroke is the prototype of a focal brain lesion, small strokes were ideal for *anatomico-clinical and pathological correlation*. No investigations were available in this era that could define the site of a lesion during life, so the key information was available only at necropsy.

During the second era (Foix to Miller Fisher, circa 1960s) clinicians and pathologists became interested in what caused the brain softenings and hemorrhages and began to investigate *disease of the blood vessels as well as their causes and frequencies*. During this era, Miller Fisher, relying on his own detailed neuropathological studies and the clinical and pathological studies of others, constructed and defined what has since become known as the "lacune hypothesis" or "lacunar concept." This concept has three aspects: (1) small deep infarcts, which are cystic after an initial acute phase, are caused by disease of a single penetrating artery; (2) the usual pathology that affects these penetrating arteries and underlies lacunes is lipohyalinosis, or microatheromas that occur within and at the orifices of these penetrating arteries; and (3) these infarcts are often associated with clinically recognizable syndromes. During this era no investigations were available that could give information about lacunes or the penetrating arteries during life. Most of the data came from necropsy examination of the brain and its arterial supply system.

The third and fourth eras are really concurrent and continue today. The third, or the era of *in vivo clinico-anatomical correlation*, was ushered in during the early 1970s when CT was introduced into clinical practice. Since then, MRI has also become available, and these two imaging techniques allow rapid and safe diagnosis of the nature and location of the brain lesions in patients with stroke. Other new diagnostic technologies, such as cardiac and vascular ultrasound and magnetic resonance angiography, make possible the identification of cardiac or arterial lesions giving rise to stroke. These newer technologies led to some surprises. Brain lesions including lacunes were often found without accompanying clinical findings. Some patients who had so-called "clinical lacunar syndromes" had brain lesions other than lacunes on CT and MRI scans. Patients with small deep infarcts consistent with lacunes were sometimes found to have cardiac and/or large artery occlusive disease suggestive of embolism. These findings led to questions about the clinical diagnosis of lacunes and the validity of the various parts of the lacunar hypothesis. These questions have in turn led to a plethora of clinical, imaging, and epidemiologic studies.

The fourth epoch relates to interest in *treatment*. Until very recently, there was little effective treatment for acute stroke. Now there are a host of new surgical, transluminal catheter, and medical therapies, many as yet not fully tested. Therapeutic trials now abound, some of which are showing very positive results for some patients with certain specific stroke subtypes. Of course, treatment depends very heavily upon diagnostic accuracy.

The mass of new information relating to small deep infarcts or lacunes has not, until now, been gathered, analyzed, or interpreted for the many physicians who care for patients with strokes. This book has been planned both to critically review the older autopsy-based literature, as well as to collect the recent imaging-based data; to try to separate the wheat from the chaff; and to refine the material into a concise, readable, user-friendly format. In order to determine where we are now and where we are headed, we need to know where we have been. To do this we have included detailed reviews of the historical evolution of the clinical and pathological concepts related to lacunes. We have also included reviews of the anatomy of the brain regions and blood vessels involved and of typical imaging appearances. Finally we have tried to concisely review recent epidemiologic data.

This book approaches small artery disease from two main starting points. Starting with clinical features, clinicians will be able to determine from Chapters 7 and 9 whether a particular presentation is known to be a lacunar syndrome and what will be the likely sites of the infarcts. Starting with a scan showing a small deep lesion, clinicians and neuroradiologists will be able to use Chapters 2 and 3 to determine the vascular territory and anatomical location of the lesion and can then use Chapter 8 to determine the likely clinical features. In addition, clinical "imagers" can use Chapters 4 and 11 to help in the interpretation of the imaging characteristics of small deep ischemic lesions, Chapters 5 and 6 to review the pathology and pathogenesis, and Chapter 12 to review the risk factors and natural history.

The review of the literature is comprehensive, including an extensive review of the French literature on small artery disease, dating back to the nineteenth century, that has not been previously published in English. It also includes a chapter on the anatomy of small brain arteries with data from some relatively inaccessible works, as well as the recent neurosurgical literature.

This book should be of major interest to stroke neurologists. Neurologists and physicians dealing with stroke patients will also find the book very useful in correlating clinical lacunar syndromes with the anatomical site and vascular territory of the causative infarct. The book should also help neuroradiologists and neuroimagers to determine the likely clinical features of small deep infarcts found on CT or MR. Neuroscientists working in the field of vascular disease will find the book a useful, in-depth, clinically-oriented review of small artery disease.

Patrick Pullicino, MD, Buffalo
Louis R. Caplan, MD, Boston
Marc Hommel, MD, Grenoble

Acknowledgments

We thank L. J. Jacobs, MD, for his support. We acknowledge Wentsing Liu, MLS and the staff of the A. H. Aaron Health Science Library for their untiring help. We also acknowledge the secretarial assistance of Nancy Harding, Lisa Paler, the secretaries of the Neurological Department of the Buffalo General Hospital, and the secretarial staffs of the Departments of Neurology at the New England Medical Center and the Centre Hospitalier Régional et Universitaire de Grenoble.

1

Historical Aspects of Lacunes and the "Lacunar Controversy"

Gérard Besson and Marc Hommel

Department of Clinical and Biological Neurosciences, Stroke Unit, Centre Hospitalier Universitaire Régional de Grenoble, Grenoble, France

Lacune is an old anatomical term that always seems to have given rise to confusions and controversies. Before Pierre Marie's work, there was confusion between lacunes and other cavities in the brain. After Pierre Marie's work there were controversies about the etiology of lacunes (i.e., infarction versus hemorrhage versus injury secondary to inflammation of the perivascular sheaths or *vaginalite destructive*). At the present time, the controversy centers on the "lacunar concept," i.e., that a lacune is caused by ischemia in the territory of a single penetrating artery. The question is whether lacunes are distinct from other small deep infarcts by clinical criteria by imaging or in terms of their pathogenesis. A knowledge of the history of the lacunar concept may help to understand why lacunes remain controversial to this day (1,2).

BEFORE PIERRE MARIE

The term lacune, which means an empty space, defines a macroscopic entity. It was first coined in 1838 by Dechambre to define small cavities caused by the resorption of small deep cerebral softenings (3). A few years before, Cruveilhier (book 20, vol 1) had described small softenings in the white matter called *petit foyers pisiformes* (small pealike foci) (4). These lesions were most likely lacunes. In 1843, Durand-Fardel (5) distinguished lacunes from another cavitary state of the brain, *l'état criblé*, which he defined in 1842 (6). État criblé was described as multiple small round holes with sharp margins, surrounded by normal brain tissue. These cavities were centered by a small blood vessel and were located in the white matter of the insula, or sometimes in the pons or medulla. They were thought to be related to a generalized dilatation of blood vessels and to cause dementia.

In the second half of the 19th and in the beginning of the 20th centuries, authors remained very imprecise about the origin of lacunes, and both ischemic and hemorrhagic etiologies were mentioned. Moreover, there was confusion between lacunes, état criblé, and other newly described cavitary lesions. Proust (7) considered *état criblé* to be an aggregation of lacunes. From the German and the Italian schools, Bizzozero (8), Obersteiner (9), Ripping (10), Arndt (11), and Pick (12) considered that *état criblé* was a dilatation of the lymphatic sheaths of small arteries. Pick, however, thought that the Virchow-Robin space was dilated in addition to the lymphatic sheaths (12). Adler, on the other hand, proposed that only the Virchow-Robin space was involved (13). In addition to describing *état criblé* (small holes surrounded by normal brain tissue), Arndt also described small holes surrounded by abnormal brain tissue (lacunes), as well as large holes with smooth margins (cerebral porosis) (11).

The term cerebral porosis was coined by Pierre Marie (14) to describe a cavitary state that was first described by Clarke (15). In cerebral porosis, the cavities are round or oval with smooth and regular margins, and are located anywhere in the brain except in the medulla oblongata (16) (Fig. 1). No vessels were found in the cavities. Their largest diameter could reach 5 cm (17). In spite of the different anatomical characteristics of cerebral porosis and *état criblé*, some confusion persisted. In his work on *état criblé*, Vassale included only cavities corresponding to cerebral porosis and not to *état criblé* (18). He suggested that cerebral porosis could be due to postmortem damage. This was first formally hypothesized by Reuling and Herring in 1899, who believed that the cavities were due to the presence of the bacillus aerogenes capsulatus (17).

In 1894, Campbell reported the brain macroscopic and microscopic findings in 50 aged insane persons (19). He found dilated perivascular spaces (*état criblé*) affecting the lenticulostriate and the lenticulo-optic arteries, as well as the arteries supplying the dentate nucleus and the upper part of the pons. The author distinguished *état criblé* from irregular small cavities formed around vessels that "occasioned the destruction of a considerable amount of nervous tissue." He noted that the walls of the blood vessels were fibrillated, and he suggested that rupture of the vessel walls might induce an effusion of blood into the perivascular spaces with resulting destruction of the surrounding tissues. The anatomical description of these cavities corresponds well with lacunes. The author did not use this term, although he did quote Durand-Fardel's book. Campbell noted that *état criblé* was common in atheromatous brains. Jacobsohn (20) and Alzheimer (21) also noted dilated perivascular spaces in atheromatous brains and found that perivascular spaces in the basal ganglia were often affected. Alzheimer noted that these irregular-shaped small cystic cavities formed around vessels and caused the destruction of nervous tissue (21). He suggested that some of these cavities were remnants of resolved perivascular hemorrhages. Probst also noted similar cavities in atheromatous brains (22) and suggested that these were due to the resorption of small cerebral softenings. Alzheimer and Probst's descriptions of small cystic cavities correspond to lacunes.

FROM PIERRE MARIE TO C. M. FISHER

In 1901, Pierre Marie (Fig. 2) defined the characteristics of lacunes in anatomical studies on 50 brains as follows (14):

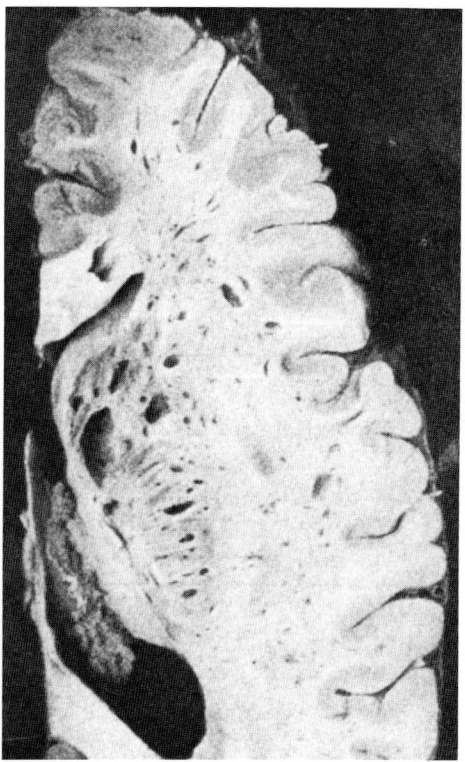

FIG. 1. Cerebral porosis. From ref. 16a, with permission.

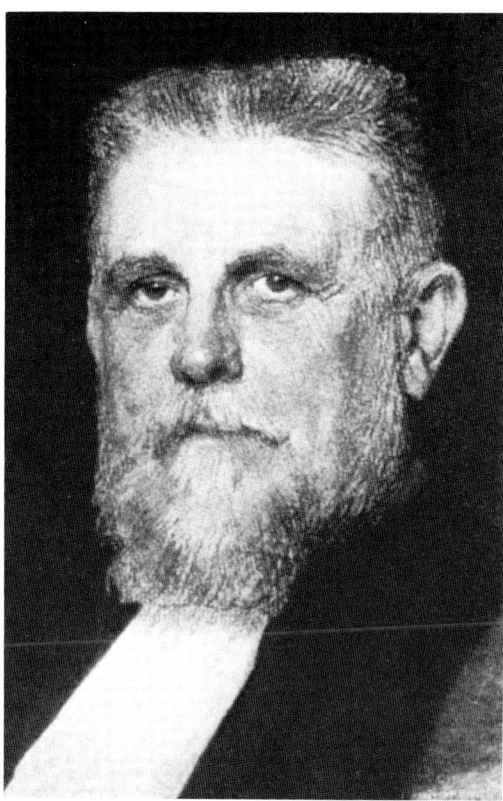

FIG. 2. Pierre Marie. From ref. 22a, with permission.

microscopical aspect: small, irregular cavities containing one or more patent vessels.
size: varied from the size of a birdseed to that of a pea or even of a haricot bean.
number: one to ten.
location: lenticular nucleus (45/50), thalamus (17/50), caudate nucleus, pons, and cerebellum. He did not find lacunes in the mesencephalon, the medulla oblongata, or the spinal cord.
age: the mean age of 26 patients was 60.5 years.
pathogenesis: Pierre Marie suggested that lacunes were due to arteriosclerosis. This might produce either a thrombotic occlusion (ischemic hypothesis of lacunes) or a decrease in cerebral blood flow. He proposed that this decrease in cerebral blood flow might lead to a dilatation of perivascular spaces, and to destruction of brain parenchyma around vessels. He thought that this process, which was called *vaginalite destructive*, might also give rise to lacunes (Fig. 3). While it is clear that Pierre Marie considered lacunes as small infarcts, he also referred to a hemorrhagic aspect of lacunes.
clinical symptoms: The most common clinical feature was acute hemiplegia without loss of consciousness, hypesthesia, hemianopia, or aphasia. Marie considered the prognosis of the hemiplegia to be good because the weakness was often incomplete and substantial recovery occurred. Thirty-two of 50 patients had one or more further strokes and in some this led to the development of a lacunar state (see chapter 9). Death occurred at a mean age of 68 years.

In the second part of this study, Pierre Marie distinguished lacunes from other cavities observed in the brain. Like Durand-Fardel, he considered *état criblé* an entity. He found that *état criblé* was mainly located in the insula and in the temporal lobe, and suggested that this condition was due to the shrinkage of the brain around vessels.

Marie commented on a peculiar form of *état criblé* that affected the lenticulostriate arteries as they penetrated the lenticular nucleus. He called this "dilatation of the perivascular spaces around the lenticulostriate arteries." This was characterized by small regular cavities centered by patent and tortuous lenticulostriate arteries with no parenchymal change. The volume of these cavities varied from the size of a lentil to that of a small haricot bean. Pierre Marie agreed that cerebral porosis was due to postmortem bacterial autolysis.

In summary, Pierre Marie established the morphological characteristics of lacunes, demonstrated the association of lacunes with an isolated hemiplegia, and noted the good prognosis of the hemiplegia. His view of pathogenesis, however, remained ambiguous.

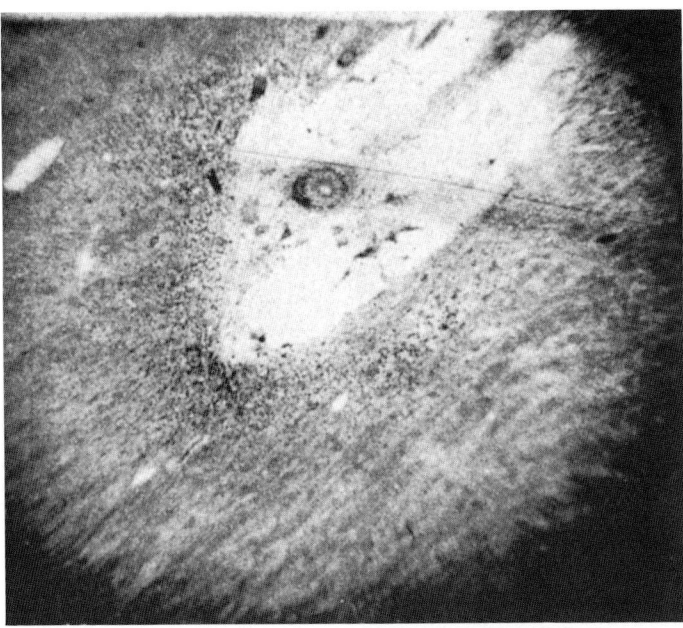

FIG. 3. *Vaginalite destructive*, showing lacune containing a patent vessel with thickened walls. Leukocytes surround the artery in its "lymphatic sheath" and are also seen around the periphery of the cavity of the lacune. From ref. 16a, with permission.

In the subsequent 30 years, several major articles failed to clarify the pathogenesis of lacunes. Between 1901 and 1926, different authors divided lacunes into three groups: an ischemic group, a *vaginalite destructive* group, and a mixed group. No author defined lacunes as being exclusively scars of old hemorrhages.

In 1901, Dupré and Devaux (23,24) studied the brain of a patient suffering from pseudobulbar palsy. The authors divided the brain cavities into four groups according to their size and their microscopical aspects:

1. large irregular cavities: containing thick-walled vessels and caused by hemorrhage or thrombosis.
2. small cavities: Three stages of evolution of these cavities, which they called lacunes, were described. The first stage consisted of a cavity formed by a central vessel surrounded by an enlarged lymphatic sheath. In the second stage, the perilymphatic spaces also became dilated. The third stage had the same characteristics as the second stage but the cavities were larger. Unlike the large cavities of group 1, all stages of the small cavities had regular outlines. Dupré and Devaux thought that these small cavities were not caused solely by ischemia because the central vessel was not occluded. They thought that *vaginalite destructive* was the likely etiology.
3. intermediate cavities: had characteristics of both the previous groups.
4. *état criblé*: was due to "parenchymal atrophy" around vessels.

In 1902, Ferrand (25) defined lacunes as areas of focal brain destruction producing cavities of varying size. This work is certainly the most important and the most complete work of the beginning of the 20th century. Ferrand studied 88 autopsies with 189 lacunes (mean = 2.3 per brain). Their size, their morphology, the clinical findings and the prognosis were the same as in Pierre Marie's description. The mean age at first stroke varied from 65 to 70 years. He distinguished three stages in the development of a lacune:

first stage: also named *lacune miliaire*, was not really a lacune but a prelacunar lesion, consisting of a rarefaction of brain tissue around an artery without a periarterial space or lacunar cavity. The arterial wall, especially the adventitia, was thickened but the artery remained patent.
second stage: This stage was characterized by the appearance of a periarterial cavity that was irregular and contained cellular fragments.
third stage: In this stage the cavity was partitioned or filled by a sclerotic scar.

Ferrand did not accept the ischemic hypothesis of the pathogenesis of lacunes because he thought that the arteries supplying lacunes were not occluded. He suggested, however, that lacunes might be produced by a sclerotic degeneration of small arteries that decreased the cerebral blood flow and led to a "chronic encephalitis" and an associated "cerebral sclerosis." He thought that the perivascular sheaths might have a pathogenetic role since he thought that the cerebrospinal fluid contained by them had an irritant effect.

Ferrand noted an association of lacunes with hypertensive heart strain but considered hypertension to be a concomitant disease, not an etiology. He found diabetes mellitus, syphilis, and uremia to be rare in lacunar patients. The description of the other cavities of the brain were the same as in Pierre Marie's work, but Ferrand wondered whether *état criblé* was really a pathological state.

In 1904, Pic and Bonnamour claimed that the signs and symptoms occurring in patients with lacunes were due to a concomitant spinal cord sclerosis (26). In the same year, Castaigne and Ferrand studied the lacunar state in patients with renal failure (27) [an association first reported by Raymond in 1885 (28)]. Castaigne and Ferrand did not propose a pathogenetic link between lacunes and renal failure, but suggested that a part of the neurological deficits of these patients might be due to lacunes. Grasset classified lacunes under cerebral infarcts (29) and proposed that arterial sclerosis induced a decrease in cerebral blood flow, which in turn gave rise to a periarterial cerebral injury or "dystrophic lacunar sclerosis." This dystrophic lacunar sclerosis was the precursor of a lacune. The lacune, which was characterized by a cavity centered by a patent vessel, contained fragments of brain tissue and blood.

Catola (16) studied 16 brains with lacunes and summarized the previous literature. He developed the *vaginalite destructive* theory without giving new ideas. The only authors of this period who opted for the ischemic hypothesis of lacunes were C. and O. Vogt (30). Other authors did not emphasize a precise etiology [Lejonne and Lhermitte (31), and Leri (32)]. In 1908, Barbe and Levy-Valensi (33) reported one case and suggested that syphilis might be an etiology; this was supported by Marie and Foix, who also reported a case due to syphilis (34).

In 1923, Foix and Nicolesco (35) distinguished lacunes from microscopic infarcts, which they described as being more regular, round, and empty, and from microscopic hemorrhages, which were linear. In keeping with Catola's hypothesis, Foix and Nicolesco suggested that lacunes were exclusively produced by *vaginalite destructive*, in three successive stages:

1. Perivascular disintegration: This stage corresponded to the first stage of Ferrand, and was also named "dysmyelinic state" by C. and O. Vogt.
2. *État criblé*: In this stage irregular perivascular cavities surrounded by indented edges appeared, particularly in the basal ganglia. Axons were distended and myelin became scarce perivascularly. This corresponded to the "*état pré-criblé*" of C. and O. Vogt.

3. Lacunar state: Lacunes were small irregular cavities with indented edges, located in the basal ganglia, especially in the putamen. These authors maintained that even if a small cavitary lesion looked like a lacune it had to be called a microscopic infarct rather than a lacune if it was outside the basal ganglia.

In 1926, Foix and Chavany claimed that lacunes were sclerotic foci due to arteriosclerosis. However, they did not consider lacunes to be infarcts (36).

By 1926 lacunes were well established as a neuropathological entity, but many unsolved questions remained. During the next 40 years, very few papers on lacunes appeared in the literature and there was no further advance in the understanding of lacunes. In 1953 Fisher noted coexisting hypertension in lacunar patients (37), but like Ferrand he thought that hypertension was only an associated factor and concluded that atherosclerosis was the main risk factor. Fisher also noted that lacunes were uncommon in normotensive patients. In 1954, Hughes et al. (38) found multiple small ischemic lesions in 15 hypertensive patients. These lesions probably corresponded to lacunes, although the authors did not use this term. The lesions involved the striatum in every case and the thalamus in 11. They occurred mainly in the territories supplied by the perforating arteries, which were narrowed but not occluded. A hemodynamic hypothesis was suggested to explain the distribution of the lesions. The same year, Moore (39) published a paper entitled "Perivascular Encephalolysis." This paper described cystic cavities centered by vessels with perivascular demyelination and cystic liquefaction necrosis. These lesions corresponded with *vaginalite destructive*, although the author did not refer to the term. He suggested that perivascular encephalolysis might be due to the development of a lytic agent in the perivascular space. This lytic agent might have resulted from an alteration of cerebral metabolism due to a systemic disease, such as diabetes mellitus.

FROM C. M. FISHER TO THE COMPUTED TOMOGRAPHY/ MAGNETIC RESONANCE ERA

Although the "ischemic" hypothesis had been put forward at the beginning of the 20th century, it was C. M. Fisher who propagated this hypothesis in the 1960s (Fig. 4).

In 1965, Fisher published a study of 1,042 autopsies, 114 (11%) of which had at least one lacune (40). He defined lacunes as small trabeculated cavities, which were the scars of softenings due to small vessel occlusions. They were located in the same areas as Pierre Marie had stated, and their size varied between 2 and 17 mm. Fisher

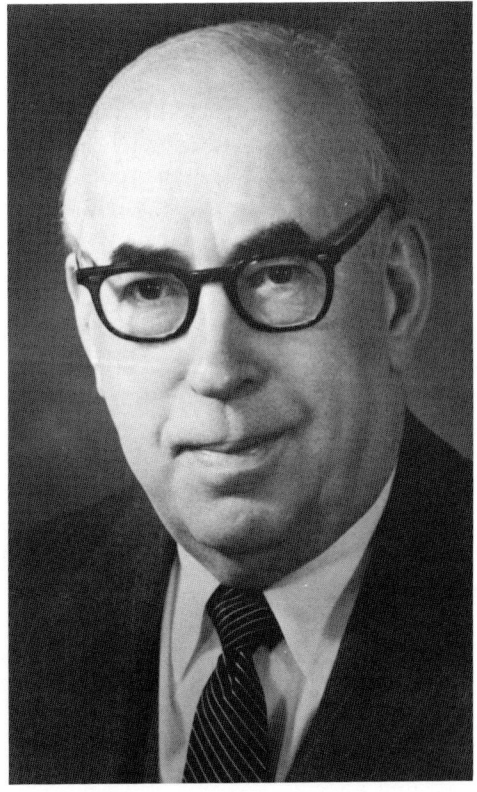

FIG. 4. C. M. Fisher, M.D.

stressed the major role of arterial hypertension in the pathogenesis of lacunes because only two patients in his series were normotensive. However, he did not rule out the possibility of embolism. In six of these patients he found vascular occlusion in the deep perforating branches of the middle cerebral, anterior cerebral, posterior cerebral, anterior choroidal, and basilar arteries. Fisher also found a correlation between the degree of intracranial atherosclerosis and the number of lacunes.

In the same year, Hughes also suggested that lacunes were small infarcts due to hypertension (41). He proposed that chronic hypertension lengthens and dilates small arteries, causing them to become tortuous. He called this process "unfolding" (see chapter 6). Two consequences might occur from unfolding: firstly, that pulsations of these tortuous arteries would clear a space around them, and secondly, that lengthening of small arteries might alter the position or angle of the ostia on the parent artery, which might reduce or even at times reverse blood flow in the unfolded artery. Both of these mechanisms could account for perivascular dilatation in *état criblé* and lacunes. This proposal revived the *vaginalite* hypothesis and again called into question the ischemic hypothesis. Prineas and Marshall (42) and Cole and Yates both supported a pathogenetic role of hypertension in lacunes (43). In 1967, Cole and Yates examined a consecutive series of 100 autopsy brains from hypertensive subjects and compared them with 100 brains from normotensive subjects, matched for age and sex. The authors used two criteria for the diagnosis of hypertension: a diastolic blood pressure of 110 mm Hg or more and heart weight of 400 g or more in a man and 350 g or more in a woman. Fifteen patients had at least one small recent infarct. Eight of these cases were in the hypertensive group, seven in the normotensive group. The size of the infarcts varied from a few millimeters to 2 cm. These authors applied the names *état criblé* and lacunar state to similar cavities centered by small vessels and they regarded both of these as enlarged perivascular spaces. They called cystic spaces containing no vessel old small infarcts. They found lacunes and *état criblé* in 38% of hypertensive patients and 9% of normotensive patients.

In 1969, Fisher used serial sections to investigate the arterial lesions underlying 50 consecutive lacunes in four hypertensive brains (44). An occlusion of the small artery supplying the territory of an infarct was found in 45 instances. He found a pathology that he called "segmental arterial disorganization" to be affecting arterioles of 40 to 200 μm diameter in 40 lacunes. Among these 40 pathological arteries, there was a local enlargement of the vessel in 31, a focal hemorrhagic extravasation in 26, and a fibrinoid deposit in 14. Connective tissue that was sometimes dissociated and contained large macrophages was present in the arteriolar walls, protruded into the lumen, and was occasionally responsible for arteriolar occlusions. Two of the remaining 10 lacunes were due to thrombosis of an asymmetric fusiform microaneurysm and three to an occlusion or stenosis due to a plaque of foam cells at the site of origin of the deep perforating artery; two were suspected to be due to a segmental disorganization of the vessel wall, one to an unidentified pink-staining material, one to an embolus, and one remained unexplained. In 1971, Fisher coined the word lipohyalinosis for this segmented arterial disorganization (45).

These seminal works defined lacunes as small infarcts (17 mm diameter or less) that occur especially in the basal ganglia, internal capsule, or pons and are due to a small vessel (200 μm diameter or less) disease called lipohyalinosis.

De Reuck and Vander Eecken used microangiography to study the angioarchitecture of the deep arteries supplying lacunes in 10 brains. These vessels arise directly from large arteries and have an unbranched end-artery anatomy (46). In the brains with lacunes, the penetrating arteries showed several narrowings and poststenotic dilatations. An occlusion of the penetrating artery was found in 24 of 30 lacunes whilst no occlusions were observed in the remaining six cases.

Although Caplan suggested that lacunes were exclusively due to hypertension (47), other causes of lacunes began to be described. Apart from lipohyalinosis, Fisher had mentioned the possibility of embolism as a cause of lacunar infarction, and this was later confirmed (48). Diabetes mellitus was suspected to be a risk factor for lacunar infarcts (49). In the early 1980s, Mohr summarized the different arterial lesions underlying lacunes as follows (50):

fibrinoid necrosis
lipohyalinosis
microatheroma involving the walls or the ostia of the penetrating arteries
microembolism
macroembolization involving multiple arteries
arteritis due to chronic meningitis, chronic neurosyphilis, or granulomatous meningitis

In 1983, Poirier et al. reported a single case of a new type of cerebral lacune that they called "expanding cerebral lacuna" (51), although a similar case had been previously reported in 1965 by Pilleri (52). Derouesné et al. subsequently reported a further case in 1987 (53). In Derouesné et al.'s case the cavity of the expanding lacune was centered by a normal vessel and was lined by a single layer of epithelial-like cells. It was located in the territory of the paramedian mesencephalic arteries and ballooned into the lateral ventricle (52).

Poirier stressed that not all lacunes were due to softenings and together with Derouesné, he suggested a new neuropathological classification of lacunes (54):

type I: old small infarcts of less than 15 to 20 mm diameter, with irregular cavities surrounded by a reactive astrocytic gliosis and containing parenchymatous fragments.
type II: old small hemorrhages of less than 15 to 20 mm in diameter. The cavities were more regular than in type I and were filled with hemosiderin containing macrophages.
type III: dilatation of perivascular spaces. These cavities were rounded and regular and were centered by a patent vessel with normal walls. The brain tissue appeared more compressed than destroyed.

According to their number and their volume, type III lacunes were divided into four varieties:

type III a: corresponded to *état criblé* (very small diameter and high number).
type III b: with the size, location, and number of type I but with the morphology of type III.
type III c: corresponded to a single dilatation of the perivascular space around a lenticulostriate artery in the inferior part of the lenticular nucleus.
type III d: giant cerebral lacune as described by Poirier et al. (53).

This classification went back to Pierre Marie since he had previously described all these subtypes of lacunes apart from type III d. On the other hand, this classification considered every small brain cavity less than 20 mm in diameter to be a lacune, whatever its etiology. In contrast with this classification, Mancardi used the term lacune only for small cavities due to ischemic necrosis (55), and he used the term cribriform cavities for cavities caused by the dilatation of perivascular spaces (i.e., *vaginalite destructive*). Recently, Challa et al. have studied the relationship between lacunes and their blood vessels (56). Their findings support Fisher's hypothesis on microvascular disease. However, they found that the most common vascular disease was a variable narrowing due to intimal hyperplasia, hyalinization, or atherosclerosis, while occlusions were uncommon. The authors suggested that the natural history of lacunar infarcts might be changing since Fisher's works, owing to antihypertensive treatment.

RECENT QUESTIONS ABOUT THE LACUNAR HYPOTHESIS. LACUNE OR SMALL DEEP INFARCT?

In summary, it must be emphasized that the lacunar concept is a pathological concept based on *single* artery disease. In addition to the pathological concept, a clinical concept has emerged that is based on neuropathological findings. In 1965, Fisher and Curry (57) coined the term pure motor hemiplegia to define the first so-called lacunar syndrome. In fact, pure motor hemiplegia and other acute lacunar syndromes had been described prior to Fisher and Curry's paper (see chapter 7). Since 1965 other lacunar syndromes have been described, some with neuropathological confirmation, others with only imaging evidence of a lacune. Over the past 130 years, the most generally accepted criterion of the lacunar concept has been that lacunar disease is a disease of single arteries. Despite the fact that modern imaging is still unable to distinguish single from multiple artery disease, imaging is being used to determine the clinical features and pathogenesis of lacunes.

Studies based on imaging assessment without pathological verification may include infarcts due to occlusion of several arteries; the etiology of the occlusion of more than one perforating artery may be completely different from the etiology of lacunes. In conclusion, if the term lacune is restricted to small deep infarcts (type I of Piorier), it is likely that many small deep infarcts seen on imaging are not what neuropathologists call lacunes.

REFERENCES

1. Poirier J, Derouesné C. Le concept de lacune cérébrale de 1838 à nos jours. *Rev Neurol* 1985;141:3–17.
2. Besson G, Hommel M, Perret J. Historical aspects of the lacunar concept. *Cerebrovasc Dis* 1991;1:306–310.
3. Dechambre A. Mémoire sur la curabilité du ramollissement cérébral. *Gaz Med Paris* 1838;6:305–314.
4. Cruveilhier J. *Atlas d'anatomie pathologique du corps humain.* Paris: JB Baillière; 1829–1842.
5. Durand-Fardel M. *Traité du ramollissement du cerveau.* Paris: JB Baillière; 1843.
6. Durand-Fardel M. Mémoire sur une altération particulière de la substance cérébrale. *Gaz Med Paris* 1842;10:23–38.
7. Proust A. Des différentes formes de ramollissement du cerveau [Thèse d'agrégation Médecine]. Paris: 1866.
8. Bizzozero G. Di alcune alterazioni dei linfatici del cervello e della pia madre. *Riv Clin Bologna* 1868;7:33–37.
9. Obersteiner H. Ueber Ectasien der Lymphgefässe des Gehirns. *Arch Pathol Anat Physiol Klin Med* 1872;55:318–323.
10. Ripping LH. Ueber die cystoide Degeneration der Hirnrinde bei paralytischen Geistesteskranken. *Allg Z Psychiatr ihre Grenzgeb* 1874;30:309–318.
11. Arndt R. Zur pathologischen Anatomie der Centralorgane des Nervensystems. *Arch Pathol Anat Physiol Klin Med* 1875;63:241–266.
12. Pick A. Uber cystöse Degeneration des Gehirns. *Arch Psychiatr Nervenkr* 1890;21:910–928.
13. Adler. Ueber einige pathologische Veränderungen an den Hirngefässen Geisteskranker. *Arch Psychiatr Nervenkr* 1875;5:77–90.
14. Marie P. Des foyers lacunaires de désintégration et de différents autres états cavitaires du cerveau. *Rev Med* 1901;21:281–298.
15. Clarke L. A case of general paralysis with examination of the brain medulla oblongata and spinal cord. *J Ment Sci* 1870:500–506.
16. Catola G. Etude clinique et anatomo-pathologique sur les lacunes de désintégration cérébrale. *Rev Med* 1904;4:778–809.
16a. Marie P. *Travaux et memoires.* Paris: Masson; 1928.
17. Reuling R, Herring AP. Cavities in the brain produced by the bacillus aerogenes capsulatus. *Bull Johns Hopkins Hosp* 1899:62–65.
18. Vassale G. Sullo stato cribroso del cervello. *Riv Sper Freniatr Med Leg Alien Ment* 1891;17:480–484.
19. Campbell AW. The morbid changes in the cerebro-spinal nervous system of the aged insane. *J Ment Sci* 1894:638–649.
20. Jacobsohn L. Ueber die schwere Form der Arteriosklerose im Centralnervensystem. *Arch Psychiatr Nervenkr* 1895;27:831–849.
21. Alzheimer A. Neuere Arbeiten über die Dementia senilis und die auf atheromatöser Gefässerkrankung basierenden 23 Gehirnkrankheiten. *Monatsschr Psychiatr Neurol* 1898:101–115.
22. Probst M. Ueber arteriosklerotische Veränderungen des Gehirns und deren Folgen. *Arch Psychiatr Nervenkr* 1901;34:570–602.
22a. Haymaker W, Schiller F. *The founders of neurology.* 2nd ed. Springfield, IL: Charles C. Thomas; 1970.

23. Dupré E, Devaux A. Foyers lacunaires de désintégration cérébrale (note sur le processus histogénique). *Rev Neurol* 1901;9:653–657.
24. Dupré E, Devaux A. Rire et pleurer spasmodiques par ramollissement nucléo-capsulaire antérieur: syndrome pseudo-bulbaire par désintégration lacunaire bilatérale des putamens. *Rev Neurol* 1901;9:919–927.
25. Ferrand J. *Essai sur l'hémiplégie des vieillards. Les lacunes de désintégration cérébrale* [Thesé Médecine]. Paris: 1902.
26. Pic A, Bonnamour S. Des troubles médullaires de l'artériosclérose. La parésie spasmodique des athéromateux. *Rev Med* 1904;2:104–133.
27. Castaigne J, Ferrand J. Paralysies urémiques et lacunes de désintégration cérébrale. *Semain Med* 1904;24:201–202.
28. Raymond F. Sur la pathogénie de certains accidents paralytiques observés chez des vieillards. Leurs rapports probables avec l'urémie. *Rev Med* 1885;5:705–738.
29. Grasset J. La cérébrosclérose lacunaire progressive d'origine artérielle. *Semain Med* 1904; 24:329–330.
30. Vogt C, Vogt O. Zur Lehre der Erkrankungen des striaren Systems. *J Psychol Neurol* 1920; 25:627–846.
31. Lejonne P, Lhermitte J. Les paraplégies d'origine lacunaire et d'origine myélopathique chez les vieillards. *Arch Gen Med* 1905;49:3073–3086.
32. Léri A. Le cerveau sénile. *Rev Neurol* 1906; 14:756–764.
33. Barbe, Levy-Valensi. Lacunes de désintégration cellulaire dans un système nerveux d'hérédosyphilitique. *Rev Neurol* 1908;16:339–340.
34. Marie P, Foix C. Formes cliniques et diagnostic de l'hémiplégie cérébelleuse syphilitique. *Semain Med* 1913;33:145–152.
35. Foix C, Nicolesco I. Grands syndromes de désintégration sénile cérébro-mésencéphalique. *Presse Med* 1923;92:957–963.
36. Foix C, Chavany JA. Palilalie syllabique. Sclérose intracérébrale en foyers disséminés. *Rev Neurol* 1926;43:61–68.
37. Fisher CM. Concerning strokes. *Can Med Assoc J* 1953;69:257–268.
38. Hughes W, Dodgson MCH, MacLennan DC. Chronic cerebral hypertensive disease. *Lancet* 1954;2:770–774.
39. Moore MT. Perivascular encephalolysis. Histopathology and pathogenesis. *Arch Neurol Psychiatry* 1954;71:344–357.
40. Fisher CM. Lacunes: small, deep cerebral infarct. *Neurology* 1965;15:774–784.
41. Hughes W. Origin of lacunes. *Lancet* 1965;2: 19–21.
42. Prineas J, Marshall J. Hypertension and cerebral infarction. *Br Med J* 1966:14–17.
43. Cole FM, Yates P. Intracerebral microaneurysms and small cerebrovascular lesions. *Brain* 1967;90:759–768.
44. Fisher CM. The arterial lesion underlying lacunes. *Acta Neuropathol* 1969;12:1–15.
45. Fisher CM. Cerebral ischemia. Less familiar types. *Clin Neurosurg* 1971;18:267–336.
46. De Reuck J, Vander Eecken H. The arterial angioarchitecture in lacunar state. *Acta Neurol Belg* 1976;76:142–149.
47. Caplan LR. Lacunar infarction: a neglected concept. *Geriatrics* 1976;31:71–75.
48. Laloux P, Brucher JM. Lacunar infarctions due to cholesterol emboli. *Stroke* 1991;22:1440–1444.
49. Alex M, Baron EK, Goldenberg S, Blumenthal HT. An autopsy study of cerebrovascular accident in diabetes mellitus. *Circulation* 1962; 25:663–673.
50. Mohr JP. Lacunes. *Stroke* 1982;13:3–11.
51. Poirier J, Barbizet J, Gaston A, Meyrignac C. Démence thalamique. Lacune expansive du territoire thalamomésencéphalique paramédian. Hydrocéphalie par sténose de l'acqueduc de Sylvius. *Rev Neurol* 1983;139:349–358.
52. Pilleri G. Über eine besondere normotone intracerebrale Gefässerkrankung ("Status cavernosus") mit Schwerpunkt im oberen Hirnstamm. *Psychiatr Neurol* 1965;150;358–382.
53. Derouesné C, Gray F, Escourolle R, Castaigne P. "Expanding cerebral lacunae" in a hypertensive patient with normal pressure hydrocephalus. *Neuropathol Appl Neurobiol* 1987;13:309–320.
54. Poirier J, Derouesné C. Cerebral lacunae. A proposed new classification. *Clin Neuropathol* 1984;3:266.
55. Mancardi GL. Neuropathologic study of lacunae and cribriform cavities of the brain. *Eur Neurol* 1989;29:16–19.
56. Challa VR, Bell MA, Moody DM. A combined hematoxylin-eosin, alkaline phosphatase and high-resolution microradiographic study of lacunes. *Clin Neuropathol* 1990;9:196–204.
57. Fisher CM, Curry B. Pure motor hemiplegia of vascular origin. *Arch Neurol* 1965;13:30–44.
58. Fisher CM. Lacunar infarcts—a review. *Cerebrovasc Dis* 1991;1:311–320.

2

The Course and Territories of Cerebral Small Arteries

Patrick M. Pullicino

Department of Neurology, State University of New York at Buffalo, Buffalo General Hospital, Buffalo, New York 14203

This chapter will be divided into three main sections:

The anterior perforating arteries
The posterior perforating arteries
The arterial supply of the brainstem

Under each section, the origin, course, site of perforation, and territory of supply will be discussed. Comparison will also be made with the structures affected by infarction in the different territories.

THE ANTERIOR PERFORATING ARTERIES

The anterior perforating arteries are a group of arteries that enter the brain through the anterior perforated substance. They can be divided into the following groups:

Anterior lenticulostriate arteries (perforators arising from the anterior cerebral artery or anterior communicating artery, and Heubner's artery)
Internal carotid artery perforators
Middle cerebral artery perforators
Medial, intermediate, and lateral lenticulostriate arteries
Anterior choroidal artery perforators

Anterior Lenticulostriate Arteries

Anterior Cerebral Artery Perforators

An average of six direct perforating arteries arise from the A_1 segment of the anterior cerebral artery (the anterior cerebral artery proximal to the anterior communicating artery) (Fig. 1) and divide to yield 22 arteries on entering the brain. The mean diameter of the perforating branches at their origin is 325 μm, narrowing to 276 μm on entering the brain (1). Most arise from the proximal part of the A_1 segment (2).

After penetrating the anterior perforated substance, these arteries supply a territory that includes the medial third of the anterior commisure, the medial globus pallidus, the posterior medial paraolfactory nuclei (2), the optic chiasm (3,4), and the suprachiasmatic portion of the hypothalamus, including the preoptic, paraventricular, and supraoptic nuclei (5), as well as the substantia innominata (6). Structures anterior to the anterior commisure are perfused in 70% of cases. These include the most medial inferior aspect of the head of the caudate and the putamen, the anterior olfactory nuclei, the septal area (7), and parts of the anterior limb of the internal capsule (8).

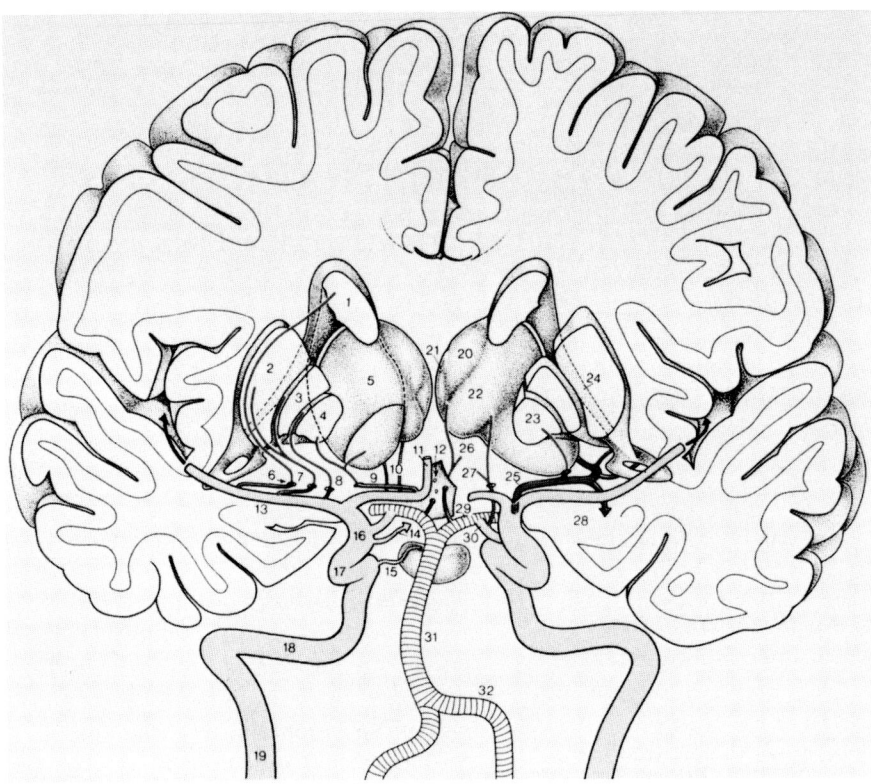

Key to arteries:
6. Lateral lenticulostriate arteries
7. Intermediate lenticulostriate arteries
8. Medial lenticulostriate arteries
9. Heubner's artery
10. Anterior lenticulostriate arteries
11. Anterior cerebral artery
13. Middle cerebral artery
14. Hypophyseal arteries
16. Internal carotid artery
25. Anterior choroidal artery
26. Paramedian thalamic artery
27. Thalamotuberal artery
29. Posterior cerebral artery
30. Posterior communicating artery
31. Basilar artery
32. Vertebral artery

FIG. 1. The perforating arteries arising from the arteries of the circle of Willis. From ref. 91, with permission.

Anterior Communicating Artery Perforators

An average of two to five penetrating arteries arise from the anterior communicating artery (9–11) and supply the optic chiasm, most anterior hypothalamus, mesial anterior commisure, lamina terminalis (10), columns of the fornix, septum pellucidum, and corpus callosum (8,9). Vincentelli et al. (11) found the following areas to be constantly vascularized by the anterior communicating artery: the lamina terminalis, hypothalamus, anterior commisure, trigone, septum pellucidum, and paraolfactory gyrus.

The structures found to be involved following basal forebrain infarction secondary to repair of a ruptured anterior communicating artery aneurysm were the septal gray, the nucleus accumbens, the nucleus of the diagonal band of Broca, and the inferior portions of the anterior limb of the internal capsule and the globus pallidus (12).

Recurrent Artery of Heubner

The recurrent artery is an artery of mean diameter of 662 μm (1) that in most cases originates at or near the site of origin of the anterior communicating artery. The artery was said to be constant in earlier works (13,14), but it may be absent in a small percentage of cases. The recurrent artery doubles back on the anterior cerebral artery, passes above the carotid bifurcation, and accompanies the middle cerebral artery into the medial part of the Sylvian fissure before penetrating the anterior perforated substance. Estimates of the number of recurrent arteries per brain vary widely. A single artery was reported in from 28% (2,15) to 85% (1,16) of hemispheres. The estimate of the frequency of double recurrent arteries varies from 12% (16) to about 50% of brains (2,15). Marinkovic et al. found a double recurrent artery to be always associated with a vascular variant or malformation of the region of the anterior communicating artery (1). Three or more arteries may be present in up to 25% of brains (2,15). A recurrent artery gives 10 branches, which divide to give 20 branches before entering the brain (2). These branches have a diameter of 354 μm on entering the brain (1) (Fig. 2). In addition to its well-known subcortical territory, the recurrent artery supplies parts of the cerebral cortex (1). The recurrent artery usually gives rise to collateral branches to the paraterminal and subcallosal gyri, the olfactory trigone and tract, the orbital operculum, the caudomedial orbitofrontal cortex (1), and the hypothalamus (15). In 20% of cases the recurrent artery gives a branch that accompanies the middle cerebral artery and supplies the frontal cortex anterior to the syl-

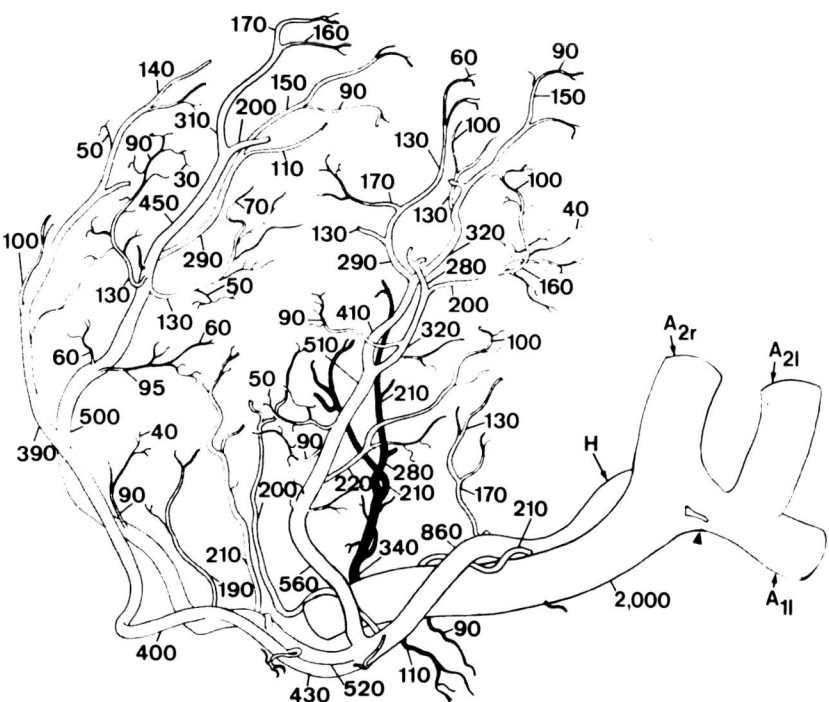

FIG. 2. Drawing of a cast of the recurrent artery of Heubner (H) and the perforating branches arising from the anterior cerebral artery giving diameters at different sites (in micrometers). From ref. 1, with permission.

vian fissure (15). Extracerebral direct anastomoses between the recurrent artery and the medial lenticulostriate arteries are present in 9–12% of cases (15,17).

The recurrent artery territory extends from the tip of the lateral ventricle to the anterior commisure in 92% of cases (8). It supplies the inferior half of the head of the caudate nucleus and putamen (6,7) and the inferior part of the anterior limb of the internal capsule constantly (18). It also supplies part of the septal nuclei, the rostrolateral part of the olfactory trigone (7), and the subcortical paramedian white matter of the orbitofrontal region. In over 50% of brains it supplies the entire anterior striatum (8). At the level of the anterior commisure it supplies the lateral part of the anterior commisure and the inferior part of the putamen. In 15% of cases it participates in the supply to the genu of the internal capsule (15).

Internal Carotid Artery Perforators

The perforating branches of the carotid artery arise from the supraclinoid (C4) portion of the carotid artery. The C4 portion of the carotid artery has three segments, each of which begins at the origin of the arterial branch after which it is named: ophthalmic, posterior communicating, or anterior choroidal (19).

About four arteries arise from the ophthalmic segment and are most commonly distributed to the hypophysis and the adjacent hypothalamus (superior hypophyseal and tuberoinfundibular arteries) (20), the optic chiasm, and less commonly the optic nerve and tract, and the premamillary floor of the third ventricle (19).

The communicating segment does not give rise to any perforating arteries in about 60% of cases. In the remainder, one to three arteries arise and supply the optic tract, premamillary part of the floor of the third ventricle, optic chiasm, infundibulum, and anterior perforated substance (19).

The choroidal segment is the most frequent site of perforating branches. These arteries are three to four in number and divide to give eight branches of mean diameter 243 μm on entering the anterior perforated substance (2,21). These arteries penetrate the anterior perforated substance just lateral to the optic chiasm and the initial part of the optic tract, and may supply the optic tract and uncus (19). The mean diameter of the intracerebral segments of these perforators is 177 μm (21).

The territory of supply includes the optic chiasm (4,22), the infundibulum (22), and occasionally the anterior border of the hypothalamus (4). Perforating branches supply the genu of the internal capsule and the adjacent parts of the globus pallidus (6), posterior limb of the internal capsule, and anterior thalamus (2,8). Rosner et al. (2) found that the territory of supply of the internal carotid perforators overlaps with that of the anterior lenticulostriates anteriorly, with the medial lenticulostriates laterally, and with the anterior choroidal perforators posteriorly.

Middle Cerebral Artery Perforators

The middle cerebral artery extends laterally from its origin, and the M_1 segment ends where it turns sharply posterosuperiorly. In 86% of cases the middle cerebral artery bifurcation occurs in the M_1 segment (2). A mean of 9–15 perforating branches arise from the middle cerebral artery (17,23), which divide to give an average of 26 branches on penetrating the brain (2) (Fig. 1). Seventeen percent to 22% of the branches arise distal to the bifurcation of the middle cerebral artery (2,17) (Figs. 3 and 4). Ninety-six percent of perforating arteries arise from the proximal 17 mm of the middle cerebral artery (17) (Fig. 5) and the perforating arteries usually take origin from the superior wall of the middle cerebral artery (17).

Twenty percent to 50% of perforating ar-

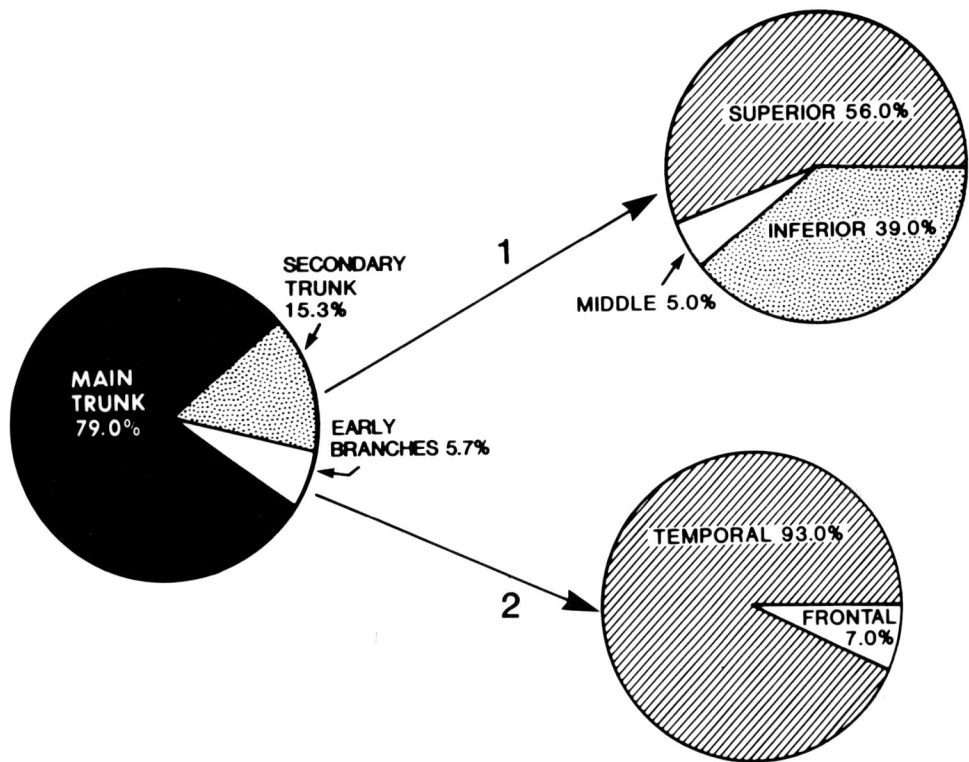

FIG. 3. Diagram showing the percentage of perforating arteries arising from the main middle cerebral artery trunk and its branches. From ref. 17, with permission.

teries arise as branches from a common stem (17,24) giving rise to up to 13 branches according to Umansky et al. (17) (Figs. 4 and 6) or 37 branches according to Rosner et al. (2). Common stems have a mean diameter of about 0.9 mm and occasionally reach the diameter of the larger cortical branches of the middle cerebral artery (17).

The mean diameter of the single arteries is 0.39 mm (17). There is a statistically significant relationship between the number and relative size of perforating arteries, that is, the greater the number of perforating arteries the smaller their diameter and *vice versa* (23).

The extracerebral segments of the middle

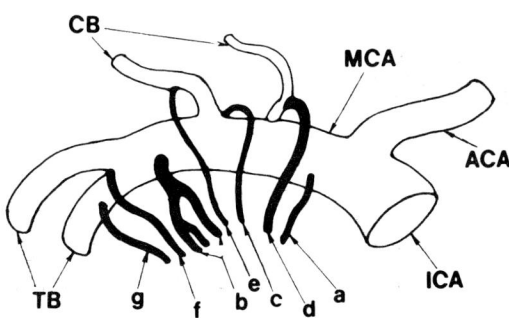

FIG. 4. Diagram showing the site of origin of perforating arteries that arise either from the proximal segment of the middle cerebral artery (MCA), either as individual arteries (**a**) or sharing a common stem (**b**). They may also arise from the cortical branches (CB) (**c–e**) or from the bifurcation or terminal branches (TB) of the MCA. From ref. 23, with permission.

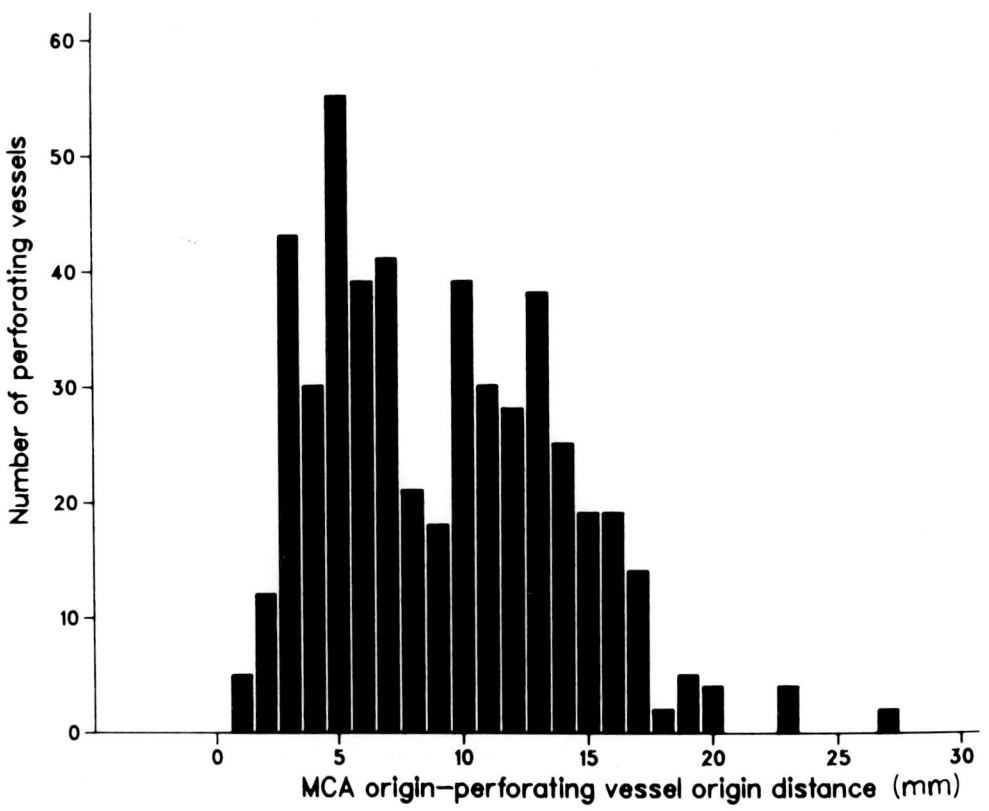

FIG. 5. Histogram showing the number of perforating arteries arising from different distances from the origin of the middle cerebral artery. From ref. 17, with permission.

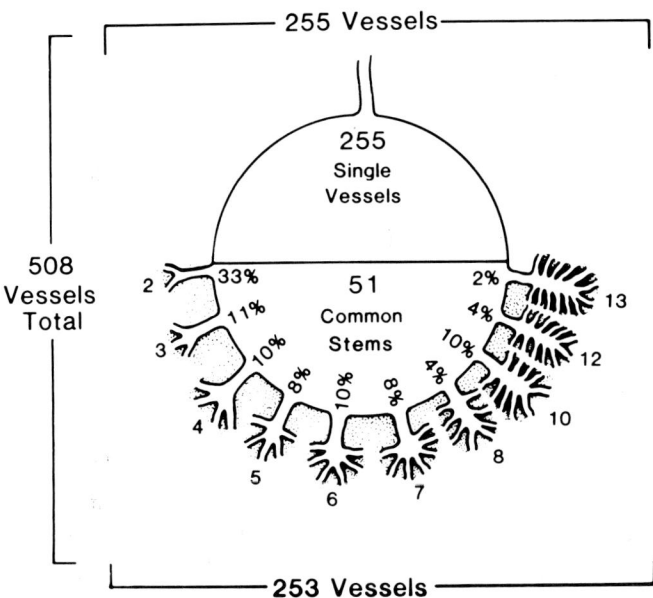

FIG. 6. Diagram showing the branching characteristics of 508 perforating arteries; 50% arise from common stems. From ref. 17, with permission.

cerebral artery perforators can be divided into three groups (2,23)—medial, intermediate, and lateral—according to their site of origin from the middle cerebral artery and their morphology.

Medial Lenticulostriate Arteries

These arteries arise from the middle cerebral artery just distal to the carotid bifurcation (Fig. 1). They are present in 50–86% of hemispheres (2,23), and are usually two in number (2,23) and give an average of four branches as they enter the anterior perforated substance (2). These arteries usually originate as single arteries, but in 17% they originate from common stems (23). In the 15% of brains in which the medial lenticulostriates are not represented, the terminal branches of the recurrent artery of Heubner replace the medial lenticulostriates (17). There is only a clear distinction between medial and lateral lenticulostriate arteries in 41% of cases (17).

The medial lenticulostriates vascularize the area lateral and posterolateral to the anterior commisure (25), the centromedial part of the putamen (26), and the lateral part of the globus pallidus (2). They also supply the inferior parts of the posterior limb of the internal capsule (26).

Intermediate Lenticulostriate Arteries

Rosner et al. (2) described an intermediate group of lenticulostriate arteries, which they found in 94% of cases. These arteries arise from the middle cerebral artery between the medial and lateral lenticulostriates. Rosner et al. reported that these arteries are characterized by a high frequency of multiple arteries arising from a common stem. Marinkovic et al., however, found that only a third of these arteries (which they called middle perforating arteries) arise from a common stem (23). There are an average of three intermediate lenticulostriate arteries, which divide to give a mean of 14 branches on entering the anterior perforated substance (2). The common stems occasionally give rise to pial arteries supplying the insular cortex (23).

The territory of supply of the intermediate lenticulostriate arteries is the anterior part of the lateral lenticulostriate territory (27).

Lateral Lenticulostriate Arteries

Shellshear (25) was the first to describe that the lateral lenticulostriates originate from the middle cerebral artery at an acute angle directed back toward the direction of blood flow. The more lateral the origin, the more acute the angle (17). The arteries describe an S-shaped course and enter the posterolateral part of the anterior perforated substance. On penetrating the cerebral substance, they course dorsomedially (18). There are an average of four to five lateral lenticulostriate arteries, which divide to yield an average of eight arteries on entering the anterior perforated substance (2,23). One or more common stems give rise to lateral lenticulostriates in over 50% of hemispheres according to Marinkovic et al. (23). The lateral lenticulostriates originate prior to the middle cerebral bifurcation in 78%, prior and distal to the bifurcation in about 20%, and solely distal to the bifurcation, including origin from the cortical branches of the middle cerebral artery, in 2% (2,23) (Fig. 4).

The territory of supply of the lateral lenticulostriates includes almost the entire length of the upper internal capsule (2,28). The lenticulostriates (probably the lateral group) contribute to the blood supply of the genu of the internal capsule (29), particularly in its anterior half (30). Superiorly, the territory of the lenticulostriates reaches up to the white matter of the corona radiata lateral to the lateral ventricles (31,32), although the paraventricular white matter suprajacent to the posterolateral thalamus is probably supplied by the posterolateral choroidal artery (32). The lateral lenticulostriates supply the optic radiations posteriorly (33). The lenticulostriates also supply the body and the upper half of the head of the caudate nucleus (28,30,31,34), as well as the putamen and globus pallidus (6).

Intracerebral Segments of Lenticulostriate Arteries

The extracerebral segments of the lenticulostriates turn sharply dorsally on entering the cerebral substance, turning through a mean angle of 69° (27) (Fig. 7). The three extracerebral divisions of the lenticulostriates (medial, intermediate, and lateral) divide into two groups intracerebrally: medial and lateral (27). The medial and lateral extracerebral divisions give rise to the medial and lateral intracerebral groups and the extracerebral intermediate lenticulostriates give rise to the anterior part of the lateral intracerebral group (27). The perforating branches are layered in an "onion-skin" fashion (28). The lateral intracerebral arteries are longer than and approximately twice the diameter of (510 μm

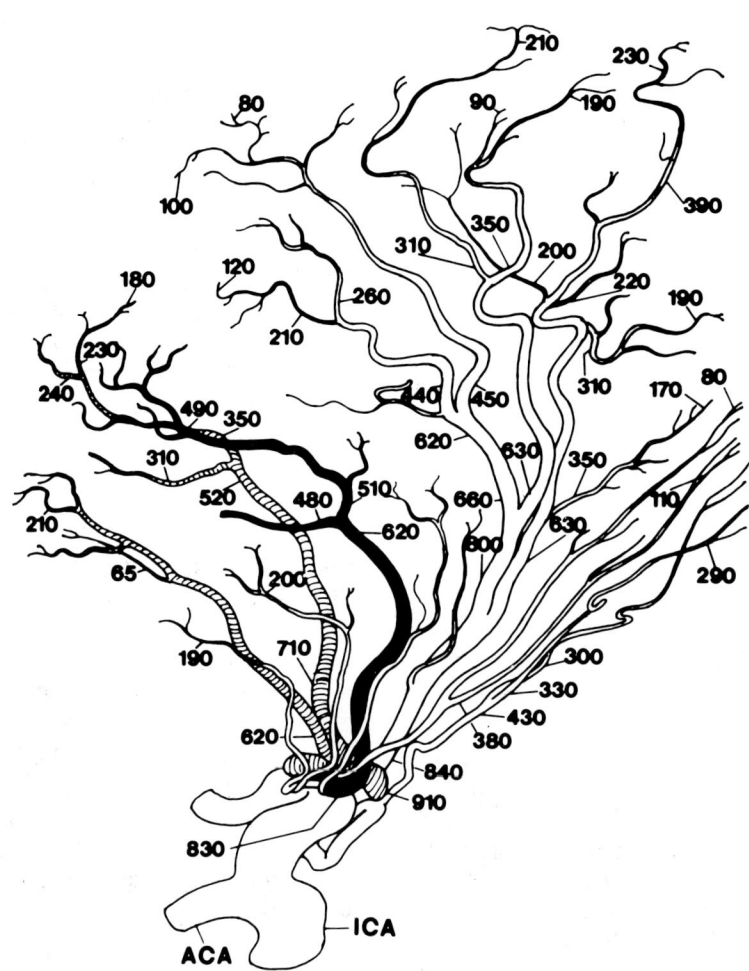

FIG. 7. Drawing of a cast of the perforating branches of the middle cerebral artery showing diameters (in micrometers) of the main stems and branches at different sites. From ref. 27, with permission.

versus 280 μm) the medial ones; 60% of their proximal stems have diameters of 500–840 μm (27).

The intracebral segments form a narrow concave fan, whose concavity is directed medially, dorsally, and posteriorly (27). The intracerebral segments can be divided into a proximal and distal portion, which are separated by a well-formed obtuse angulation of the artery (mean value 111°) (27). Two types of collateral branches are given off intracerebrally from the proximal portions: longitudinal, which run parallel to the parent artery and whose mean diameter is 155 μm (27), and transverse, whose mean diameter is 105 μm. The distal portions also give off collateral branches and terminal branches. First-, second-, third-, and fourth-order branching occurs proximal to the capillaries.

The mean diameter of the intracerebral segments just proximal to their terminal divisions is 470 μm (lateral stems) and 260 μm (medial stems) (27). Distal intracerebral stems give off large (300–350 μm), middle-sized (90–200 μm), and small (50–90 μm) branches. Fourth-order branches have a caliber of about 30 μm (27).

Marinkovic et al. have measured the ramification zone of perforating arteries at different points. This is the greatest anteroposterior and lateral diameter occupied by all the branches of a single artery. Their findings are listed in Table 1 (see also Fig. 7).

TABLE 1. *Ramification zone of perforating arteries*

	AP (mm)	Lat (mm)
Smallest collateral branches	2.6	1.4
Larger collateral branches	8.9	5.5
Terminal stem of a lateral intracerebral artery	23.0	13.0
Distal portion of a lateral intracerebral artery	30.0	15.5
Distal portion of a medial intracerebral artery	11.0	4.4
Proximal portion of a lateral intracerebral artery	37.9	15.5
Whole lateral perforating artery	41.6	15.5
Common stem giving rise to multiple perforating arteries	53.0	41.0

AP, anteroposterior; Lat, lateral.

Anterior Choroidal Artery

The anterior choroidal artery arises from the carotid artery in over 77% of cases, but occasionally arises from the middle cerebral artery (35,36) or from the posterior communicating artery (37). It courses along the lateral border of the optic tract and goes posteriorly and laterally to reach the temporal horn of the lateral ventricle, which it supplies. The average diameter of this artery is about 1 mm (37). In about 4% of hemispheres there are two or three anterior choroidal arteries (38) and it may rarely be absent (36).

The anterior choroidal artery gives perforating branches to the anterior perforated substance in about 90% of cases (2) (Figs. 1 and 8), with two branches to the anterior perforated substance, which divide to give an average of six branches on entry into the brain (2). There are free anastomoses between the anterior choroidal territory and the posterior cerebral circulation (posterolateral choroidal artery) (7,30,36) at two main sites: over the lateral geniculate body (39,40) and over the thalamus by way of the choroid plexus (41). In addition, there are anastomoses with the posterior communicating artery and middle cerebral arteries (42).

The superficial territory of the anterior choroidal includes the optic tracts (4,22) and optic radiation, and the medial temporal lobe, including the anterior parts of the hippocampus, uncus (38%) (43), piriform cortex, and posterior part of the amygdaloid nucleus (44). It also supplies the middle third of the cerebral peduncle (44%) and of the substantia nigra (30,34,42), and according to Khan, the ventral part of the midbrain tegmentum (45), and according to Abbie, the medial half of the lateral geniculate body (34,42).

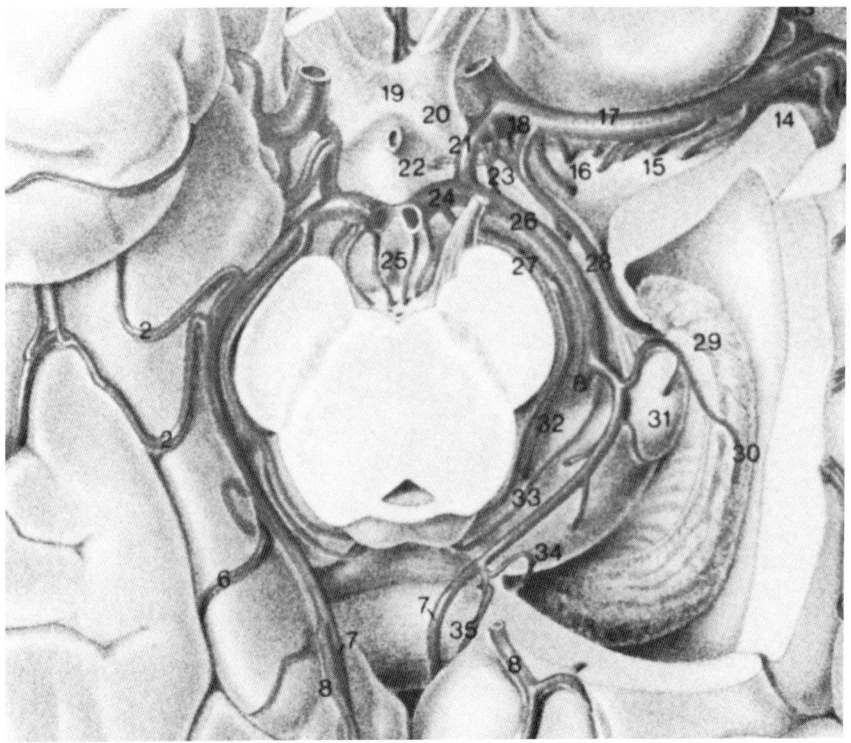

Key to selected arteries:
15. Lateral lenticulostriate arteries
16. Medial lenticulostriate arteries
17. Middle cerebral artery
18. Perforators from the internal carotid and proximal anterior cerebral artery
21. Posterior communicating artery
23. Thalamotuberal artery
24. P_1 segment of posterior cerebral artery
25. Paramedian mesencephalic arteries
26. P_2 segment of posterior cerebral artery
27. Collicular artery
28. Anterior choroidal artery
29. Choroidal branches of anterior choroidal artery
30. Posterolateral choroidal artery
31. Lateral geniculate body
33. Posteromedial choroidal artery
34. Thalamogeniculate arteries

FIG. 8. Basal view of the circle of Willis and of the branches of the posterior cerebral artery. From ref. 91, with permission.

The perforating territory includes the lower portion of the posterior limb of the internal capsule [supplying the posterior two thirds (34,44)] and the retrolenticular part of the internal capsule, including the optic radiations (6,41) and auditory radiations (26), the medial globus pallidus (6) (75% of cases), and the superficial part of the ventrolateral thalamus (34,41,42) (37%). It also may supply the upper lateral part of the red nucleus (42), the upper part of the subthalamic nucleus, the H_2 field of Forel, and the zona incerta (26,41). Its territory does not extend up as far as the margin of the lateral ventricle, and does not include the corona radiata (43). The extent of the anterior choroidal supply varies inversely with the extent of neighboring territories. The anterior choroidal may supply the genu and anterior third of the internal capsule if the posterior communicating artery is small, and according to Abbie, if the anterior choroidal artery is small the territory of the posterior communicating artery (thalamotuberal artery) may supply the posterior limb of the internal capsule (42).

This variability also affects the supply of the anterior choroidal to the substantia nigra, the red nucleus, and the subthalamic nucleus (42).

Infarcts in the territory of the anterior choroidal seen at autopsy are of a smaller size than would be expected from injection studies (43). The posterior limb of the internal capsule and the medial globus pallidus are always involved (46–48). Less frequently, infarction of the thalamus (48), optic tract, and cerebral peduncle is seen (43).

THE POSTERIOR PERFORATING ARTERIES

Nomenclature for thalamic nuclei is according to Van Buren and Borke (49).

Posterior Communicating Artery

The posterior communicating artery gives rise to an average of seven branches of diameter 100–600 μm (37). There are three types of branches according to Percheron (50): hypothalamic arterioles, pedunculo-subthalamic arterioles, and the thalamotuberal artery.

Hypothalamic Arteries

The territory of supply of these arteries is variable but extends from the infundibulum anteriorly in 12% of cases (51), to the mammillary bodies posteriorly, and includes the posterior hypothalamus (4) and the optic tract in 12% (51). The superior hypophyseal arteries and tuberoinfundibular arteries arise from the internal carotid artery and supply the hypophysis and adjacent hypothalamus (20). A branch to the mamillary bodies can also arise from the paramedian thalamic arteries or from the P_1 segment of the posterior cerebral artery (52,53). Anastomoses appear to be frequent among hypothalamic arteries and are most common between the tuberoinfundibular branches (20).

Pedunculo-subthalamic Arteries

These arteries have a variable territory but may include part of the cerebral peduncle, the fields of Forel, the zona incerta, and the subthalamic nucleus (50). The territory of these arteries varies inversely with that of the anterior choroidal artery.

Thalamotuberal Artery

The thalamotuberal artery (thalamic polar artery, anterior internal optic artery of Duret, premamillary pedicle of Foix, and Hillemand) usually originates from the middle third of the posterior communicating artery (37), or rarely from the P_1 segment of the posterior cerebral artery (Fig. 9). It is present in 60–80% of cases (37,50). This artery is always single and penetrates the brain lateral to the mammillary body and ascends vertically to the inferior border of the thalamus. Its average diameter is 600 μm (37).

Its area of supply varies inversely with the territory of the paramedian thalamic arteries (50) and of the anterior choroidal artery (42). It includes the reticular nucleus and lateropolar nuclei, part of the dorso-oral and ventro-oral nuclei, the medial nucleus, and part of the mammillothalamic tract (34,50,54). It also supplies the genu of the internal capsule (26) and the most anterior portion of the posterior limb of the internal capsule (30,55). Its area of supply does not include the anterior nuclei of the thalamus (50).

Posterior Cerebral Artery

The posterior cerebral artery is divided into P_1 and P_2 segments. The P_1 segment extends from its origin to the posterior communicating artery origin. The P_2 segment extends from the posterior communicating

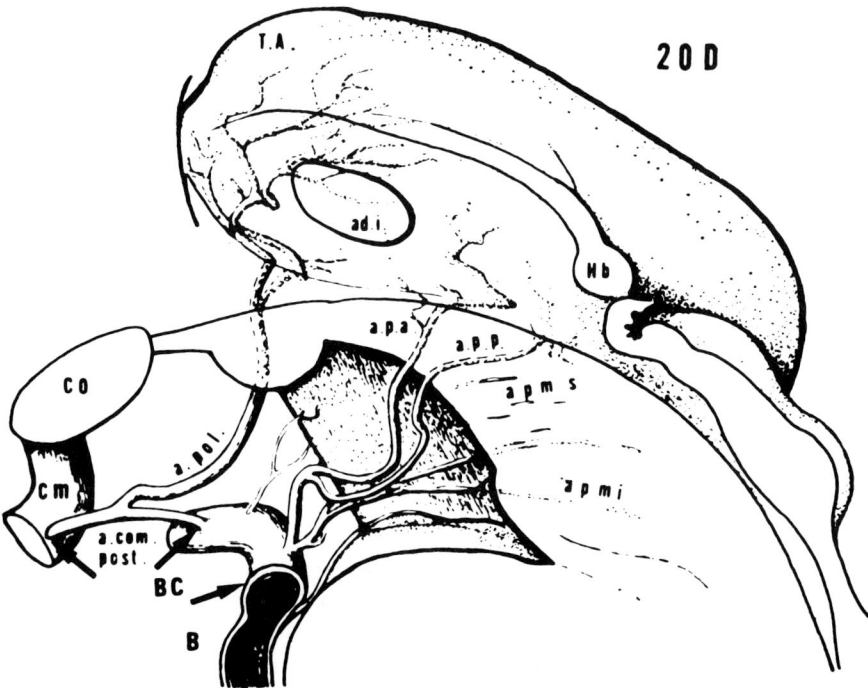

FIG. 9. Drawing of a superimposed dissection and radiograph to show the thalamotuberal artery (a.pol.) arising from the posterior communicating artery (a.com.post.) and supplying the anterior thalamus. The paramedian thalamic (a.p.a., a.p.p.) and the superior and inferior mesencephalic arteries (a.p.m.s., a.p.m.i.) arising from the P_1 segment of the posterior communicating artery. From ref. 50, with permission.

artery origin to the posterior aspect of the midbrain (Fig. 8).

The proximal or P_1 segment gives rise to the paramedian thalamic and mesencephalic arteries (94%) (53), the collicular (80%) and accessory collicular (86%) arteries (56), the posteromedial choroidal artery (60%), the peduncular and hippocampal arteries, and to direct branches to the mesencephalic tegmentum (37,57).

The distal or P_2 (56,57) segment gives rise to the proximal (51–83%) posterolateral choroidal artery and the posterolateral thalamic (distal posterolateral choroidal) artery (20%) (56,57), the thalamogeniculate arteries (80%) (58), the proximal (40–54%) and distal (41%) posteromedial choroidal arteries, the paramedian thalamic or mesencephalic arteries (6%) (53), the collicular (20%) or accessory collicular (14%) artery (56), and to anterior (29%), middle (30%), and posterior (29%) hippocampal arteries, and peduncular and splenial arteries.

Paramedian Thalamic and Mesencephalic Arteries

(Also called the interpeduncular perforators, thalamoperforating arteries, posterior internal optic arteries of Duret, retromamillary pedicle of Foix and Hillemand, or the posterior perforating arteries of Gillilan.)

These arteries can be divided into three groups according to the site at which they perforate the brain in the interpeduncular fossa (45,52). The interpeduncular fossa is the space limited by the mamillary bodies anteriorly, the anterior part of the mesencephalic tegmentum posteriorly, the cerebral peduncles laterally, and the upper part of the pons inferiorly. The posterior perforated substance (PPS) is a triangular area of gray matter located behind the mamillary bodies. The paramedian thalamic arteries penetrate the anterior half of the PPS, the superior paramedian mesencephalic arteries penetrate the posterior half of the PPS, and the inferior paramedian mesencephalic arteries penetrate the posterior third of the interpeduncular fossa, inferior to the PPS (52) (Fig. 10).

The average number of paramedian arteries is two to five. One (95%) or two (5%) common stems giving rise to an average of five perforating arteries are present in 88% of brains (53,56)

The individual penetrating arteries originate from the P_1 segment of the posterior cerebral artery in 94% of cases and from the P_2 segment in 6% (53). The branch nearest the basilar bifurcation is the largest in 56% of cases (37). The P_1 segment on one side may give off no perforating branches, with all the perforating arteries being given off from one side (56). The mean diameter of the arteries just distal to their origin is 389 μm (53). In 30% of cases individual arteries may take origin from the collicular and accessory collicular artery or from the posteromedial choroidal artery (53). The common stems always arise from the P_1 segment close to the bifurcation. The diameter of the common stems was 612 μm (53).

The territory of supply of the common stems was restricted to the thalamic (30%) or mesencephalic (14%) territory ipsilaterally in 44% of cases. In 56% of cases the stems supplied both of these territories, ipsilaterally in 35% and bilaterally in 20% (52).

There are an average of four to five collateral branches to the cerebral peduncle (52). Marinkovic et al. found a supply from the paramedian perforators to the mamillary bodies in 26% (53). Branches to the oculomotor nerve are present in 15–71% (52,53). Sixty percent to 80% of cases had extracerebral anastomoses between the perforating arteries (52,53,59,60).

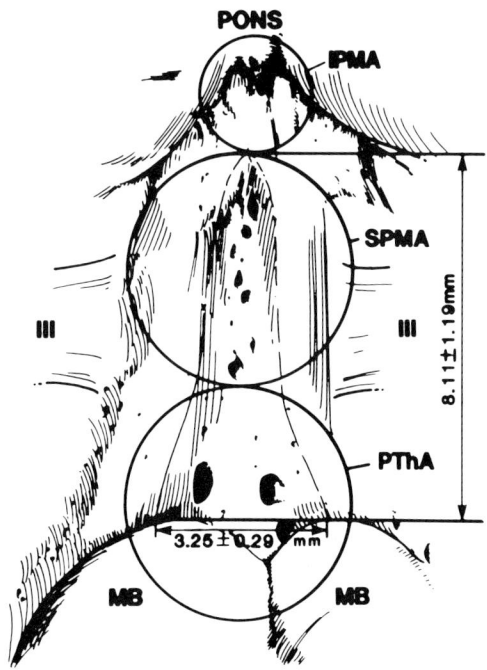

FIG. 10. Drawing of the interpeduncular fossa to show the entrance points of the superior (SPMA) and inferior (IPMA) mesencephalic arteries and of the paramedian thalamic arteries (PThA). MB, mammillary body. From ref. 52, with permission.

Inferior Paramedian Mesencephalic Arteries

These arteries usually originate from the P_1 segment of the posterior cerebral artery but may originate from the basilar bifurcation (45,61). They often originate separately from the other paramedian arteries (61). These arteries supply the inferior paramedian midbrain (52), including the medial margin of the cerebral peduncles, the medial part of the substantia nigra, and the medial part of the tegmentum, ventral to the medial longitudinal fasciculus (45).

The lower midbrain structures that are commonly affected by paramedian infarcts include the medial longitudinal fasciculus, the central tegmental tract, the supratrochlear and fourth nerve nuclei, and the decussation of the superior cerebellar peduncles (54).

Superior Paramedian Mesencephalic Arteries

These arise higher up and more laterally on the P_1 segment than the inferior mesencephalic arteries. Although these arteries may arise from the P_1 segment ipsilateral to their territory of supply, the P_1 segment of the posterior cerebral artery often supplies both sides of the midbrain, either because the mesencephalic arteries may arise from the contralateral P_1 or because individual arteries terminate by giving branches to both sides of the midline (particularly in the region of the third nerve nucleus) (61). This contralateral supply may be total or partial. The superior mesencephalic arteries may arise on a common stem with the paramedian thalamic arteries or independently (52,61) (Fig. 11).

These arteries penetrate the posterior PPS and remain close to the midline but have slightly divergent curves (53) (Fig. 12). The longer rami are smaller than the thalamic paramedian arteries and measure 176 μm in diameter (53). The territory of the short rami includes the midbrain tegmentum ventral and lateral to the medial longitudinal fasciculus, the medial part of the red nucleus, the decussation of the superior cerebellar peduncle, the interpeduncular nucleus, the central tegmental tract, and the medial part of the medial lemniscus (45,61). The longer central rami supply the anterior periaqueductal gray matter, as well as the trochlear, oculomotor, and dorsal tegmental nuclei, the interstitial nucleus of Cajal, the nucleus of the posterior commissure (45), and the rostral interstitial nucleus of the medial longitudinal fasciculus (MLF) (62).

The lateral part of the anteromedial midbrain territory is supplied by short penetrating arteries arising from the collicular artery (63). These supply the lateral part of the red nucleus and part of the medial lemniscus.

The upper midbrain structures that are commonly affected in paramedian infarcts are (a) at the most rostral midbrain level, the third nerve nucleus, the Edinger-West-

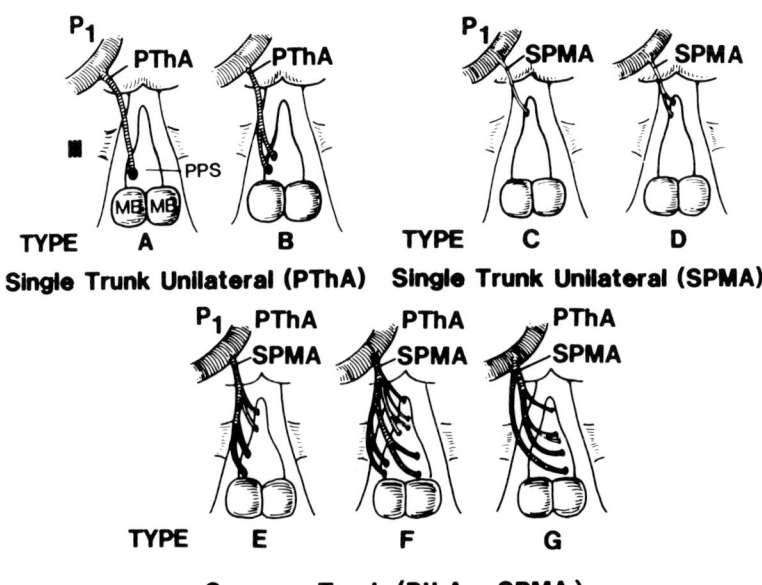

FIG. 11. Drawing showing how the paramedian thalamic arteries (PThA) and the superior mesencephalic arteries (SPMA) may either arise separately (**A–D**) or by a common trunk that penetrates unilaterally or bilaterally (**E–G**). From ref. 52, with permission.

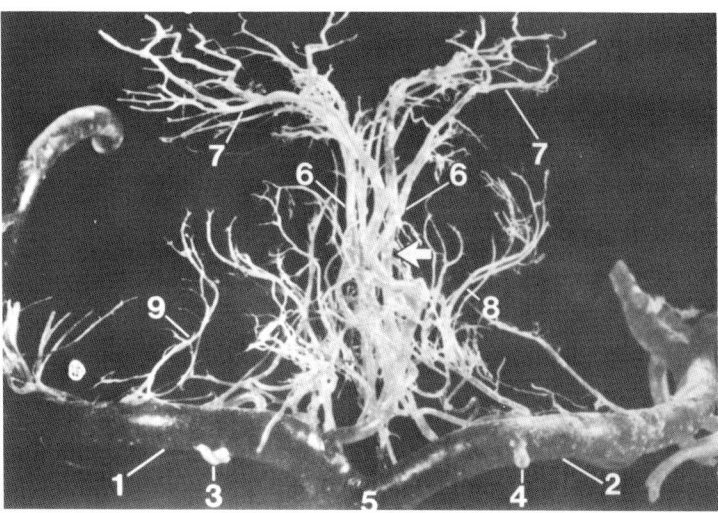

FIG. 12. Corrosion specimen of cast of perforating branches of the posterior cerebral artery. 1, 2: Posterior cerebral arteries. 3, 4: Posterior communicating arteries. 5: Basilar artery. 6: Paramedian mesencephalic and thalamic arteries (long rami). 7: Distal portions. 8: Short rami of the paramedian mesencephalic arteries. 9: Direct branch to the cerebral peduncle. From ref. 53, with permission.

phal nucleus, the nuclei of the reticular formation, the medial longitudinal fasciculus, the medial part of the red nucleus, and the pars compacta of the substantia nigra (54); and (b) at an upper midbrain level, the medial longitudinal fasciculus, the superior cerebellar peduncle, and the inferior pole of the third nerve nucleus (54).

Paramedian Thalamic Arteries

According to Percheron (61), each thalamus is usually supplied by one artery that arises from the P_1 segment, but in about 50% of cases this artery divides into two, either extra- or intracerebrally, before reaching the thalamus (Fig. 13).

The thalami have an independent blood supply from the ipsilateral P_1 in 50% of cases (61), but a common bilateral supply from one side, not necessarily from a common stem, is present in 44%. Occasionally there is a common supply to both thalami from an arcade that originates from both P_1 segments (61) (Fig. 13).

The thalamic arteries are larger and longer than the mesencephalic arteries, and their mean diameter is 332 μm (53). The diameter of the distal part of the intracerebral segments of these arteries is 227 μm (53) and the diameter of their terminal stems is 189 μm (53). These arteries remain paramedian in their initial intraparenchymal course, just anterior to the red nucleus. They then incline outward to follow the floor of the third ventricle, passing above the red nucleus, superiorly and laterally.

These arteries have a subthalamic territory and a thalamic territory. The subthalamic territory is small and is contiguous with that of the mesencephalic arteries. It includes the region of the superior red nucleus. The thalamic territory is very variable in its anteroposterior extent, depending largely on the territory of the thalamotuberal artery. When the thalamotuberal artery is present, the anterior limit of the paramedian territory is the mamillothalamic fasciculus. The paramedian territory includes part of the medial nucleus, the

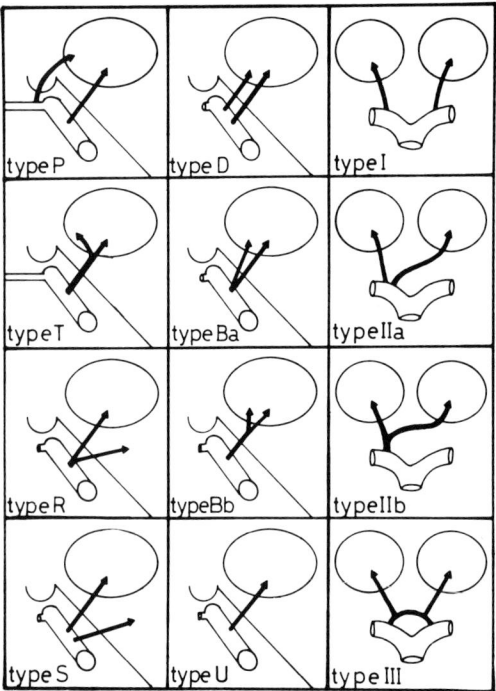

FIG. 13. Diagrams showing variations in the paramedian thalamic artery (PTA) supply to the thalamus. Types P and T show the anterior thalamus supplied by the thalamotuberal artery and by the PTA. The PTA may be double (type D), or bifurcate outside (Ba) or within (Bb) the thalamus, or may be single (U). There may be a bilateral symmetrical origin (type I), or arteries to both thalami may arise from one P_1 segment (IIa), by a common trunk (IIb), or by an arcade (III). From ref. 61, with permission.

parafascicular nucleus, the intralamellary nucleus, the fasciculus retroflexus, the central nucleus, the inferior paraventricular region, and the internal ventro-oral nuclei. The superior limit of the paramedian territory varies with the territory of the posteromedial choroidal artery and inferolaterally the territory abuts on and varies with the size of the territory of the collicular arteries.

In more than 75% of paramedian thalamic infarcts, the thalamic structures involved include the median, central, parafascicular, and intralamellary nuclei. In more than 50% there is also involvement of the dorsocaudal, and the internal ventro-oral and ventrocaudal nuclei (54).

Thalamogeniculate Arteries

The thalamogeniculate arteries arise from the posterior cerebral artery P_2 segment in 80% of cases (58) (Figs. 8 and 14). They perforate the inferior surface of the medial geniculate body (100%), pulvinar (80%), brachium of the superior colliculus (53%), or lateral geniculate body (12%) (58). They terminate in the posterior portion of the lateral thalamic nuclear mass (37,41). The posterior cerebral arteries give origin to an average of two to five thalamogeniculate arteries (56,58). The mean caliber of these arteries is 346 μm (58). These arteries most often originate as individual arteries, but common stems with a mean diameter of 583 μm are present in 33% (58). Collateral branches may supply the medial geniculate body, pulvinar, brachium of the superior colliculus, cerebral peduncle, or lateral geniculate body (58). Anastomoses usually with the posteromedial choroidal artery are present in 67% (58).

According to Schlesinger, the thalamogeniculate arteries supply the majority of the ventrocaudal nucleus, the dorsocaudal nucleus, the lateral parts of the medial pulvinar nucleus, the medial nucleus, the central nucleus, and the parafascicular nucleus. They also supply the reticular nucleus and the zona incerta and give small rami to the posterior limb of the internal capsule (41).

Posterolateral Choroidal Artery

The posterolateral choroidal arterial system is a system of arteries that arise from the distal part of the P_2 segment (Figs. 8, 14, and 15). The most constant artery passes laterally through the choroidal fissure and upward over the pulvinar to supply the choroid plexus of the temporal horn and the glomus of the choroid plexus in the atrium of the lateral ventricle (56). It anastomoses with branches of the anterior choroidal artery over the lateral geniculate body

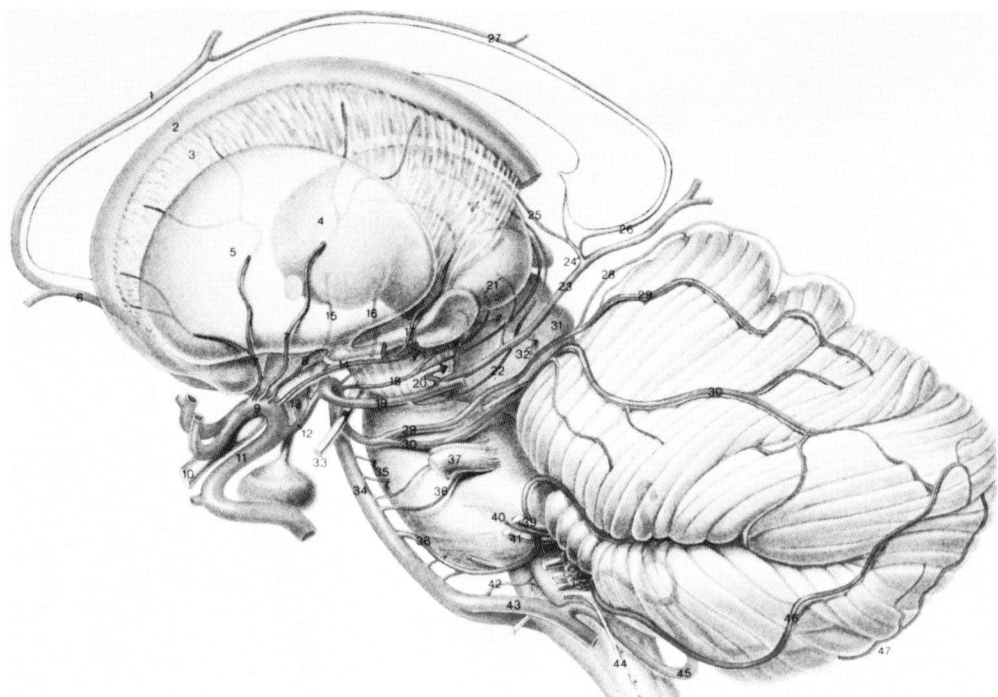

FIG. 14. The perforating arteries supplying the basal ganglia, thalamus, and brainstem. From ref. 91, with permission.
Key:
7. Lateral lenticulostriate arteries
8. Medial lenticulosriate arteries
9. Middle cerebral artieres
18. Posteromedial choroidal artery
19. Posterior cerebral artery
20. Posterolateral choroidal artery
21. Thalamogenticulate artery
29. Superior cerebellar artery (medial branch)
30. Superior cerebellar artery (lateral branch)
34. Basilar artery
35. Paramedian pontine arteries
36. Inferolateral pontine artery
38. Anterior inferior cerebellar artery
43. Basilar artery
45. Posterior inferior cerebellar artery (PICA)
46. PICA (lateral branch)
47. PICA (medial branch)

(30,36,45). A single posterolateral choroidal artery may be present [only 9% of cases (64)] and gives branches to the temporal lobe, the hippocampus, the thalamus and, the choroid plexus. However, these structures may be supplied by separate arteries. Most commonly there are two arteries [79% (64)], a posterolateral choroidal artery and a posterolateral thalamic artery [or distal posterolateral choroidal artery (57)] (Fig. 15).

The posterolateral choroidal artery (64) [also called the proximal posterolateral choroidal artery (57)] is present in 91% of cases (57). Its mean diameter is 500 μm and it usually arises from the P_2 segment [51–83% of cases (56,57)]. It otherwise arises from a branch of the posterior cerebral, most commonly the parieto-occipital (56).

The posterolateral thalamic artery (64) arises more distally on the P_2 segment and has a mean diameter of 500 μm (57), and may be multiple [up to five in number (57)]. It is not a true choroidal artery since it only supplies the thalamus and gives no branches to the choroid plexus (64), but it ascends up over the posterior pulvinar.

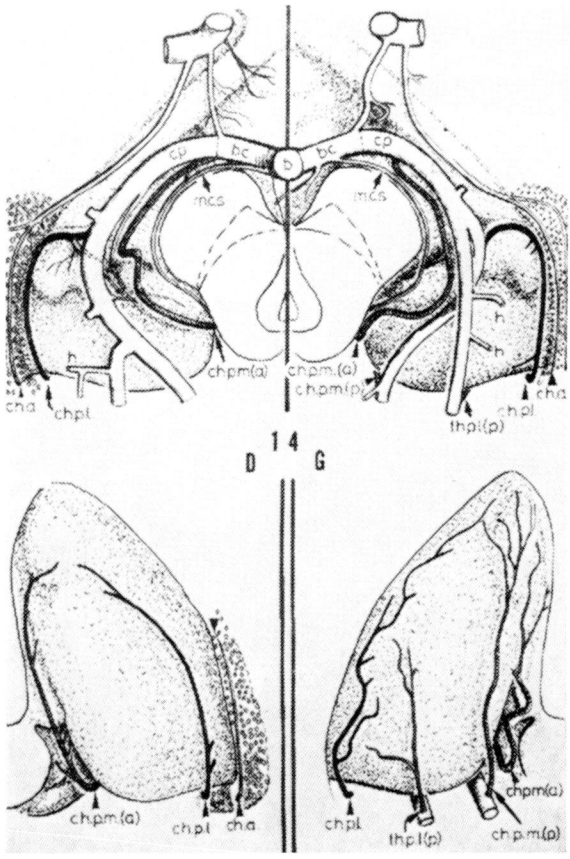

FIG. 15. Drawing showing two common arrangements of the posteromedial and posterolateral choroidal arteries. The upper part of the figure shows the upper midbrain and inferior thalami from below and the lower part of the figure is a view of the thalami from above. The inferior and superior views of the same thalamus are on the same side of the drawing. Key: cha, anterior choroidal artery; chpl, posterolateral choroidal artery; chpm(a) and chpm(p), posteromedial choroidal arteries; thpl(p), posterolateral thalamic artery; mcs, collicular artery. From ref. 64, with permission.

Posteromedial Choroidal Artery

The posteromedial choroidal artery arises from the posteromedial aspect of the proximal P_1 segment, encircles the midbrain medial to the trunk of the posterior cerebral, passes under the medial geniculate body and pulvinar, turns forward around the posteromedial border of the pulvinar, joins the choroid plexus just above the habenula, and continues anteriorly on the superior border of the thalamus (56,64) (Figs. 8 and 15). Most commonly [51–76% (57,64)] there is a single posteromedial choroidal artery (also called the proximal posteromedial choroidal artery), which takes origin from the P_1 segment in 60% of cases and the P_2 segment in 40–54% (56,57). This artery supplies the cerebral peduncle, the substantia nigra, the peripheral part of the tegmentum of the midbrain [including parts of the medial lemniscus and the spinothalamic tracts (45)], the geniculate bodies, the ventral part of the brachium of the inferior colliculus, the cranial part of the superior colliculus (45,63), the pretectal nucleus, the cranial part of the mesencephalic nucleus and tract of the trigeminal nerve, and the cranial dorsolateral periaqueductal gray (45). It also supplies the pulvinar and medial thalamus up to and including the anterior nuclei (32,41,65), the tela choroidea of the third ventricle, and the choroid plexus of the lateral ventricle (56). Anastomoses occur with the posterolateral choroidal artery and the collicular artery lateral to the midbrain and with the collicular arteries and the superior cerebellar arteries on the dorsal aspect of the midbrain (45,60).

In 21–47% (57,64) of cases there is a second (distal) posteromedial choroidal artery that takes origin from the P_2 segment in 41% of cases (57), or further posteriorly.

Devic et al. reported a posteromedial choroidal infarct at autopsy (66). The infarct involved the midbrain tectum, the superior colliculus, and the medial thalamus extending to the anterior nuclei.

Percheron (32) has described an artery that arises from the posteromedial choroidal artery just anterior to the medial geniculate body and penetrates the thalamus and supplies the anterodorsal and anteroprincipal nuclei and the posterior part of the median nucleus. He named this the oblique inferolateral artery.

Splenial Artery

Arteries supplying the splenium of the corpus callosum were present in all cases examined by Zeal and Rhoton (56). They arise from one of the branches of the posterior cerebral artery, most commonly the parieto-occipital (56). Anastomosis of this artery with the branches of the pericallosal artery occurs just anterior to the tip of the splenium of the corpus callosum.

Peduncular Branches

The anterolateral territory of the midbrain is supplied by arteries entering the cerebral peduncle. The main supply is from the collicular and accessory collicular (52,56) arteries, the posteromedial choroidal arteries and to a lesser extent from the superior cerebellar (45,67), the anterior choroidal, and the posterior cerebral arteries [an average of three branches from the P_2 segment of the posterior cerebral artery (37,57)]. Branches may also arise from the posterior communicating artery or even the basilar artery (45,67).

Hippocampal Arteries

The uncus and ventral surface of the parahippocampal gyrus is supplied by the uncal and parahippocampal arteries. These originate from the anterior choroidal artery (100%), internal carotid artery (59%), middle cerebral artery (65%), and the posterior cerebral artery (47%) (68). The dorsal surface of the parahippocampal gyrus and the hippocampus is supplied by the hippocampal arteries, which are divided into anterior (one or two in number, caliber 500 μm), middle [present in 94% of cases (57) (one artery, caliber 500 μm)] and posterior (one artery, caliber 500 μm) (57). They arise from the posterior cerebral artery (68) or the posterolateral choroidal artery (64).

Tegmental Branches

Direct rami to the mesencephalic tegmentum from the posterior cerebral artery are said to be relatively constant (37). These may also occasionally arise from the collicular artery (45).

THE ARTERIAL SUPPLY OF THE BRAINSTEM

The arteries supplying the brainstem can be subdivided in three main ways:

1. According to their point of penetration into the brainstem, into four groups (63): anteromedial, anterolateral, lateral (short circumferential), and posterior (long circumferential) (22).
2. According to the territory of supply in the brainstem, which can also be divided into anteromedial, anterolateral, lateral, and posterior territories (63) (see Chapter 3).
3. According to territories supplied by the larger named arteries: basilar, posterior cerebral, superior cerebellar, vertebral, anterior inferior cerebellar, and posterior inferior cerebellar.

Midbrain

Anteromedial Territory

See superior and inferior paramedian mesencephalic arteries.

Anterolateral Territory

See peduncular branches.

Lateral and Posterior Territories

The lateral territory of the midbrain includes a large number of small arteries penetrating the lateral midbrain that arise, in order of importance, from the superior cerebellar artery, the collicular artery, and the posteromedial choroidal artery. These arteries supply the lateral lemniscus, the central tegmental tract, and the surrounding reticular formation (63) (Fig. 16).

Collicular and Accessory Collicular Arteries

(Quadrigeminal, pedunculoquadrigeminal, or superior circumferential mesencephalic artery; long and short circumflex mesencephalic arteries.)

The accessory collicular arteries arise from the P_1 (86%) or the P_2 (14%) (56) segment of the posterior cerebral artery and are present in 66% of hemispheres (56). They course around the midbrain supplying small perforating branches to the cerebral peduncle and the substantia nigra, and 74% of arteries that arise from the P_1 segment terminate at the posterolateral border of the cerebral peduncle (52). Those arteries arising from the P_2 segment supply only the geniculate bodies, the midbrain tegmentum (56), and the lateral segment of the superior colliculus (63). These arteries have a mean diameter of 260–600 μm, and there are an average of one to two arteries per brain (52,56).

The collicular arteries, which are present in 96% of hemispheres, arise from the P_1 (80%) or the P_2 (20%) segments of the posterior cerebral artery (56) and encircle the midbrain to reach the quadrigeminal plate, giving small branches to the tegmentum of the midbrain, the geniculate bodies, and the cerebral peduncle (52,56) (Fig. 16). There are an average of two to three collicular arteries of diameter 650–700 μm per brain (52,56). This artery divides into two terminal branches at the level of the inferior colliculus and ends by supplying the superior colliculi (63). The collicular artery may penetrate the oculomotor nerve early in its course (69).

The collicular arteries give rise to anterolateral, lateral, and posterior branches to the brainstem (63), but also (20% of 20 brains) may supply the anteromedial territory, including the oculomotor nucleus (45). The anterolateral branches are numerous and penetrate the lower part of the cerebral peduncle, near the pontomesencephalic junction (63). The lateral branches supply the lateral surface of the lower midbrain. Frequent anastomoses occur between the collicular arteries and branches of the posteromedial choroidal artery above and the superior cerebellar artery below (60,63). The posterior branches form a dense network over the surface of the superior colliculi (63). The territory of the posterior branches varies inversely with the territories of the posteromedial choroidal and the superior cerebellar arteries (63).

Superior Cerebellar Artery

The superior cerebellar artery arises from the basilar artery, just below the pontomesencephalic sulcus (63), near the origin of the posterior cerebral artery (37) (Figs. 14 and 16). It is divided into (a) the anterior pontine segment between the pons and the clivus, (b) the ambient segment lateral to the brainstem, and (c) the quadrigeminal segment within the quadrigeminal cistern. The anterior pontine and ambient segments give rise to an average of four penetrating arteries, supplying the brainstem (37). The superior cerebellar artery divides into a lateral and medial branch, usually in the anterior pontine segment, but the course and mode of division are variable (70). The lateral superior cerebellar artery curves to reach the lateral margin of the cerebellar hemisphere. The medial superior cerebellar artery curves around the lateral surface of the midbrain (ambient and quadrigeminal segments) to reach the colliculi (63,71).

The superior cerebellar artery gives rise to lateral and posterior branches to the brainstem. The lateral branches are divided into superior and inferior groups. The superior lateral perforators arise from both the medial and lateral superior cerebellar artery and supply the posterior part of the lateral pontine tegmentum (63), also giving branches to the midbrain, including the most caudal portion of the cerebral peduncle (45,67). The inferior lateral perforators arise mainly from the lateral superior cerebellar artery. Some of these arteries supply the superolateral pontine tegmentum, including the superior cerebellar peduncle, the lateral lemniscus, the spinothalamic tract, the central tegmental tract, and the locus ceruleus (70–72), and others enter the cerebellum and supply the dentate nucleus (73).

The posterior branches reach the posterior surface of the pons and midbrain and supply the inferior colliculus (72), parts of the medial lemniscus [also supplied by anteromedial basilar penetrators (74)], spinothalamic tracts, lateral lemniscus, mesen-

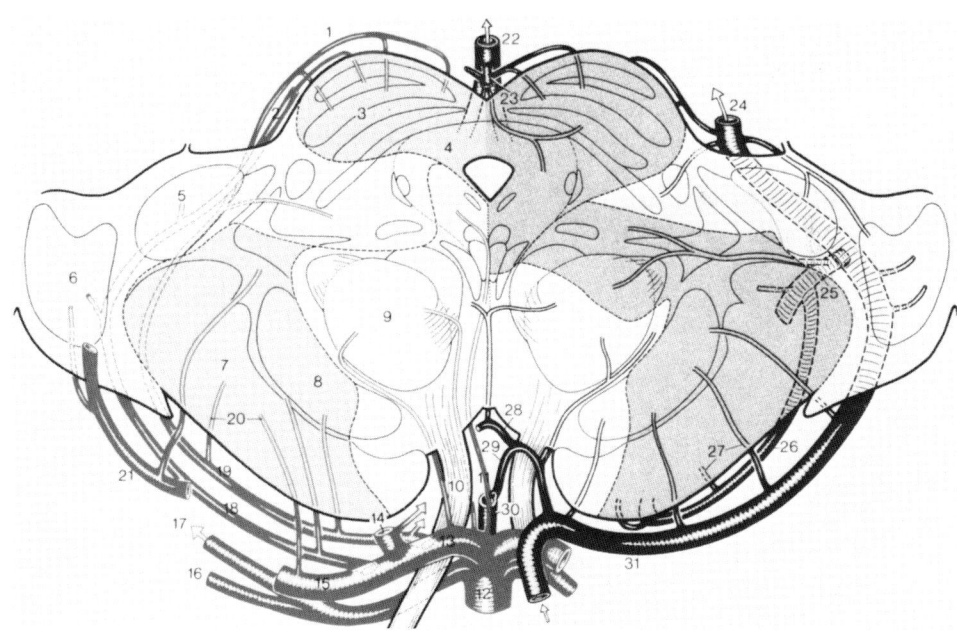

Key:
1. Collicular artery
2. Posteromedial choroidal artery
11. Superior paramedian mesencephalic arteries
12. Basilar artery
13. P_1 segment of posterior cerebral artery
14. Posterior communicating artery
15. P_2 segment of posterior cerebral artery
16. Superior cerebellar artery (lateral branch)
17. Superior cerebellar artery (medial branch)
18. Posteromedial choroidal artery
19. Collicular artery
20. Peduncular arteries
21. Anterior choroidal artery

FIG. 16. Perforating arteries of the midbrain (shown on the left half of the figure). From ref. 91, with permission.

cephalic nucleus, and tract of the trigeminal nerve (45). They also supply the reticulospinal tract and the fibers of the fourth cranial nerve (63,70,72), and anastomose with branches of the collicular artery.

The sensory loss in superior cerebellar infarction is a dissociated hemihypalgesia and hypothermesthesia in keeping with involvement of the spinothalamic tracts, but this is not constant (74). Involvement of the entire medial lemniscus is uncommon (74). Amarenco and Hauw (75) noted involvement of the following brainstem structures in 28 superior cerebellar artery territory infarcts: superior cerebellar peduncle and lateral lemniscus (43%), spinothalamic tract (36%), mesencephalic trigeminal tract (29%), central tegmental tract (21%), locus ceruleus (18%), middle cerebellar peduncle and inferior colliculus (11%), periaqueductal gray matter (7%), and trochlear decussation (4%).

Pons

Anteromedial and Anterolateral Territories

Basilar Artery

The basilar artery originates near the pontomedullary junction and terminates near the pontomesencephalic junction (Fig. 15). The average diameter below the superior cerebellar artery is 4.1 mm (37). Multiple perforating arteries arise from the posterior and lateral surfaces. An average of eight branches of 100–500 μm in diameter arise from the upper centimeter (37). The inferior paramedian mesencephalic arteries may take origin from the top of the basilar artery (45,61). The basilar artery gives rise to anteromedial and anterolateral perforators. It also gives rise to short circumferential branches, the superolateral and inferolateral pontine arteries, and to a long circumferential branch, the anterior inferior cerebellar artery (AICA). The basilar artery bifurcates as far caudal as the 1.3 mm below the pontomesencephalic junction and as far rostral as the mamillary bodies (37,76).

Branches of the basilar artery may supply the cerebral peduncle (45,67). Anteromedial pontine arteries arise from the basilar artery, either directly or by trunks common to arteries of the lateral arterial group. Anastomoses are found between arteries on the same side of the midline (63). The superficial course of the lowest branches is the longest (63).

There are two types of anteromedial penetrating artery (Fig. 17). The longer arteries reach the floor of the fourth ventricle and supply the median zone of the pontine tegmentum. The shorter arteries supply the medial parts of the corticospinal tracts (63). The long anteromedial arteries supplying the inferior part of the pontine tegmentum reach the tegmentum along a curved upward path and supply the abducens nucleus, the medial longitudinal fasciculus, and the caudal pontine reticular nuclei (63). The long anteromedial arteries supplying the superior part of the pontine tegmentum curve down in the tegmentum to supply the medial longitudinal fasciculus and oral pontine reticular nuclei.

Anterolateral pontine arteries (77) are numerous small branches of the anteromedial arteries (63). Some of these arteries supply the anterior surface of the corticospinal tract, but most supply the lateral part of the corticospinal tract, the pontine nuclei, and may supply the medial lemniscus (63).

Lateral Territory

The lateral pontine arteries ramify over the middle cerebellar peduncle. These arteries can be divided into three areas according to their site of penetration in relation to the trigeminal nerve root (anterior, inferior, or posterior) (63) (Figs. 15 and 17).

The anterior area is supplied by the lateral pontine arteries, usually two in number, the superolateral pontine artery, and

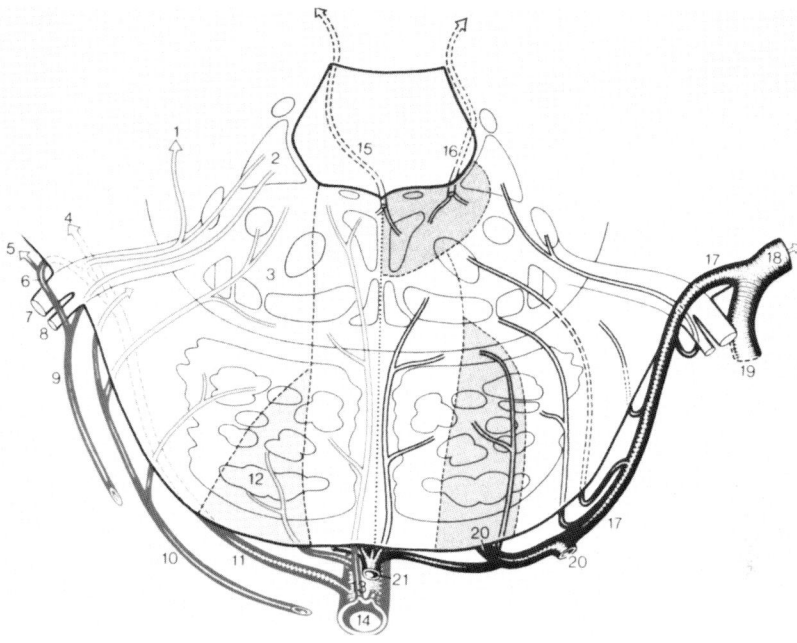

Key:
9. Superolateral pontine artery
10. Inferolateral pontine artery
11. Anterior inferior cerebellar artery
14. Basilar artery

FIG. 17. Perforating arteries of the pons (shown on the left half of the figure). From ref. 91, with permission.

the inferolateral pontine artery. These arteries usually arise directly from the basilar artery (63), but the inferolateral pontine artery may arise from the AICA (73). The superolateral and inferolateral pontine arteries ramify above and below the roots of the trigeminal nerve, respectively. The superolateral pontine artery often anastomoses with the inferolateral pontine artery (63).

The lateral pontine arteries have multiple branches that supply a relatively small area of the pons, including the pontine nuclei, the tegmentum, the lateral lemniscus and its nucleus (this is supplied by the AICA in the lower pons), the motor trigeminal nucleus, and the central tegmental tract. The more medial lateral pontine arteries supply the lateral corticospinal tract and the more lateral arteries supply the trigeminal root and the principal sensory and motor trigeminal nuclei (which may also be supplied by the AICA) (63).

The inferior area of the lateral pons is supplied by branches of the AICA (63) and also by the lateral pontine arteries (77). Fisher has shown an infarct in this area (that was an upward extension of a medullary infarct) to be supplied by a branch of the posterior inferior cerebellar artery (PICA) (78).

Anterior Inferior Cerebellar Artery

The AICA is present in 96% of cases (79) and takes origin from the basilar artery at the junction of the middle and inferior thirds (76), but can arise from the PICA or from a common trunk with that artery, and may vary considerably in size (80). It courses laterally, posteriorly, and inferiorly, goes under the trigeminal nerve, crosses the sixth cranial nerve, reaches the cerebellopontine angle, loops around the seventh/eighth nerve complex to reach the flocculus (79), and continues over the middle part of the cerebellar hemisphere (70) (Figs. 15 and 17).

The territory of the AICA varies inversely with that of the PICA, and when that artery is small the AICA may supply most of its territory. There is frequently an asymmetry between the territory of the AICA on the two sides (72). The AICA gives rise to the internal auditory artery in 80% of cases (79) and divides into two branches. The first courses over the anteromedial cerebellar hemisphere and anastomoses with the PICA, and the second ramifies over the middle cerebellar peduncle and supplies branches to this structure and to the lateral part of the pons (70). There are two types of branches to the pons from the AICA (63,80):

1. Branches that enter the pons superior to the pontomedullary sulcus with a central rostral course that supply the lateral pontine tegmentum. According to Duvernoy, the AICA supplies a clearly defined area consisting of the superior olivary nucleus, the facial nucleus, the lateral lemniscus, and occasionally the lateral parts of the abducens nucleus and the central tegmental tract. Autopsy correlations of AICA infarcts generally show a more extensive wedge-shaped area that includes the eighth nerve, the spinal trigeminal tract and nucleus, the inferior cerebellar peduncle, and part of the vestibular nuclei (70,80,81).
2. Branches that supply the middle cerebellar peduncle and course upward toward the trigeminal nerve and anastomose with the inferolateral pontine artery (a branch of the basilar artery), occasionally giving rise to this artery. The AICA may also anastomose with the superolateral pontine artery (a branch of the basilar artery) to form an arterial circle around the roots of the trigeminal nerve (63) (Fig. 17). These branches may supply the principal sensory trigeminal nucleus and the superior vestibular nucleus (63).

The posterior area of the lateral pons is supplied by branches of the superior cerebellar artery. These are small arteries supplying the lateral part of the upper pontine tegmentum, including the oral pontine reticular nuclei, the central tegmental tract, the lateral lemniscus, part of the superior cerebellar peduncle, and the locus ceruleus (63).

Posterior Territory

The posterior pontine surface is supplied by branches of the medial superior cerebellar artery. These arteries penetrate the superior cerebellar peduncle and supply this structure as well as the mesencephalic trigeminal tract and the locus ceruleus (63).

Medulla

Anteromedial Territory

The anteromedial medullary arteries are divided into superior and inferior subgroups. The inferior subgroup of arteries are small and few in number and arise from the anterior spinal artery. The superior subgroup are larger and more numerous arteries and arise from the terminal segments of the vertebral arteries and from the rami that form the anterior spinal artery. Anastomoses are often present in these two groups of arteries (63,82) (Fig. 18). The anteromedial medullary arteries increase in length from caudal to cranial levels (83).

The terminal branches of the longer cranial arteries reach the floor of the fourth ventricle in the superior medulla and they supply the hypoglossal nucleus, the medial lemniscus, the central reticular formation, and the dorsal accessory olivary nucleus (63). The shorter more caudal anteromedial arteries supply the medial accessory olivary nucleus and the medial part of the oli-

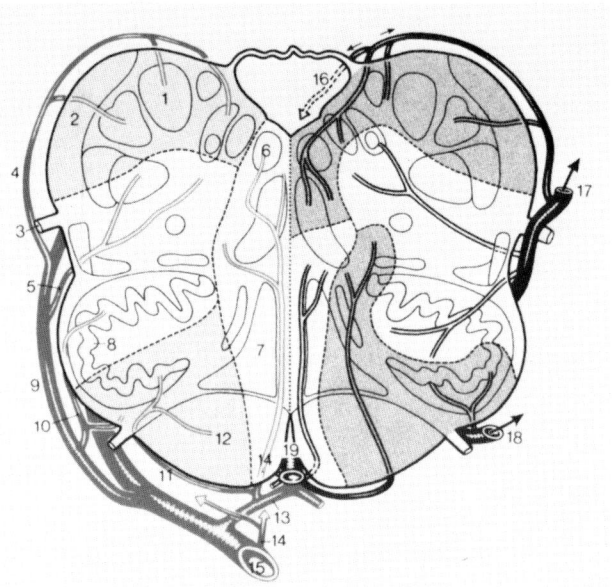

Key:
9. Posterior inferior cerebellar artery
13. Anterior spinal artery
15. Vertebral artery

FIG. 18. Perforating arteries of the medulla (shown on the left half of the figure). From ref. 91, with permission.

vary nucleus, but they do not reach the floor of the fourth ventricle (63).

Anterolateral Territory

The anterolateral medullary territory was first described by Gillilan (72). There are differences in the nomenclature and extent of this territory. According to Duvernoy, the arteries supplying this territory are penetrating arteries that mostly arise from the anteromedial group of arteries and supply most of the pyramids and the medial part of the olive (63) (Fig. 18). He groups the short circumferential arteries, including the "olivary arteries" (84), which are direct branches from the vertebral artery, in the lateral medullary territory.

Other authors recognize an olivary territory that is supplied by the olivary arteries (83–85). This territory does not include the pyramids and includes the whole of the olive (83,85), and may include the spinothalamic tract (85,86) (Ch. 3, Section 24). The size of the olivary territory varies inversely with that of the lateral and anteromedial territory. De Smet et al. noted that infarcts in the olivary territory have the shape of a pyramid, with its base uppermost. They described a "total" olivary territory infarct extending through several craniocaudal levels, due to occlusion of the "inferior short circumferential olivary arteries" and a "minimum" infarct involving only the most rostrolateral portion of the olive due to occlusion of the "superior short circumferential olivary arteries" (85).

Lateral Territory

The arteries of the lateral group arise mainly from the vertebral artery and from the initial segment of the basilar artery. The lateral group of arteries are the short circumferential arteries, and these can be divided into four subgroups (inferior, middle, superior, and posterior) according to their position in relation to the roots of the glossopharyngeal and vagus nerves.

All the lateral arteries except the posterior group have short and long penetrating arteries. The short arteries supply the white matter tracts (spinothalamic and spinocerebellar). The long arteries supply the deeper regions and reach the floor of the fourth ventricle in the superior part of the medulla, and form part of the vascular supply of the hypoglossal, vagal, solitary tract, and in some cases the vestibular nuclei (63). Laterally they supply the spinal trigeminal nucleus, and medially the lateral part of the inferior olivary nucleus, the dorsal accesory olivary nucleus, and the central reticular formation (63,85).

Arteries of the inferior subgroup arise from the vertebral artery or the posterior inferior cerebellar artery and reach the inferior pole of the olive and the inferior cerebellar peduncle.

The middle subgroup is the most important and is made up of one to three branches from the vertebral artery or posterior inferior cerebellar artery (63). Some of these branches supply the olive and may extend to the anterolateral sulcus, taking over the territory of the anterolateral group (85).

The superior subgroup is composed of two groups of arteries, the first arising from the initial segment of the basilar artery and the second from the anterior inferior cerebellar artery (63).

The posterior subgroup arteries are branches of a trunk that originates from the anterior inferior cerebellar artery and penetrates the medulla lateral to the glossopharyngeal and vagus nerves (63). Several anastomoses connect the posterior group with the other groups (63). Their territory comprises the inferior cerebellar peduncle, the cuneate nucleus, and sometimes the spinal trigeminal nucleus in the inferior medulla (63) and the dorsal and ventral cochlear nuclei, the superior part of the cuneate nucleus, and the medial and inferior vestibular nuclei in the inferior medulla (63).

Structures affected in 80% of lateral medullary territory infarcts include the spinothalamic tract, the ventral spinocerebellar tract, the spinal trigeminal tract and nucleus, the nucleus ambiguus, and the lateral reticular formation (83).

Posterior Inferior Cerebellar Artery

The PICA usually arises from the vertebral artery but its site of origin from this artery is very variable (71). The PICA may also originate directly from the basilar artery or from a common trunk with the AICA. In 7% of cases the vertebral artery terminates in the PICA, the remainder of the vertebral artery being hypoplastic or absent. In 15% of cases it is absent and hypoplastic in 5% (70).

After arising from the vertebral artery, the PICA courses laterally and downward on the medulla (Fig. 15). It then loops caudally on the lateral surface of the medulla and ascends in the sulcus, separating the medulla from the tonsil of the cerebellum. It then makes a cranial loop over the tonsil and descends under the inferior vermis. The common trunk gives rise to a medial branch and a lateral branch at a variable level between the first two loops. The posterior inferior cerebellar artery supplies the lateral and posterior parts of the medulla, but the supply to the lateral medulla is inconstant, being the main supply in only 22% of cases and absent in 50% of cases (70,87). The PICA also gives rise to the arteries of the choroid plexus of the fourth ventricle (82).

Posterior Territory

The medial branch of the PICA gives rise to branches that together with the posterior spinal artery supply the posterior medulla (88). The PICA supply to the posterior medulla is constant (70,89). Its territory includes the middle and inferior vestibular nuclei, the inferior cerebellar peduncle, the gracile and cuneate nuclei, the inferior parts of the solitary tract and its nucleus, the vagal nucleus, the spinal trigeminal nucleus, and the area postrema (63,70). The arteries of the posterior group are absent from the superior or open part of the medulla (63).

Infarcts in this territory involve the vestibular nuclei, the gracile and cuneate nuclei, the cochlear nuclei, the nucleus solitarius, and the dorsal vagal nucleus (83).

REFERENCES*

1. Marinkovic S, Milisavljevic M, Kovacevic M. Anatomical bases for surgical approach to the initial segment of the anterior cerebral artery. Surg Radiol Anat 1986;8:7–18.
2. Rosner SS, Rhoton AL Jr, Ono M, Barry M. Microsurgical anatomy of the anterior perforating arteries. J Neurosurg 1984;61:468–485.
3. Perlmutter D, Rhoton AL Jr. Microsurgical anatomy of the anterior cerebral-anterior communicating-recurrent artery complex. J Neurosurg 1976;45:259–272.
4. Lazorthes G, Poulhes J, Gaubert J. Les artères et les territoires vasculaires de l'hypothalamus. Presse Med 1956;64:1701–1703.
5. Ostrowski AZ, Webster JE, Gurdjian ES. The proximal anterior cerebral artery: an anatomic study. Arch Neurol 1960;3:661–664.
6. Alexander L. The vascular supply of the striopallidum. Proc Assoc Res Nerv Ment Dis 1942;21:77–132.
7. Kaplan HA, Ford DH. The brain vascular system. Amsterdam: Elsevier; 1966.
8. Dunker RO, Harris AB. Surgical anatomy of the proximal anterior cerebral artery. J Neurosurg 1976;44:359–367.
9. Crowell RM, Morawetz RB. The anterior communicating artery has significant branches. Stroke 1977;8:272–273.
10. Marinkovic S, Milisavljevic M, Marinkovic A. Branches of the anterior communicating artery. Microsurgical anatomy. Acta Neurochir 1990;106:78–85.
11. Vincentelli F, Lehman G, Caruso G, Grisoli F, Rabehanta P, Gouaze A. Extracerebral course of the perforating branches of the anterior communicating artery: microsurgical anatomical study. Surg Neurol 1991;35:98–104.
12. Phillips S, Sangalang V, Sterns G. Basal forebrain infarction. Arch Neurol 1987;44:1134–1138.
13. Heubner O. Zur Topographie der Ernahrungsgebiete der einzelnen Hirnarterien. Centralbl Med Wiss 1872;10:817–821.
14. Lazorthes G, Gaubert J, Poulhes J. La distribution centrale et corticale de l'artère cérébrale antérieure. Etude anatomique et incidences neurochirurgicales. Neurochirurgie 1956;2:237–253.
15. Gorczyca W, Mohr G. Microvascular anatomy of Heubner's recurrent artery. Neurol Res 1987;9:259–264.
16. Gomes F, Dujovny M, Umansky F, et al. Microsurgical anatomy of the recurrent artery of Heubner. J Neurosurg 1984;60:130–139.
17. Umansky F, Gomes FB, Dujovny M, et al. The perforating branches of the middle cerebral artery. J Neurosurg 1985;62:261–268.
18. Kaplan HA. The lateral perforating branches of the anterior and middle cerebral arteries. J Neurosurg 1965;23:305–310.
19. Gibo H, Lenkey C, Rhoton AL Jr. Microsurgical anatomy of the supraclinoid portion of the internal carotid artery. J Neurosurg 1981;55:560–574.
20. Marinkovic SV, Milisavljevic MM, Marinkovic ZD. Microanatomy and possible clinical significance of anastomoses among hypothalamic arteries. Stroke 1989;20:1341–1352.
21. Marinkovic S, Milisavljevic M, Marinkovic ZD. The perforating branches of the internal carotid artery: the microsurgical anatomy of their extracerebral segments. Neurosurgery 1990;26:472–479.
22. Lazorthes G, Gouaze A, Salamon G. Les artères centrales du cerveau. In: Vascularisation et circulation de l'encéphale. Paris: Masson; 1976:154–182.
23. Marinkovic SV, Kovacevic MS, Marinkovic JM. Perforating branches of the middle cerebral artery. J Neurosurg 1985;63:266–271.
24. Vincentelli F, Caruso G, Andriamamonjy C, et al. Etude micro-anatomique des branches collatérales perforantes de l'artère cérébrale moyenne. Neurochirurgie 1990;36:3–15.
25. Shellshear JI. The basal arteries of the forebrain and their functional significance. J Anat 1920;55:27–35.
26. Ghika JA, Bogousslavsky J, Regli F. Deep perforators from the carotid system. Arch Neurol 1990;47:1097–1100.
27. Marinkovic SV, Milisavljevic MM, Kovacevic MS, Stevic ZD. Perforating branches of the middle cerebral artery. Stroke 1985;16:1022–1029.
28. Herman LH, Ostrowski AZ, Gurdjian ES. Perforating branches of the middle cerebral artery. Arch Neurol 1963;1:32–34.
29. Manelfe C, Clanet M, Gigaud M, Bonafé A, Guiraud B, Rascol A. Internal capsule: normal anatomy and ischemic changes demonstrated by computed tomography. AJNR 1981;2:149–155.
30. Beevor CE. On the distribution of the different

---

*This reference list is a combination of references from chapters 2 and 3.

arteries supplying the human brain. *Philos Trans R Soc Lond [Biol]* 1909;200:1–55.
31. De Reuck J. La limite du territoire profond de l'artère Sylvienne chez l'homme. *Acta Anat* 1969;74:30–35.
32. Percheron G. Les artères du thalamus humain. Les artères choroidiennes. *Rev Neurol (Paris)* 1977;133:547–558.
33. Duret H. Recherches anatomiques sur la circulation de l'encéphale. *Arch Physiol Norm Pathol* 1874;1:60–91.
34. Abbie AA. The anatomy of capsular vascular disease. *Aust Med J* 1937;2:564–568.
35. Herman LH, Fernando OU, Gurdjian ES. The anterior choroidal artery: an anatomical study of its area of distribution. *Anat Rec* 1966;154:95–102.
36. Carpenter MB, Noback CR, Moss ML. The anterior choroidal artery. *Arch Neurol Psych* 1954;71:714–722.
37. Saeki N, Rhoton AL Jr. Microsurgical anatomy of the upper basilar artery and the posterior circle of Willis. *J Neurosurg* 1977;46:563–578.
38. Hussein S, Renella RR, Dietz H. Microsurgical anatomy of the anterior choroidal artery. *Acta Neurochir* 1988;92:19–28.
39. Abbie AA. The blood supply of the lateral geniculate body with a note on the morphology of the choroidal arteries. *J Anat* 1933;67:491–521.
40. Rhoton AL Jr, Fujii K, Fradd B. Microsurgical anatomy of the anterior choroidal artery. *Surg Neurol* 1979;12:171–187.
41. Schlesinger B. *The upper brainstem in the human. Its nuclear configuration and vascular supply.* Berlin: Springer-Verlag; 1976.
42. Abbie AA. The clinical significance of the anterior choroidal artery. *Brain* 1933;56:233–246.
43. Mohr JP, Steinke W, Timsit SG, Sacco RL, Tatemichi TK. The anterior choroidal artery does not supply the corona radiata and lateral ventricular wall. *Stroke* 1991;22:1502–1507.
44. Beevor CE. the cerebral arterial supply. *Brain* 1908;30:403–425.
45. Khan NM. *The blood supply of the midbrain in man and monkey* [PhD Thesis]. London: University of London, 1969.
46. Foix C, Chavany H, Hillemand P, Schiff-Wertheimer M. Oblitération de l'artère choroidienne antérieure. Ramolissement de son territoire cérébral. Hémiplégie, hémianesthésie, hémianopsie. *Bull Soc Ophthalmol* 1925;27:221–223.
47. Buge A, Escourolle R, Hauw JJ, Rancurel G, Gray F, Tempier P. Syndrome pseudobulbaire aigu par infarctus bilatéral. Limite du territoire des artères choroidiennes antérieures. *Rev Neurol (Paris)* 1979;135:313–318.
48. Poppi U. Sindrome talamo-capsulare per rammollimento nel territorio dell'arteria coroidea anteriore. *Riv Patol Nerv Ment* 1928;33:505–542.
49. Van Buren JM, Borke RC. *Variations and connection of the human thalamus. Vol 1. The nuclei and cerebral connections of the human thalamus.* Berlin: Springer; 1972.
50. Percheron G. Les artères du thalamus humain. I. Artère et territoire thalamiques polaires de l'artère communicante postérieure. *Rev Neurol (Paris)* 1976;132:297–307.
51. Vincentelli F, Caruso G, Grisoli F, Rabehanta P, Andriamamonjy C, Gouaze A. Microsurgical anatomy of the cisternal course of the perforating branches of the posterior communicating artery. *Neurosurgery* 1990;26:824–831.
52. Pedroza A, Dujovny M, Ausman JI, et al. Microvascular anatomy of the interpeduncular fossa. *J Neurosurg* 1986;64:484–493.
53. Marinkovic S, Milisavljevic M, Kovacevic M. Interpeduncular perforating branches of the posterior cerebral artery. *Surg Neurol* 1986;26:349–359.
54. Castaigne P, Lhermitte F, Buge A, Escourolle R, Hauw JJ, Lyon-Caen O. Paramedian thalamic and midbrain infarcts: clinical and neuropathological study. *Ann Neurol* 1981;10:127–148.
55. Takahashi S, Goto K, Fukasawa H, Kawata Y, Uemura K, Yaguchi K. Computed tomography of cerebral infarction along the distribution of the basal perforating arteries. Part II: thalamic arterial group. *Radiology* 1985;155:119–130.
56. Zeal AA, Rhoton AL Jr. Microsurgical anatomy of the posterior cerebral artery. *J Neurosurg* 1978;48:534–559.
57. Milisavljevic M, Marinkovic S, Marinkovic Z, Malobabic S. Anatomic basis for surgical approach to the distal segment of the posterior cerebral artery. *Surg Radiol Anat* 1988;10:259–266.
58. Milisavljevic MM, Marinkovic SV, Gibo H, Puskas LF. The thalamogeniculate perforators of the posterior cerebral artery: the microsurgical anatomy. *Neurosurgery* 1991;28:523–530.
59. Marinkovic SV, Milisavljevic MM, Kovacevic MS. Anastomoses among the thalamoperforating branches of the posterior cerebral artery. *Arch Neurol* 1986;43:811–814.
60. Milisavljevic M, Marinkovic S, Lolic-Draganic V, Djordjevic L. Anastomoses in the territory of the posterior cerebral arteries. *Acta Anat* 1986;127:221–225.
61. Percheron G. Les artères du thalamus humain. II. Artères et territoires thalamiques paramedians de l'artère basilaire communicante. *Rev Neurol (Paris)* 1976;132:309–324.
62. Pierrot-Deseilligny C, Chain F, Gray F, Serdaru M, Escourolle R, Lhermitte F. Parinaud's syndrome. *Brain* 1982;105:667–696.
63. Duvernoy HM. *Human brainstem vessels.* Berlin: Springer-Verlag; 1978.
64. Percheron G. Les artères du thalamus humain. Les artères choroidiennes. *Rev Neurol (Paris)* 1977;133:533–545.
65. Plets C, De Reuck J, Vander Eecken H, Van Den Bergh R. The vascularization of the human thalamus. *Acta Neurol Belg* 1970;70:687–770.
66. Devic M, Michel F, Lenglet JP. Nystagmus re-

tractorius, paralysie de la verticalité, aréflexie pupillaire et anomalie de la posture du regard par ramollissement dans la territoire de la choroidienne postérieure. *Rev Neurol (Paris)* 1964;110:399–404.
67. Alezais, D'Astros L. La circulation artérielle du pédoncule cérébral. *J Anat Physiol* 1892;28:519–528.
68. Marinkovic SV, Milisavljevic MM, Vuckovic VD. Microvascular anatomy of the uncus and the parahippocampal gyrus. *Neurosurgery* 1991;29:805–814.
69. Milisavljevic M, Marinkovic S, Lolic-Draganic V, Kovacevic M. Oculomotor, trochlear, and abducens nerves penetrated by cerebral vessels. *Arch Neurol* 1986;43:58–61.
70. Amarenco P, Hauw JJ. Anatomie des artères cérébelleuses. *Rev Neurol (Paris)* 1989;145:267–276.
71. Foix C, Hillemand P. Les artères de l'axe encéphalique jusqu'au diencéphale inclusivement. *Rev Neurol (Paris)* 1925;32:705–739.
72. Gillilan LA. The correlation of the blood supply to the human brain stem with clinical brain stem lesions. *J Neuropathol Exp Neurol* 1964;23:78–108.
73. Stephens RB, Stilwell DL. *Arteries of the human brain.* Springfield, IL: Charles C. Thomas; 1969.
74. Davison C, Goodhart SP, Savitsky N. The syndrome of the superior cerebellar artery. *Arch Neurol Psychol* 1935;33:1143–1174.
75. Amarenco P, Hauw JJ. Cerebellar infarction in the territory of the superior cerebellar artery. *Neurology* 1990;40:1383–1390.
76. Stopford JSB. The arteries of the pons and medulla oblongata. *J Anat Physiol* 1916;50:131–164.
77. Stopford JSB. The arteries of the pons and medulla oblongata: part II. *J Anat Physiol* 1916;51:255–280.
78. Fisher CM, Tapia J. Lateral medullary infarction extending to the lower pons. *J Neurol Neurosurg Psychiatry* 1987;50:620–624.
79. Lazorthes G. *Vascularisation et circulation cérébrales.* Paris: Masson; 1961.
80. Atkinson WJ. The anterior inferior cerebellar artery. *J Neurol Neurosurg Psychiatry* 1949;12:137–151.
81. Amarenco P. The spectrum of cerebellar infarctions. *Neurology* 1991;41:973–979.
82. Duret H. Artères nourricières du bulbe rachidien. *Arch Physiol Norm Pathol* 1873;5:97–113.
83. Hauw JJ, Der Agopian P, Trelles L, Escourolle R. Les infarctus bulbaires. *J Neurol Sci* 1976;28:83–102.
84. Böhne C. Uber die arterielle Blutversorgung der Medulla oblongata. *Z Anat Entwickl-Gesch* 1927;84:760–776.
85. DeSmet Y, Brucher JM, Gonsette RE. L'infarctus du territoire olivaire du bulbe. *Rev Neurol (Paris)* 1984;140:559–566.
86. Hiller F. The vascular syndromes of the basilar and vertebral arteries and their branches. *J Nerv Ment Dis* 1952;116:988–1016.
87. Escourolle R, Hauw JJ, Der Agopian P, Trelles L. Les infarctus bulbaires. *J Neurol Sci* 1976;28:103–113.
88. Goodhart SP, Davison C. Syndrome of the posterior inferior and anterior inferior cerebellar arteries and their branches. *Arch Neurol Psychol* 1936;35:501–524.
89. Foix C, Hillemand P, Schalit. Irrigation du bulbe. *C R Soc Biol (Paris)* 1925;92:33–35.
90. DeArmond SJ, Fusco MM, Dewey MM. *Structure of the human brain. A photographic atlas.* 2nd ed. New York: Oxford University Press; 1976.
91. Nieuwenhuys R, Voogd J, van Huijsen C. *The human central nervous system. A synopsis and atlas.* Berlin: Springer-Verlag; 1981.
92. Fix JD. *Atlas of the human brain and spinal cord.* Rockville, MD: Aspen; 1987.
93. Damasio HA. A computed tomographic guide to the identification of cerebral vascular territories. *Arch Neurol* 1983;40:138–142.
94. Takahashi S, Goto K, Fukasawa H, Kawata Y, Uemura K, Suzuki K. Computed tomography of cerebral infarction along the distribution of the basal perforating arteries. Part 1: striate arterial group. *Radiology* 1985;155:107–118.
95. Savoiardo M, Bracchi M, Passerini A, Visciani A. The vascular territories in the cerebellum and brainstem: CT and MR study. *AJNR* 1987;8:199–209.
96. Frisen L, Holmegaard L, Rosencrantz M. Sectorial optic atrophy and homonymous, horizontal sectoranopia: a lateral choroidal artery syndrome? *J Neurol Neurosurg Psychiatry* 1978;41:374–380.
97. Frisen L. Quadruple sectoranopia and sectorial optic atrophy: a syndrome of the distal anterior choroidal artery. *J Neurol Neurosurg Psychiatry* 1979;42:590–594.
98. Fisher CM. Lacunar infarct of the tegmentum of the lower lateral pons. *Arch Neurol* 1989;46:566–567.
99. Jagiella WM, Sung JH. Bilateral infarction of the medullary pyramids in humans. *Neurology* 1989;39:21–24.
100. Matsumoto S, Okuda B, Imai T, Kameyama M. A sensory level on the trunk in lower lateral brainstem lesions. *Neurology* 1988;38:1515–1519.

3

Diagrams of Perforating Artery Territories in Axial, Coronal and Sagittal Planes

Patrick M. Pullicino

Department of Neurology, State University of New York at Buffalo, Buffalo General Hospital, Buffalo, New York 14203

The diagrams in this chapter are based on a series of normal axial, coronal, and sagittal magnetic resonance (MR) scans. The anatomical detail is based on three main sources: DeArmond, Fusco, and Dewey's *Structure of the Human Brain* (90), Nieuwenhuys, Voogd, and van Huijzen's *The Human Central Nervous System* (91), and Fix's *Atlas of the Human Brain and Spinal Cord* (92).

The broad outlines of the vascular territories were taken from published vascular territory diagrams, including those of Beevor (44), Lazorthes et al. (22), Khan (45), Duvernoy (63), Manelfe et al. (29), Damasio (93), Rosner et al. (2), Takahashi et al. (55,94), Savoiardo et al. (95), Amarenco et al. (70), and Ghika et al. (26). This was complemented by the references quoted in this and the previous chapter. In particular, the thalamic territories were largely based on the injection studies of Percheron (32,50,61,64) and the brainstem territories on those of Duvernoy (63).

The limits of the vascular territories shown are an estimate, based on the literature, of the most common situation. Since there is some variation of the limits of all vascular territories, these diagrams should only be used as a guide to the likely supply of a particular structure. The footnotes on each page mention some of the more common variations that are likely to be found, and the anatomy chapter (Chapter 2) gives further details and references.

Figure 1 shows the location of the diagrams on a mid-sagittal or mid-axial scan. Each diagram is based on an enlargement of the central portion of the MR scan slice illustrated beside it.

The supraterritorial vascular territories are illustrated from pages 43 to 57 and the brainstem vascular territories from pages 58 to 71.

The reference list for this chapter is the same as for the previous chapter.

Abbreviations used in the vascular keys are as follows:

ACA	anterior cerebral artery
AComA	anterior communicatory artery
MCA	middle cerebral artery
ICA	internal carotid artery
PCA	posterior cerebral artery
SCA	superior cerebellar artery
AICA	anterior inferior cerebellar artery
PICA	posterior inferior cerebellar artery

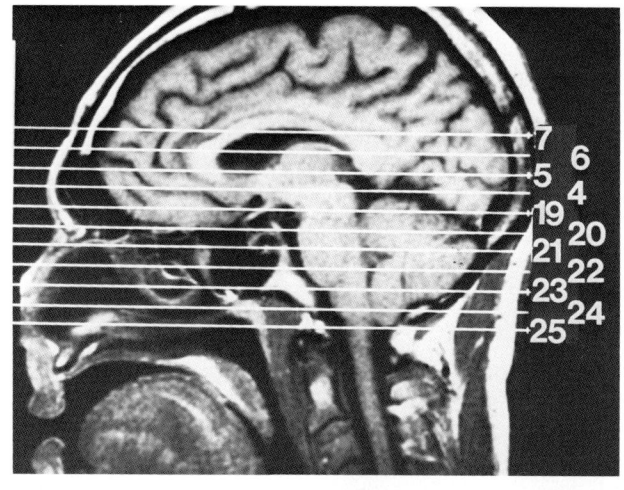
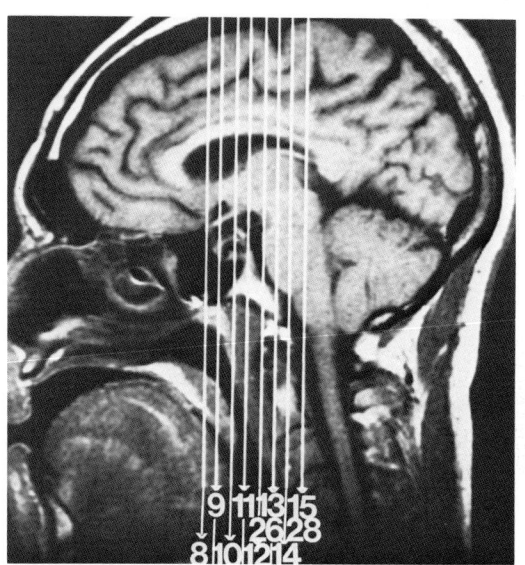
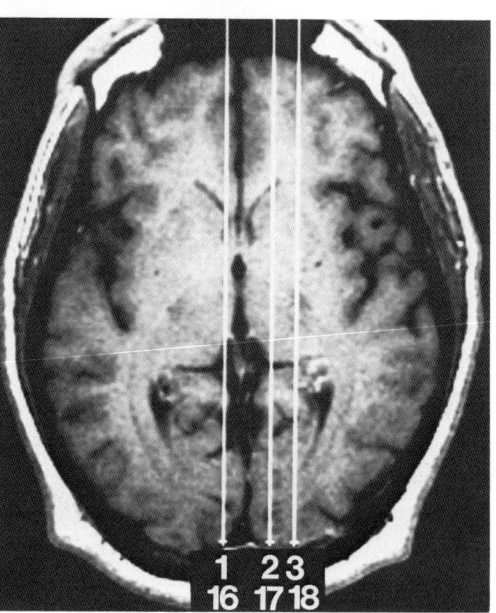

FIG. 1. Position of the axial (**A**), coronal (**B**), and sagittal (**C**) sections in this chapter. The numbers show the site of the respective sections.

SUPRATENTORIAL TERRITORIES

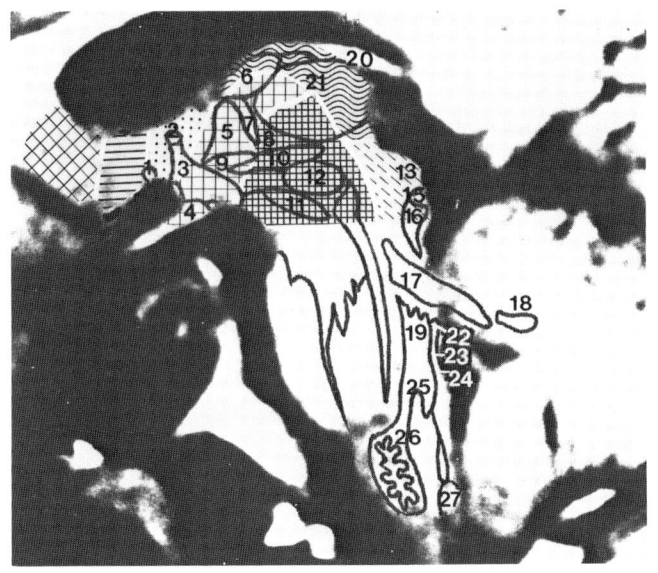
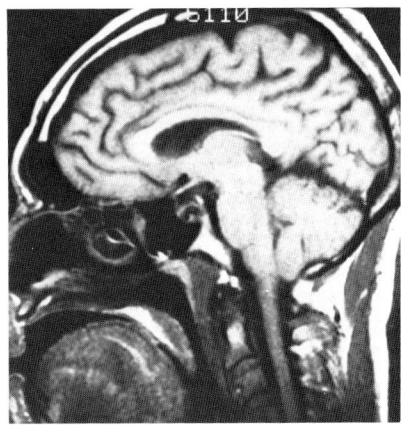

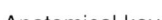 Heubner's A ≡ ACA perforators ⋮⋮⋮ AComA perforators
⊞ PComA/Thalamotuberal A ▦ Paramedian thalamic A ≋ Posteromed Choroidal A
⫶⫶ Collicular A

Anatomical key:
1. Diagonal band and nucleus of Broca
2. Anterior commissure
3. Hypothalamus
4. Optic tract
5. Lateropolar nucleus (ventral anterior nucleus)
6. Anteroprincipal nucleus (anterior nuclear group)
7. Mamillothalamic tract
8. Ventrolateral formation (ventral lateral nucleus)
9. Zona incerta
10. Prerubral tract (fields of Forel)
11. Substantia nigra
12. Red nucleus
13. Superior colliculus
14. Medial lemniscus
15. Nucleus of inferior colliculus
16. Lateral lemniscus
17. Superior cerebellar peduncle
18. Globose nucleus
19. Central tegmental tract
20. Fornix
21. Medial nucleus (dorsomedial nucleus)
22. Locus ceruleus
23. Genu of facial nerve
24. Abducens nucleus
25. Facial nucleus
26. Inferior olive
27. Cuneate nucleus

SECTION 1. Sagittal scan near midline.

The hypothalamus is supplied from anterior to posterior by the anterior communicating artery (8), the posterior communicating artery, and the paramedian thalamic arteries (4).

The thalamotuberal artery supplies the mamillothalamic tract as well as the anterior thalamus (50). The posteromedial choroidal artery courses over the top of the thalamus to reach the anterior thalamus.

The paramedian thalamic and paramedian superior and inferior mesencephalic arteries supply a continuous fan-shaped area from the midbrain to the region of the mamillothalamic tract (53,61).

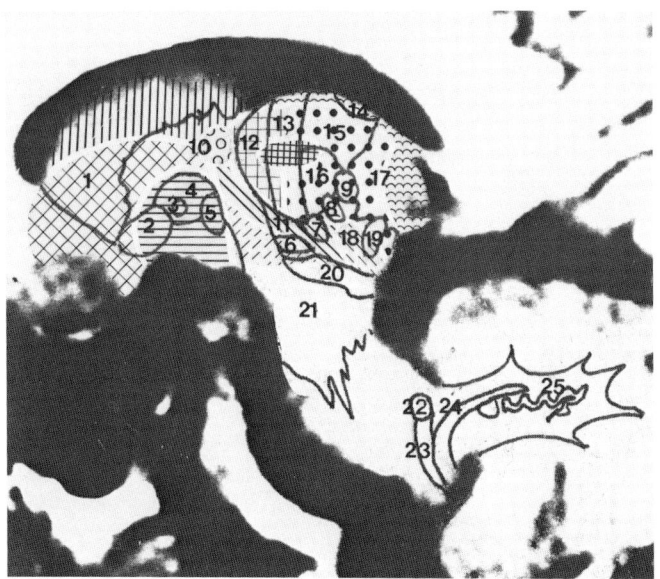
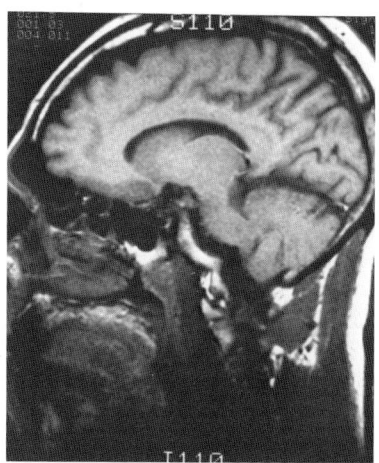

⧖⧗ Heubner's A ≡ ACA perforators ⋰⋰ MCA (medial territory)

|||| MCA (lateral territory) ⧅ AChoroidal A ∘○ ICA perforators

⊞ Thalamotuberal A ⊞ Paramedian thalamic A ∶∶ Thalamogeniculate A

≋ Posterolat Choroidal A ⦚ Collicular A

Anatomical key:
1. Head of caudate nucleus
2. Putamen
3. Anterior commissure
4. Globus pallidus
5. Lenticular fasciculus
6. Subthalamic nucleus
7. Superior cerebellar peduncle
8. Ventrocaudal nuclei (ventral posteromedial nuclei)
9. Central nucleus (centromedian nucleus)
10. Genu of internal capsule
11. Zona incerta
12. Lateropolar nucleus (ventral anterior nucleus)
13. Ventrolateral formation (ventral lateral nucleus)
14. Dorsal superficial nucleus (lateral dorsal nucleus)
15. Dorsocaudal nucleus (lateral posterior nucleus)
16. Ventrocaudal nucleus (ventral posterolateral nucleus)
17. Pulvinar
18. Medial lemniscus
19. Medial geniculate body
20. Substantia nigra
21. Cerebral peduncle
22. Principal sensory nucleus of trigeminal nerve
23. Spinal trigeminal tract
24. Inferior cerebellar peduncle
25. Dentate nucleus

SECTION 2. Sagittal scan through medial geniculate body.

The region of the anterior commissure is supplied by the anterior cerebral artery perforators just lateral to the midline (8). The tip of one of the "rabbit ears" (see Section 13) of the paramedian thalamic territory is seen surrounded by other thalamic territories (61). The thalamotuberal artery supplies the genu of the internal capsule, but this territory may be taken over by the anterior choroidal artery if the posterior communicating artery is small (42). The anterior choroidal territory may extend into the lateral diencephalic region as shown here (26).

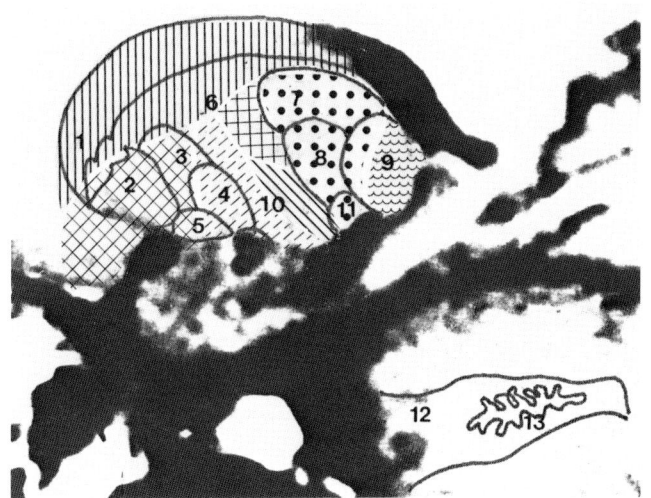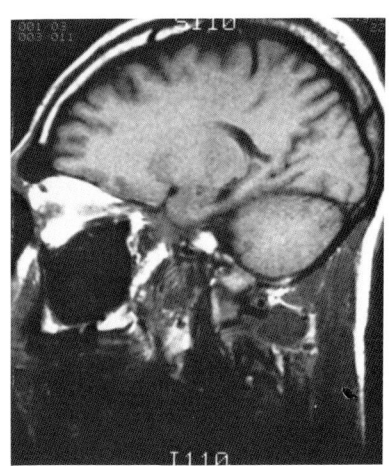

⊠ Heubner's A	∥∥∥ MCA (lateral territory)	⫽ MCA (medial territory)
⊞ Thalamotuberal A	⟋⟍ A Choroidal A	∷ Thalamogeniculate A
≋ Posterolat Choroidal A		

Anatomical key:
1. Head of caudate nucleus
2. Putamen
3. Globus pallidus, lateral segment
4. Globus pallidus, medial segment
5. Substantia innominata and nucleus basalis of Meynert
6. Genu of internal capsule
7. Dorsocaudal nucleus (lateral posterior nucleus)
8. Ventrocaudal nucleus (ventral posterolateral nucleus)
9. Pulvinar
10. Cerebral peduncle
11. Middle cerebellar peduncle
12. Dentate nucleus

SECTION 3. Sagittal scan through genu of internal capsule.

The vascularization of the genu of the internal capsule is variable (29). The perforators from the internal carotid supply part of the genu and may supply the adjacent parts of the globus pallidus (6), anterior thalamus, and posterior limb of the internal capsule (2). Heubner's artery territory includes the inferior half of the head of the caudate nucleus and, in 15% of cases it contributes to the supply of the genu of the internal capsule (15).

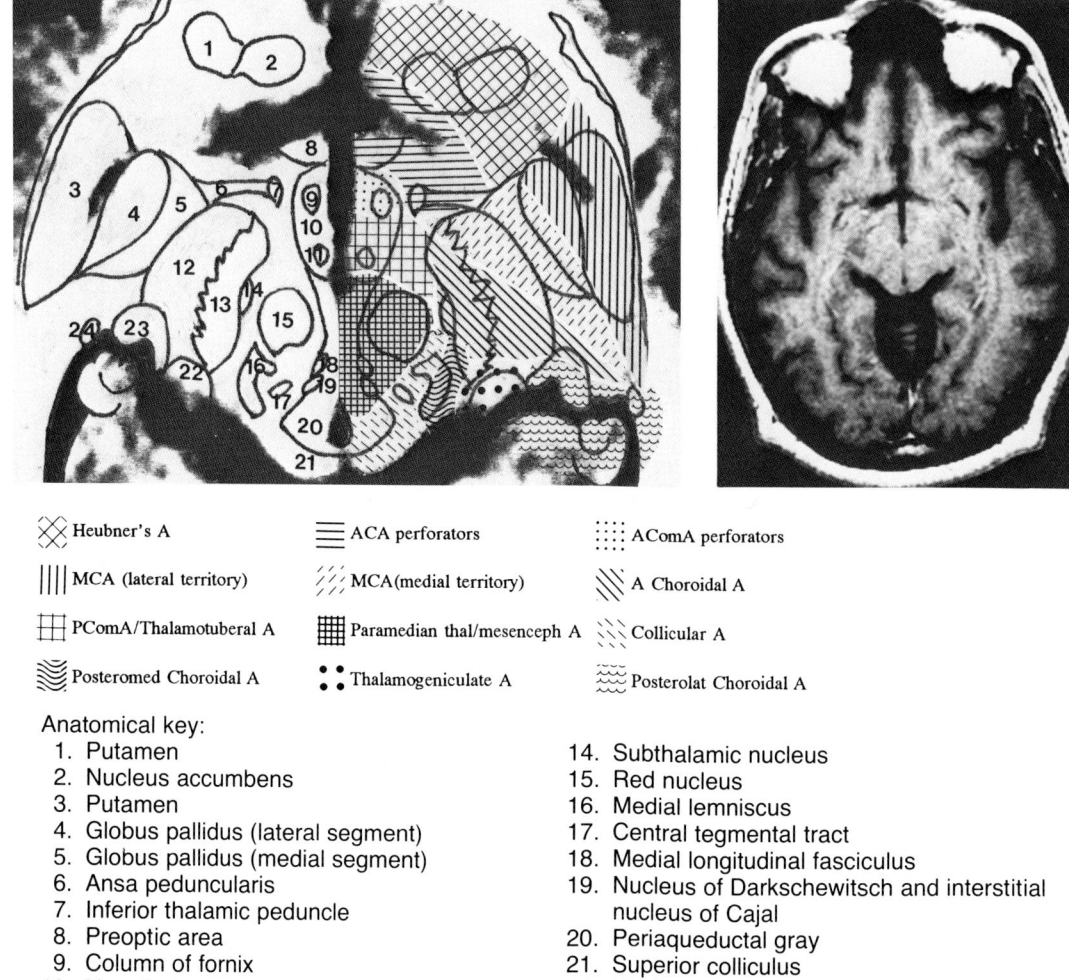

Pattern	Artery	Pattern	Artery	Pattern	Artery
⋈	Heubner's A	≡	ACA perforators	⋮⋮	AComA perforators
‖‖	MCA (lateral territory)	∕∕∕	MCA (medial territory)	⟍⟍	A Choroidal A
⊞	PComA/Thalamotuberal A	⊞	Paramedian thal/mesenceph A	⋰⋰	Collicular A
≋	Posteromed Choroidal A	∶∶	Thalamogeniculate A	≈	Posterolat Choroidal A

Anatomical key:
 1. Putamen
 2. Nucleus accumbens
 3. Putamen
 4. Globus pallidus (lateral segment)
 5. Globus pallidus (medial segment)
 6. Ansa peduncularis
 7. Inferior thalamic peduncle
 8. Preoptic area
 9. Column of fornix
10. Hypothalamus
11. Mamillothalamic tract
12. Cerebral peduncle
13. Substantia nigra
14. Subthalamic nucleus
15. Red nucleus
16. Medial lemniscus
17. Central tegmental tract
18. Medial longitudinal fasciculus
19. Nucleus of Darkschewitsch and interstitial nucleus of Cajal
20. Periaqueductal gray
21. Superior colliculus
22. Medial geniculate body
23. Lateral geniculate body
24. Tail of caudate nucleus

SECTION 4. Scan through diencephalon.

The paramedian mesencephalic/thalamic territory extends to the lateral superior red nucleus (61). The medial longitudinal fasciculus and its rostral interstitial nucleus is supplied by long and short paramedian mesencephalic arteries (63).

The medial lemniscus and spinothalamic tracts at this level are supplied by both the collicular arteries and the posteromedial choroidal artery, which supply the peripheral part of the upper midbrain tegmentum (45).

The anterior choroidal artery may also supply the upper parts of the red nucleus and of the subthalamic nucleus (26), but this territory is variable (42). It supplies the middle third of the cerebral peduncle and substantia nigra and the medial part of the lateral geniculate body (42). The lateral part is supplied by the posterolateral choroidal artery.

The hypothalamus is supplied by branches from the posterior communicating artery in the region of the mamillothalamic tract (50). The paramedian part of the most anterior hypothalamus and the columns of the fornix, however, are supplied by penetrating arteries arising from the anterior communicating artery (8). The anterior hypothalamus lateral to this and the septal area are supplied by penetrators arising from the anterior cerebral artery (8). This is more clearly seen on the sagittal view (Section 1).

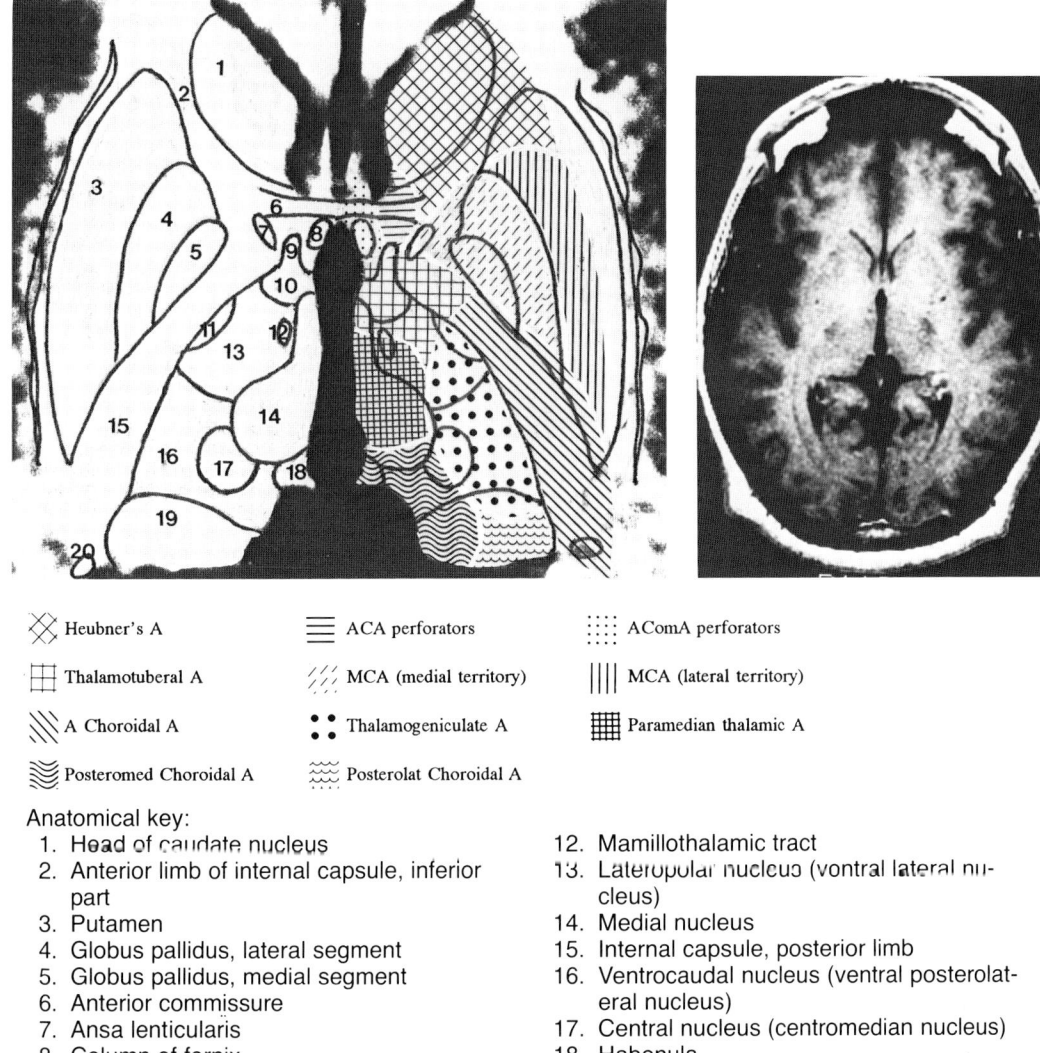

⊠ Heubner's A	≡ ACA perforators	⋮⋮⋮ AComA perforators
⊞ Thalamotuberal A	⁄⁄⁄ MCA (medial territory)	‖‖‖ MCA (lateral territory)
⦀ A Choroidal A	∶∶ Thalamogeniculate A	▦ Paramedian thalamic A
≋ Posteromed Choroidal A	≈≈ Posterolat Choroidal A	

Anatomical key:
1. Head of caudate nucleus
2. Anterior limb of internal capsule, inferior part
3. Putamen
4. Globus pallidus, lateral segment
5. Globus pallidus, medial segment
6. Anterior commissure
7. Ansa lenticularis
8. Column of fornix
9. Inferior thalamic peduncle
10. Fascicular nucleus of thalamus
11. Thalamic fasciculus
12. Mamillothalamic tract
13. Lateropolar nucleus (ventral lateral nucleus)
14. Medial nucleus
15. Internal capsule, posterior limb
16. Ventrocaudal nucleus (ventral posterolateral nucleus)
17. Central nucleus (centromedian nucleus)
18. Habenula
19. Pulvinar
20. Caudate nucleus, tail

SECTION 5. Scan through midthalamus.

The scan plane goes through the anterior commissure anteriorly and the midthalamus posteriorly. The thalamogeniculate arteries supply the lower two thirds of the lateral nuclear mass of the thalamus; they may send small branches to the posterior limb of the internal capsule (41).

According to Shellshear (25), the anterior commissure is the dividing line between five arterial territories. The most medial part of the anterior commissure is supplied by perforators from the anterior communicating artery; lateral to that is the anterior cerebral artery perforator territory (8). The artery of Heubner supplies the outermost part of the anterior commissure [in addition to the inferior part of the head of the caudate, anterior limb of internal capsule, and inferior putamen (8)]. Posterolateral to the anterior commissure is the medial lenticulostriate territory with the anterior choroidal and posterior communicating territories posteromedially.

The posterior two thirds of the internal capsule is supplied by the anterior choroidal artery. This territory may extend medially to include the lateral part of the thalamus (41).

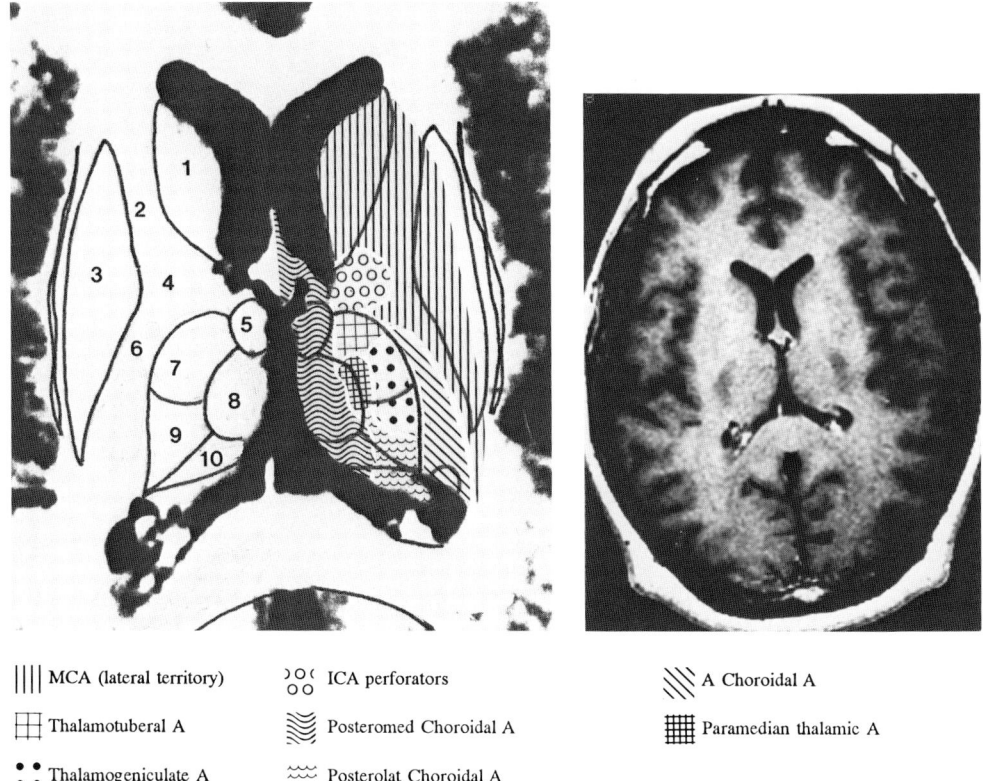

‖‖ MCA (lateral territory)	∘∘ ICA perforators	⦸ A Choroidal A
⊞ Thalamotuberal A	≋ Posteromed Choroidal A	▦ Paramedian thalamic A
∷ Thalamogeniculate A	∼ Posterolat Choroidal A	

Anatomical key:
1. Head of caudate nucleus
2. Anterior limb of internal capsule
3. Putamen
4. Genu of internal capsule
5. Anteroprincipal nucleus (anterior nuclear group)
6. Posterior limb of internal capsule
7. Ventrolateral formation (ventral lateral nucleus)
8. Medial nucleus (dorsomedial nucleus)
9. Dorsocaudal nucleus (lateral posterior nucleus)
10. Pulvinar

SECTION 6. Scan through genu of internal capsule.

The arterial supply of the genu is variable (29). It is supplied by perforators from the internal carotid medially (6), the thalamotuberal artery posteriorly (55), and the lenticulostriates anteriorly (30). In addition it may be supplied by Heubner's artery or by the anterior choroidal artery if the territories of these arteries are large (29).

The internal carotid perforators may also supply the anterior thalamus and posterior limb of the internal capsule (2). The posteromedial choroidal artery supplies the medial thalamus extending to the anteroprincipal (anterior) nucleus (32).

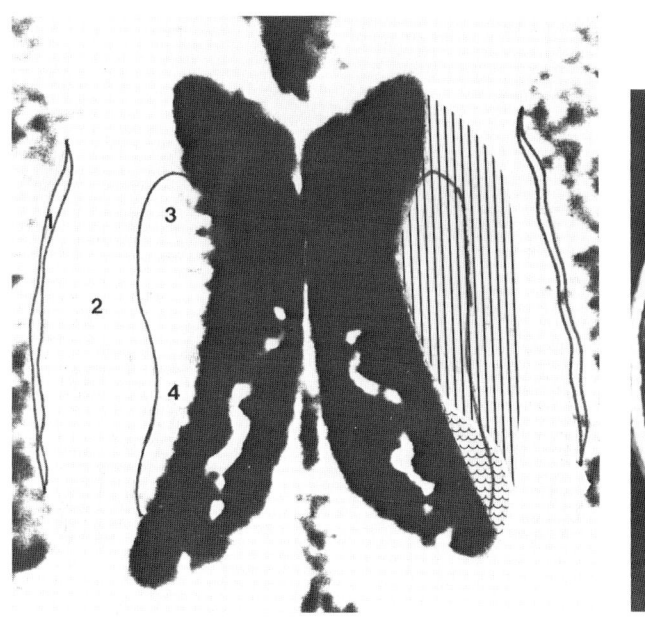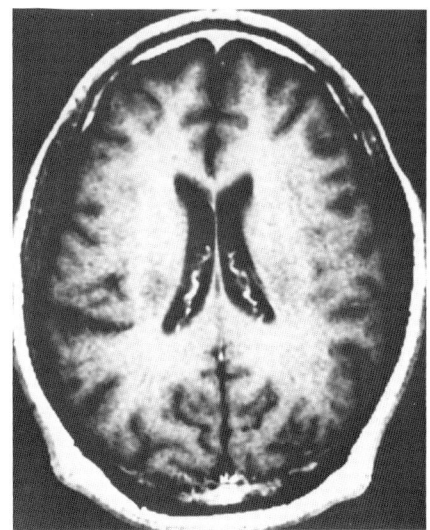

|||| MCA (lateral territory)   ～～ Posterolat Choroidal A

Anatomical key:
1. Claustrum
2. Junction of internal capsule and corona radiata
3. Head of caudate nucleus
4. Body of caudate nucleus

SECTION 7. Scan through bodies of lateral ventricles.

The lateral lenticulostriate arteries supply the white matter at the outer margins of the lateral ventricles. This is the junctional region between the internal capsule and the corona radiata (31). The lateral ventricular margin suprajacent to the posterolateral thalamus is probably supplied by the posterolateral choroidal artery (32).

SMALL ARTERIAL TERRITORIES

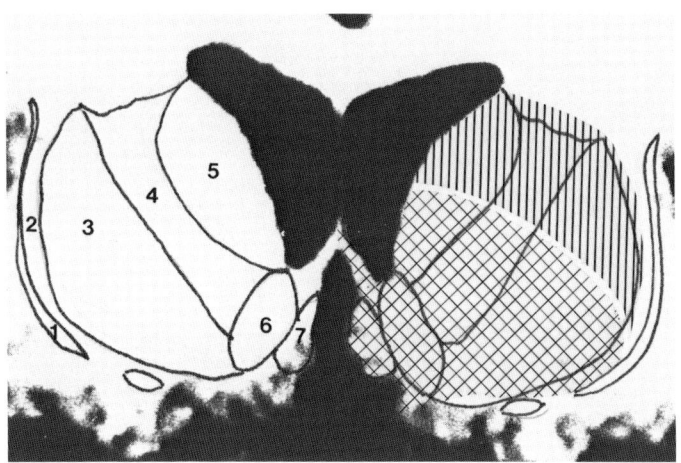
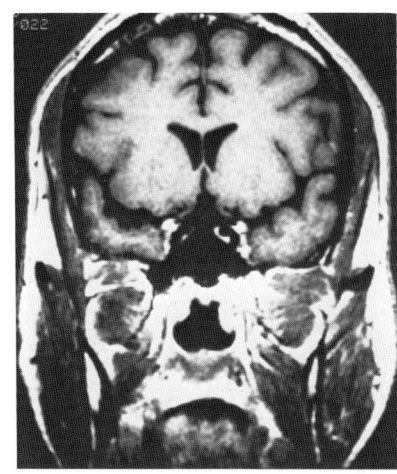

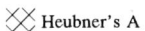 Heubner's A |||| MCA (lateral territory)

Anatomical key:
1. Claustrum
2. External capsule
3. Putamen
4. Anterior limb of internal capsule
5. Head of caudate nucleus
6. Nucleus accumbens septi
7. Paraterminal gyrus

SECTION 8. Coronal scan through head of caudate nucleus.

Heubner's artery supplies the inferior half of the head of the caudate nucleus and putamen and the lower part of the anterior limb of the internal capsule (6), as well as the most anterior part of the septal nuclei (7).

SMALL ARTERIAL TERRITORIES

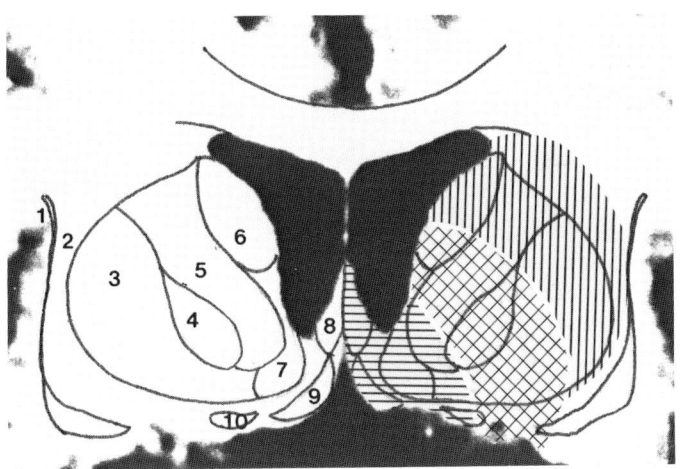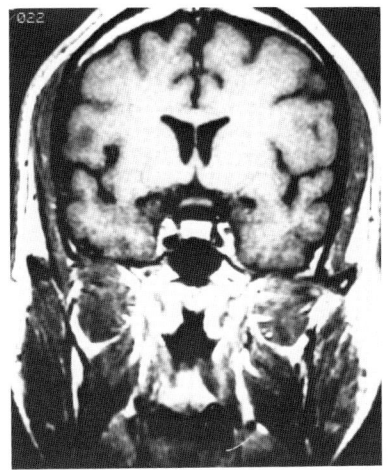

|||| MCA (lateral territory) ⊗ Heubner's A ≡ ACA perforators

Anatomical key:
1. Claustrum
2. External capsule
3. Putamen
4. Globus pallidus
5. Anterior limb of internal capsule
6. Head of caudate nucleus
7. Nucleus accumbens septi
8. Septal nuclei
9. Subcallosal area
10. Anterior olfactory nucleus

SECTION 9. Coronal scan through septal area.

The territory of the anterior cerebral artery perforators lies medial to the territory of Heubner's artery (8). It includes the septal nuclei, the anterior olfactory nucleus, and parts of the anterior limb of the internal capsule and putamen (7).

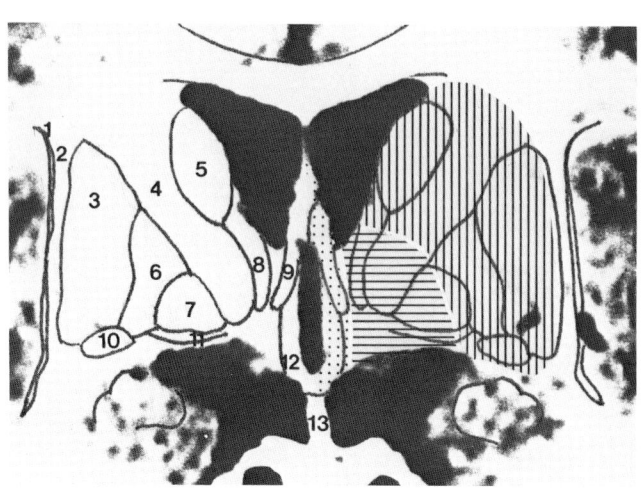
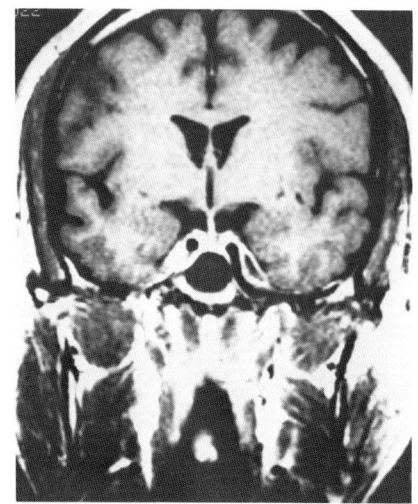

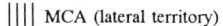 MCA (lateral territory)   ≡ ACA perforators   ⋮⋮⋮ AComA perforators

Anatomical key:
1. Claustrum
2. External capsule
3. Putamen
4. Anterior limb of internal capsule
5. Head of caudate nucleus
6. Globus pallidus, lateral segment
7. Globus pallidus, medial segment
8. Inferior thalamic peduncle
9. Fornix
10. Anterior commissure
11. Ansa peduncularis
12. Anterior hypothalamus
13. Infundibulum

SECTION 10. Coronal scan through columns of fornix.

Perforating arteries from the anterior communicating artery supply the most anterior part of the hypothalamus and the columns of the fornix (8). Lateral to this is the territory of the perforators that arise from the anterior cerebral arteries. In this section they supply the medial globus pallidus and the lowermost part of the anterior limb of the internal capsule (8).

SMALL ARTERIAL TERRITORIES

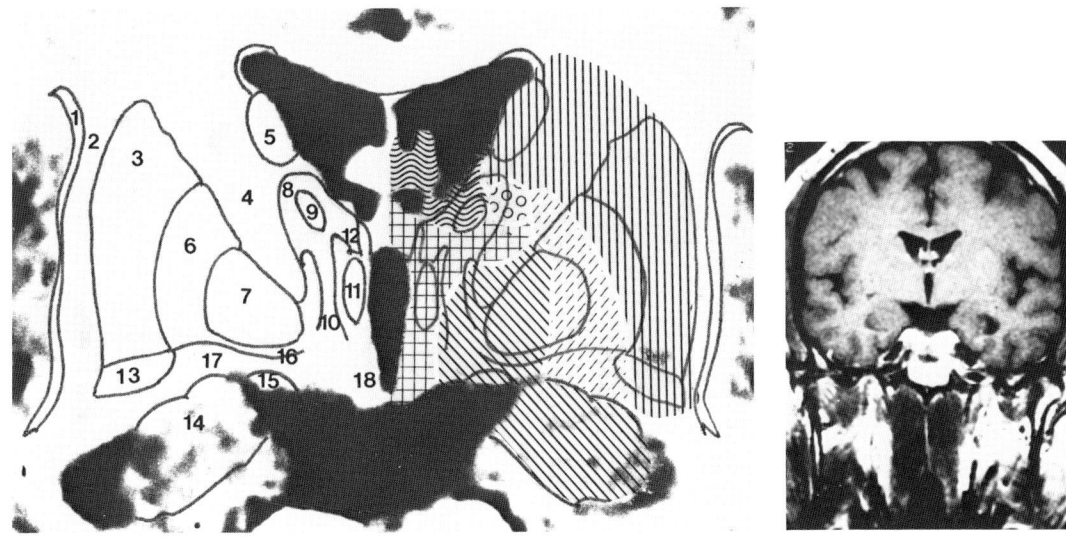

‖‖‖ MCA (lateral territory)	⁄⁄⁄ MCA (medial territory)	∘∘∘ ICA perforators
≋ Posteromed Choroidal A	⊞ PComA/Thalamotuberal A	⦸ A Choroidal A

Anatomical key:
1. Claustrum
2. External capsule
3. Putamen
4. Genu of internal capsule
5. Body of caudate nucleus
6. Globus pallidus, lateral segment
7. Globus pallidus, medial segment
8. Reticular nucleus of thalamus and anterior thalamic peduncle
9. Anteroprincipal nucleus (anterior nuclear group)
10. Inferior thalamic peduncle
11. Fornix
12. Stria medullaris
13. Anterior commissure
14. Amygdaloid nucleus
15. Optic tract
16. Ansa lenticularis
17. Substantia Innominata
18. Hypothalamus

SECTION 11. Coronal scan through genu of internal capsule.

The blood supply to the genu of internal capsule is outlined in Section 6. The thalamotuberal artery supplies the hypothalamus (4) as well as the anterolateral part of the thalamus, excluding the anterior nucleus, which is supplied by the posteromedial choroidal artery (32). The anterior choroidal artery has a perforating territory and also supplies the uncus.

SMALL ARTERIAL TERRITORIES

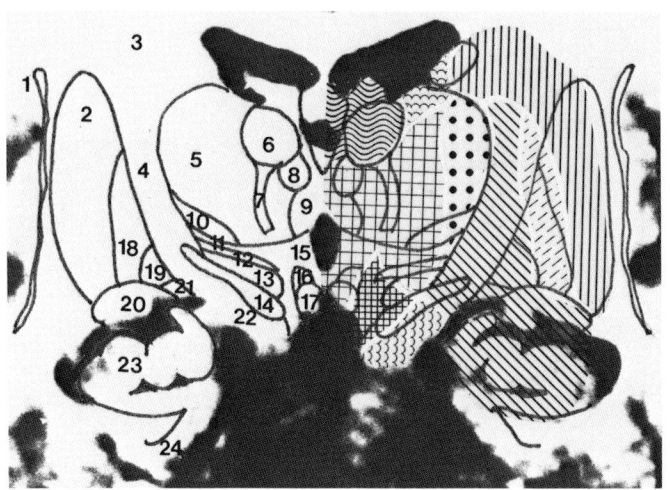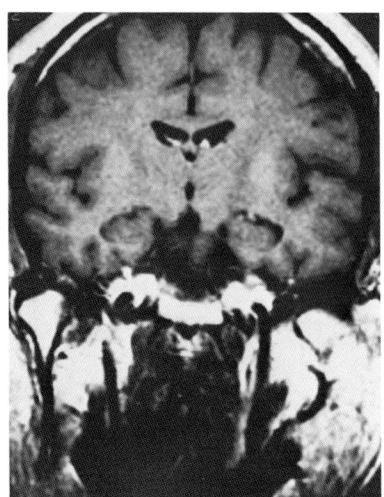

‖‖‖ MCA (lateral territory)	⁄⁄⁄ MCA (medial territory)	⦈⦈ A Choroidal A
•• Thalamogeniculate A	≋ Posterolat Choroidal A	⦇ Posteromed Choroidal A
╬ PComA/Thalamotuberal A	▦ Paramedian Thalamic A	⦃⦃ Anterolateral Midbrain territory

Anatomical key:
1. Claustrum
2. Putamen
3. Corona radiata
4. Posterior limb of internal capsule
5. Ventrolateral formation (ventral lateral nucleus)
6. Anteroprincipal nucleus (anterior nuclear group)
7. Mamillothalamic tract
8. Medial nucleus (dorsomedial nucleus)
9. Parafascicular nucleus (midline nuclear group)
10. H_1 Field of Forel/thalamic fasciculus
11. Zona incerta
12. H_2 Field of Forel/lenticular fasciculus
13. Subthalamic nucleus
14. Substantia nigra
15. Posterior hypothalamus
16. Mamillothalmic tract
17. Mamillary body
18. Globus pallidus, lateral segment
19. Globus pallidus, medial segment
20. Amygdaloid nucleus
21. Optic tract
22. Cerebral peduncle
23. Pes hippocampi
24. Parahippocampal gyrus

SECTION 12. Coronal scan through anterior thalamus.

The anterior thalamus, including the mamillothalamic tract, is usually supplied by the thalamotuberal artery that arises from the posterior communicating artery. If this artery is absent, its territory is taken over by the paramedian thalamic arteries (50). Smaller branches from the posterior communicating artery supply the hypothalamus, including the mamillary bodies.

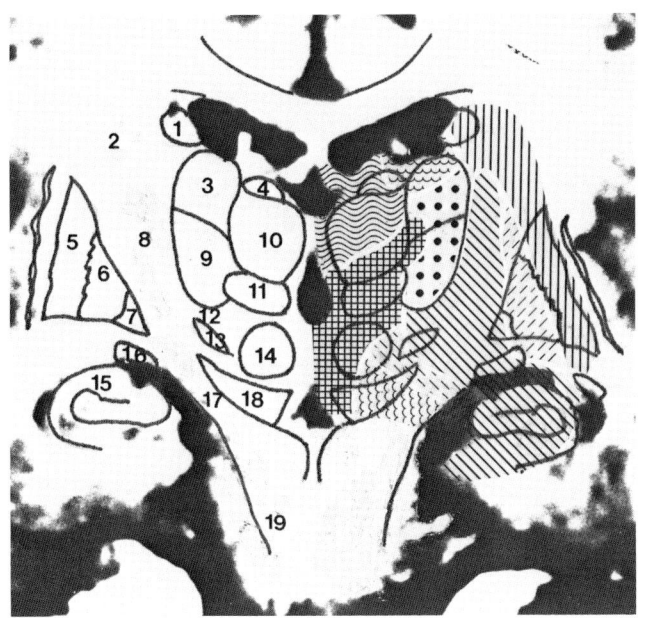
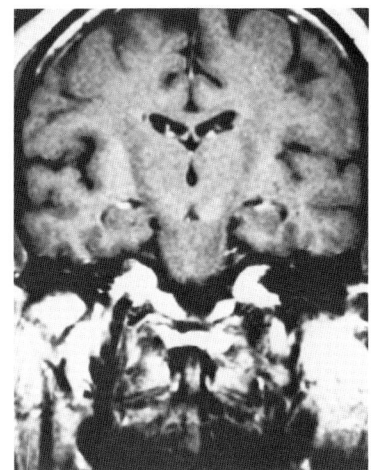

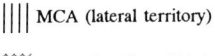 MCA (lateral territory)	MCA (medial territory)	A Choroidal A
Posterolat Choroidal A	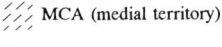 Posteromed Choroidal A	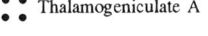 Thalamogeniculate A
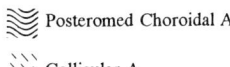 Paramedian Thalamic A	Collicular A	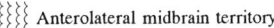 Anterolateral midbrain territory

Anatomical key:
1. Body of caudate nucleus
2. Corona radiata
3. Dorsocaudal nucleus (lateral posterior nucleus)
4. Dorsal superficial nucleus (lateral dorsal nucleus)
5. Putamen
6. Globus pallidus, lateral segment
7. Globus pallidus, medial segment
8. Posterior limb of internal capsule
9. Ventrocaudal nucleus (ventral posterolateral nucleus)
10. Medial nucleus (dorsomedial nucleus)
11. Parafascicular nucleus
12. Zona incerta
13. Subthalamic nucleus
14. Red nucleus
15. Hippocampal formation
16. Optic tract
17. Cerebral peduncle
18. Substantia nigra
19. Pyramidal tract (pons)

SECTION 13. Coronal scan through red nucleus.

The typical "rabbit ear" shape of the paramedian thalamic territory is seen extending laterally from the midline toward the dorsocaudal (lateral posterior) nucleus (61). The blood supply to the subthalamic region is variable (42) but the paramedian territory probably extends to the lateral part of the red nucleus superiorly. The zona incerta and the subthalamic nucleus are here shown supplied by the anterior choroidal artery (41), but the thalamotuberal artery (50) and the collicular artery (32) may also supply the subthalamic nucleus.

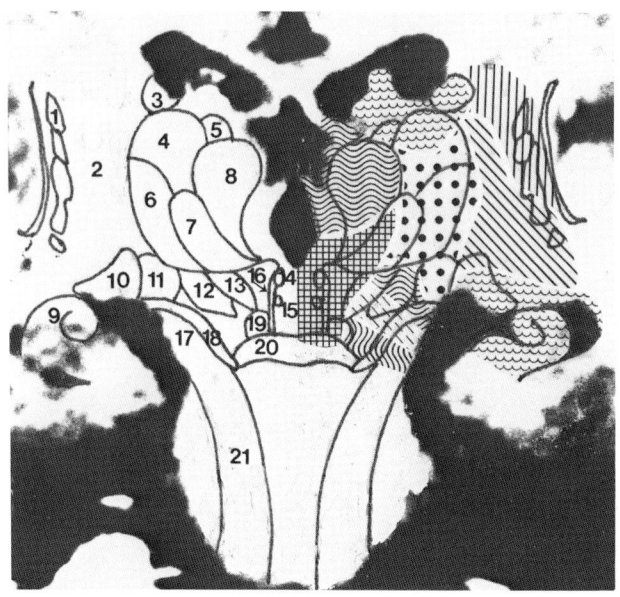 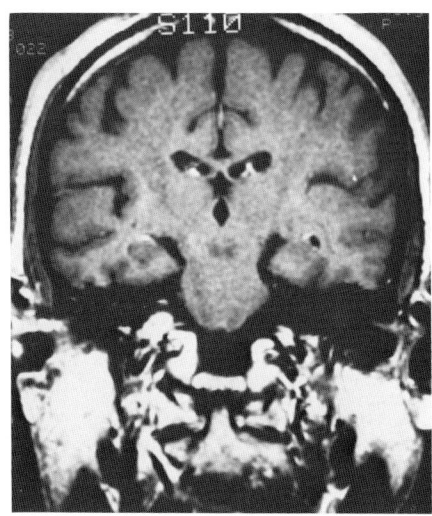

‖‖ MCA (lateral territory)	A Choroidal A	Posterolat Choroidal A
Posteromed Choroidal A	Thalamogeniculate A	Paramedian thalamic A
Collicular A	Anterolateral midbrain territory	

Anatomical key:
1. Putamen
2. Posterior limb internal capsule
3. Body of caudate nucleus
4. Dorsocaudal nucleu (lateral posterior nucleus)
5. Dorsal superficial nucleus (lateral dorsal nucleus)
6. Ventrocaudal nucleus (ventral posterolateral nucleus)
7. Central (centromedian) nucleus
8. Medial nucleus (dorsomedial nucleus)
9. Hippocampal formation
10. Lateral geniculate body
11. Medial geniculate body
12. Medial lemniscus
13. Superior cerebellar peduncle
14. Nucleus of Darkschewitsch and interstitial nucleus of Cajal
15. Accessory oculomotor nucleus
16. Medial longitudinal fasciculus
17. Cerebral peduncle
18. Substantia nigra
19. Central tegmental tract
20. Decussation of superior cerebellar peduncle
21. Pyramidal tract (pons)

SECTION 14. Coronal scan through geniculate bodies.

The lateral part of the lateral geniculate body is supplied by the posterolateral choroidal artery and the medial part by the anterior choroidal artery (39). This arrangement is said to underlie two different syndromes of infarction of the lateral geniculate body (96,97). The superior thalamus is supplied by the posteromedial and posterolateral choroidal arteries in the posterior thalamus, and the posterolateral choroidal extends up alongside the lateral ventricular wall (32).

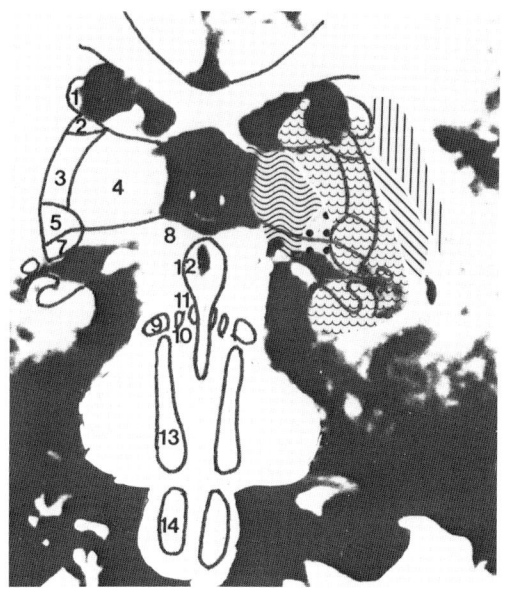 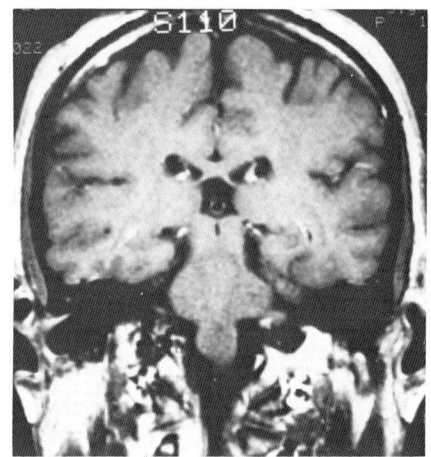

‖‖ MCA (lateral territory)	＼ A Choroidal A	≋ Posterolat Choroidal A
≋ Posteromed Choroidal A	∴ Thalamogeniculate A	

Anatomical key:
1. Body of caudate nucleus
2. Dorsocaudal nucleus (lateral posterior nucleus)
3. Lateral pulvinar nucleus
4. Medial pulvinar nucleus
5. Pulvinar nucleus
6. Tail of caudate nucleus
7. Lateral geniculate body
8. Superior colliculus
9. Superior cerebellar peduncle
10. Central tegmental tract
11. Medial longitudinal fasciculus
12. Periaqueductal gray matter
13. Medial lemniscus
14. Pyramidal tract (medulla)

SECTION 15. Coronal scan through pulvinar.

The pulvinar is supplied by the posterolateral and posteromedial choroidal arteries, which arch up over the posterior thalamus (32,55).

BRAINSTEM TERRITORIES

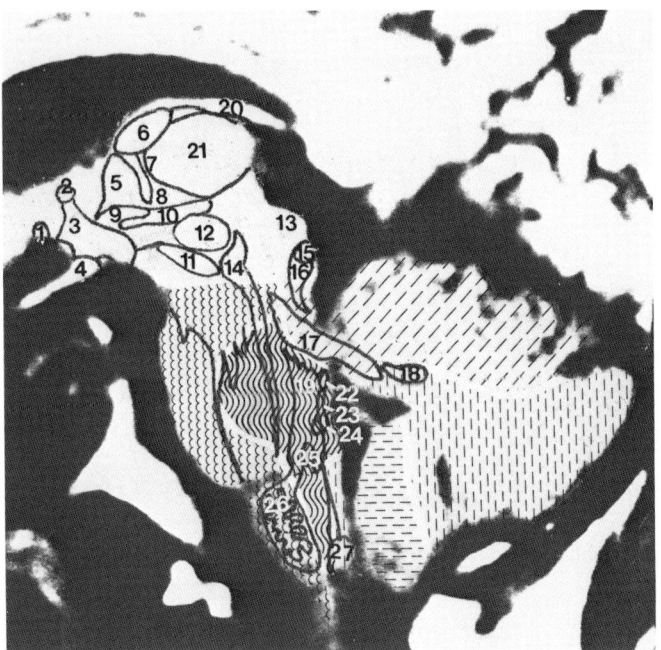
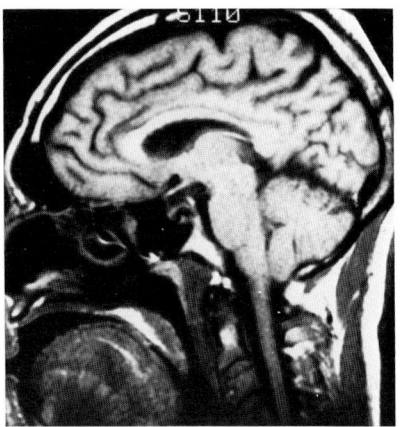

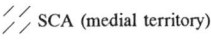 SCA (medial territory)   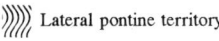 Lateral pontine territory   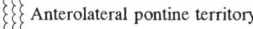 Anterolateral pontine territory

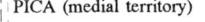 PICA (medial territory)   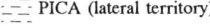 PICA (lateral territory)

Anatomical key:
1. Diagonal band and nucleus of Broca
2. Anterior commissure
3. Hypothalamus
4. Optic tract
5. Lateropolar nucleus (ventral anterior nucleus)
6. Anteroprincipal nucleus (anterior nuclear group)
7. Mamillothalamic tract
8. Ventrolateral formation (ventral lateral nucleus)
9. Zona incerta
10. Prerubral tract (fields of Forel)
11. Substantia nigra
12. Red nucleus
13. Superior colliculus
14. Medial lemniscus
15. Nucleus of inferior colliculus
16. Lateral lemniscus
17. Superior cerebellar peduncle
18. Globose nucleus
19. Central tegmental tract
20. Fornix
21. Medial nucleus (dorsomedial nucleus)
22. Locus ceruleus
23. Genu of facial nerve
24. Abducens nucleus
25. Facial nucleus
26. Inferior olive
27. Cuneate nucleus

SECTION 16. Sagittal scan near midline.

The base of the pons is supplied by perforating branches from the basilar artery. The medial lemniscus can be seen extending down through the lateral territory of the brainstem. The superior cerebellar peduncle is supplied by the superior cerebellar artery.

SMALL ARTERIAL TERRITORIES

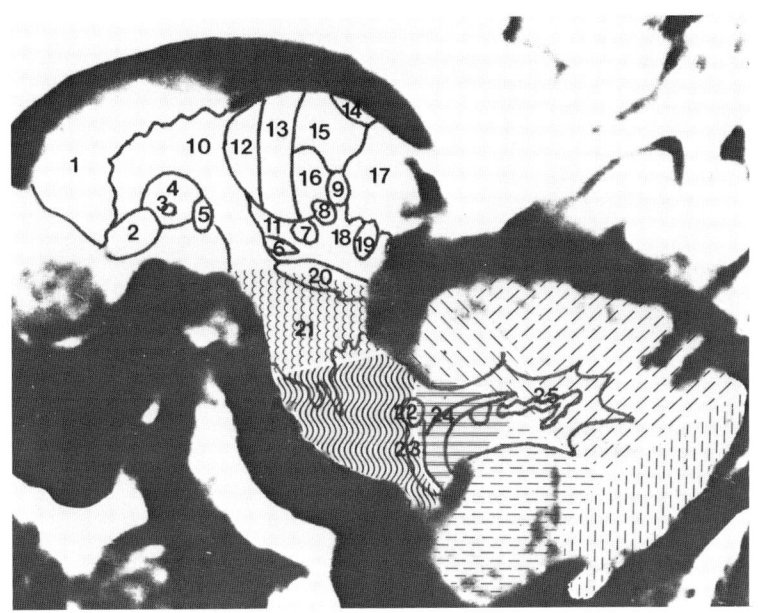
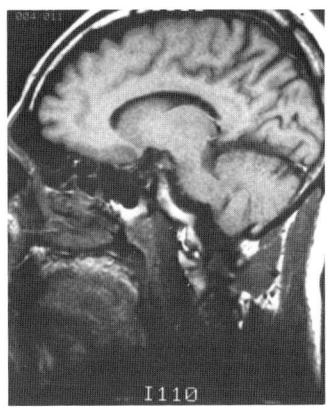

///(Lateral pontine territory   ≡ AICA   }}} Anterolateral pontine territory

\\ SCA (lateral territory)   // SCA (medial territory)   --- PICA (lateral territory)

||| PICA (medial territory)

Anatomical key:
1. Head of caudate nucleus
2. Putamen
3. Anterior commissure
4. Globus pallidus
5. Lenticular fasciculus
6. Subthalamic nucleus
7. Superior cerebellar peduncle
8. Ventrocaudal nuclei (ventral posteromedial nuclei)
9. Central nucleus (centromedian nucleus)
10. Genu of internal capsule
11. Zona incerta
12. Lateropolar nucleus (ventral anterior nucleus)
13. Ventrolateral formation (ventral lateral nucleus)
14. Dorsal superficial nucleus (lateral dorsal nucleus)
15. Dorsocaudal nucleus (lateral posterior nucleus)
16. Ventrocaudal nucleus (ventral posterolateral nucleus)
17. Pulvinar
18. Medial lemniscus
19. Medial geniculate body
20. Substantia nigra
21. Cerebral peduncle
22. Principal sensory nucleus of trigeminal nerve
23. Spinal trigeminal tract
24. Inferior cerebellar peduncle
25. Dentate nucleus

SECTION 17. Sagittal scan through lateral pons.

The different cerebellar territories are seen to meet in the region of the dentate nucleus, which is probably a deep watershed territory. The anterior inferior cerebellar artery is seen supplying the lateral pons (41).

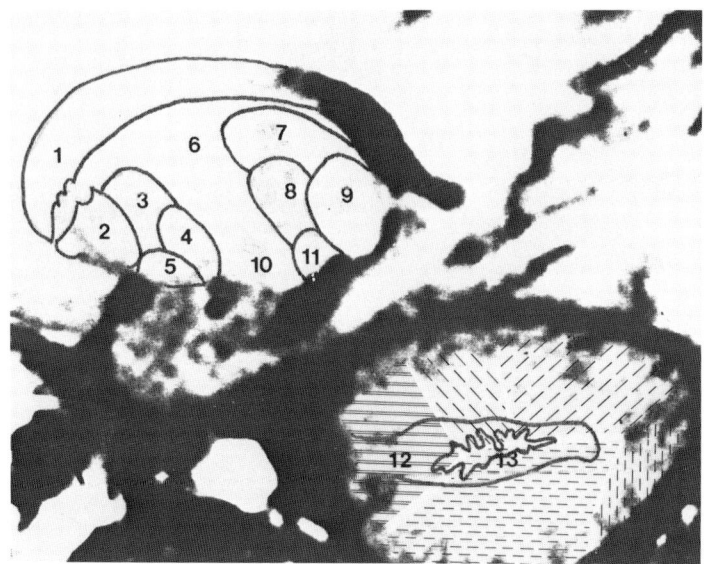
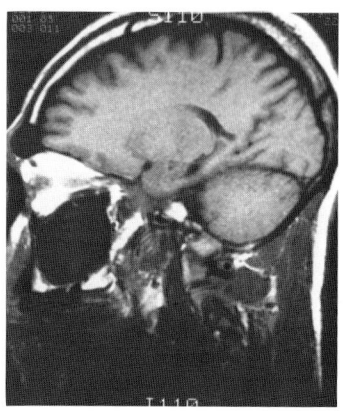

 AICA   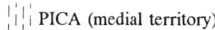 SCA (lateral territory)   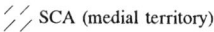 SCA (medial territory)

PICA (lateral territory)   PICA (medial territory)

Anatomical key:
1. Head of caudate nucleus
2. Putamen
3. Globus pallidus, lateral segment
4. Globus pallidus, medial segment
5. Substantia innominata and nucleus basalis of Meynert
6. Genu of internal capsule
7. Dorsocaudal nucleus (lateral posterior nucleus)
8. Ventrocaudal nucleus (ventral postero-lateral nucleus)
9. Pulvinar
10. Cerebral peduncle
11. Middle cerebellar peduncle
12. Dentate nucleus

SECTION 18. Sagittal scan through dentate nucleus.

The lateral cerebellar territories are shown in sagittal section (81).

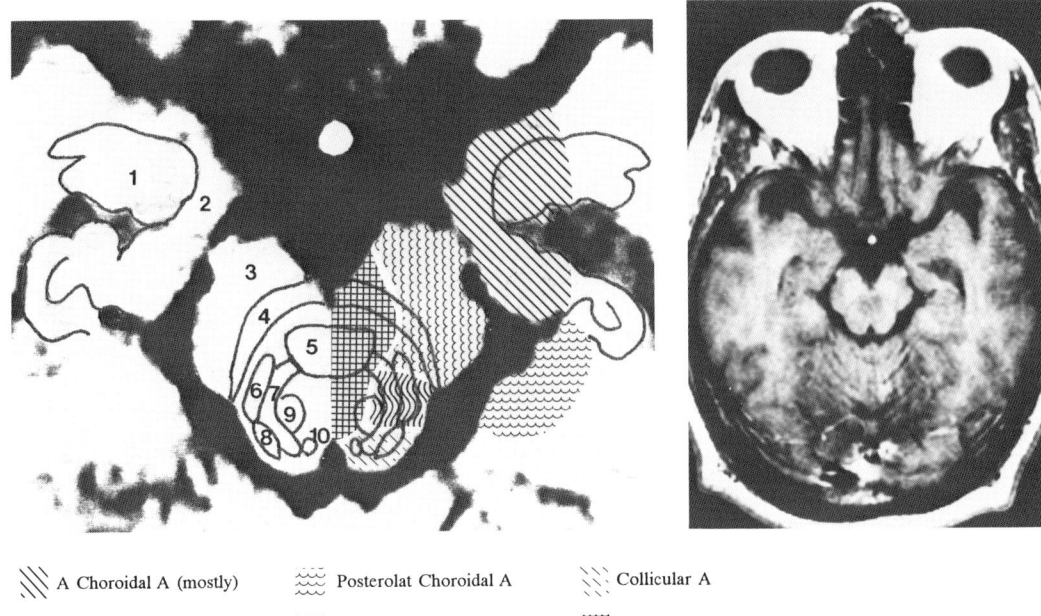

⧅ A Choroidal A (mostly)	≈≈ Posterolat Choroidal A	⧅ Collicular A
⦀ Lateral midbrain territory	}}}} Anterolateral territory	▦ Inferior paramedian mesenceph A

Anatomical key:
1. Amygdaloid nucleus
2. Uncus
3. Cerebral peduncle
4. Substantia nigra
5. Decussation of the superior cerebellar peduncle
6. Medial lemniscus
7. Superior cerebellar peduncle
8. Lateral lemniscus
9. Central tegmental tract
10. Locus ceruleus

SECTION 19. Scan through caudal midbrain.

The anteromedial territory at this level is supplied by the inferior paramedian mesencephalic arteries arising from both the P_1 segment of the posterior cerebral artery and from the tip of the basilar artery (45,61). The oculomotor nucleus, which is just above the plane of this section, is also in the anteromedial territory. The posterior territory is supplied by the collicular arteries, but there is free anastomosis with the superior cerebellar arteries below and the size of these two territories varies inversely with each other. The lateral territory is supplied mainly by the collicular arteries but also by direct branches from the posterior cerebral artery (37).

The cerebral peduncles (anterolateral territory) are supplied anteriorly by the pedunculo-subthalamic branches of the posterior communicating artery (50), the middle third by the anterior choroidal artery, and the posterior third by the accessory collicular and collicular arteries (52). Direct branches also arise from the posterior cerebral artery (37).

Anteriorly the uncus and the hippocampus are supplied by the anterior choroidal artery and by branches from the middle cerebral, internal carotid, and posterior cerebral arteries (19,43,68). More posteriorly, the hippocampus and medial temporal lobe are supplied by the posterolateral choroidal artery (64,68).

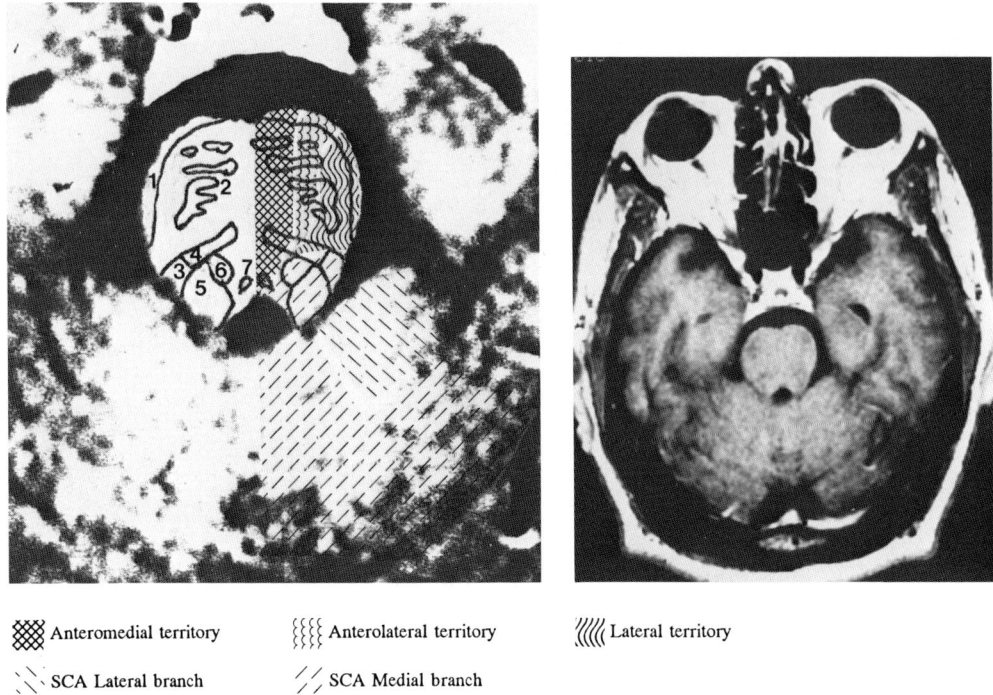

Anatomical key:
1. Middle cerebellar peduncle
2. Pyramidal tract
3. Lateral lemniscus
4. Medial lemniscus
5. Superior cerebellar peduncle
6. Central tegmental tract
7. Medial longitudinal fasciculus

SECTION 20. Axial scan through rostral pons.

The anteromedial territory is supplied by paramedian perforators from the basilar artery.

The lateral territory at this level is supplied by the superolateral pontine artery, a branch of the basilar artery.

The lateral superior pontine tegmentum (posterior territory) is supplied by the superior cerebellar artery. This includes the superior cerebellar peduncle, the lateral lemniscus, and the spinothalamic tract and part of the medial lemniscus (45,63). This artery also supplies the caudal two thirds of the inferior colliculus (45). The medial longitudinal fasciculus and fourth nerve nuclei (not shown) are supplied by the anteromedial penetrators from the basilar artery (63).

SMALL ARTERIAL TERRITORIES

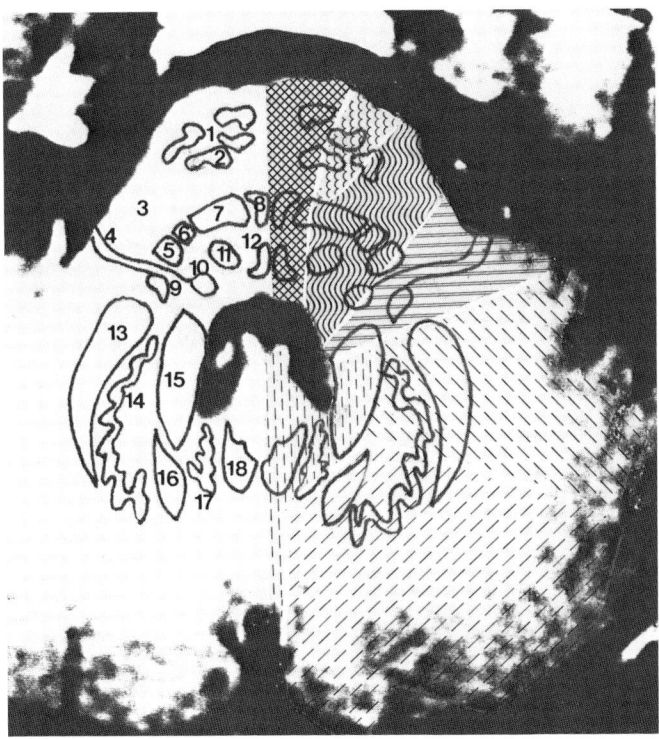
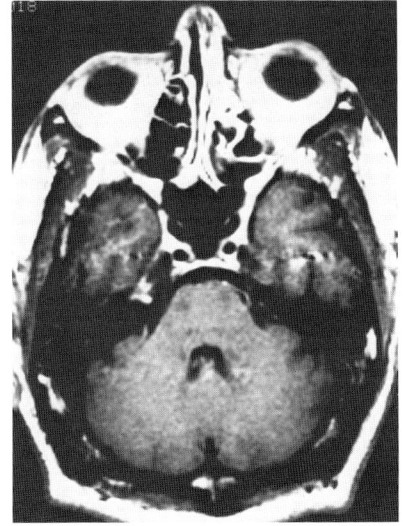

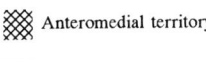 Anteromedial territory   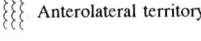 Anterolateral territory   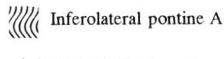 Inferolateral pontine A

≡ AICA   ＼＼ SCA Lateral branch   ／／ SCA Medial branch

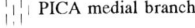 PICA medial branch

Anatomical key:
1. Pyramidal tract
2. Pontine nuclei
3. Middle cerebellar peduncle
4. Motor and sensory trigeminal nerve roots
5. Anterior spinocerebellar tract
6. Lateral lemniscus
7. Medial lemniscus
8. Pontine tegmental reticular formation and raphe nuclei
9. Principal sensory trigeminal nucleus
10. Trigeminal motor nucleus
11. Central tegmental tract
12. Medial longitudinal fasciculus
13. Inferior cerebellar peduncle
14. Dentate nucleus
15. Superior cerebellar peduncle
16. Emboliform nucleus
17. Globose nucleus
18. Fastigial nucleus

SECTION 21. Axial scan through midpons.

The lateral pons at this level can be divided by the roots of the trigeminal nerve into anterior, posterior, and inferior areas. The inferior area begins at the trigeminal root and extends inferiorly. It includes the trigeminal root and the middle cerebellar peduncle and it is supplied by the AICA. The anterior area is supplied by the inferolateral pontine artery, a branch of the basilar (63). The posterior area is supplied by the superior cerebellar artery.

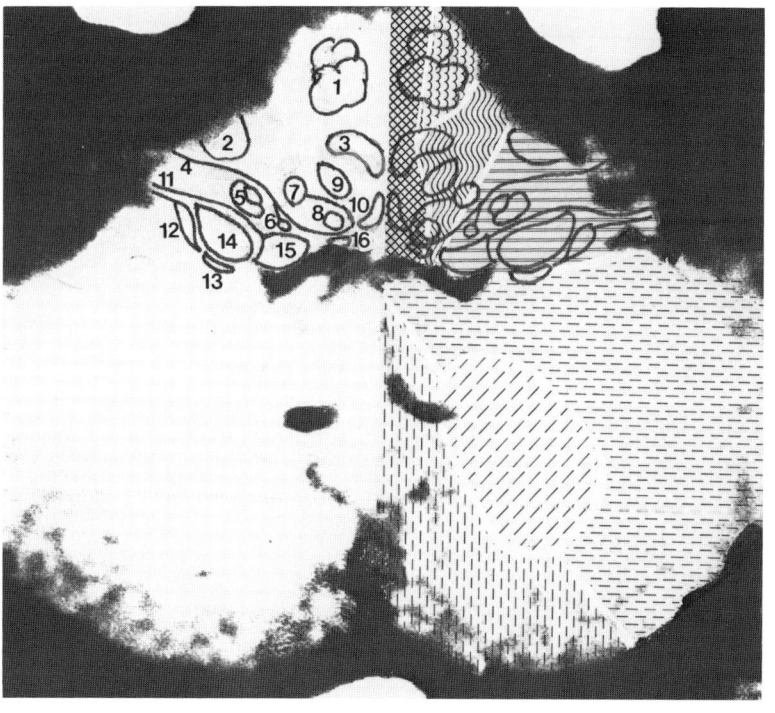
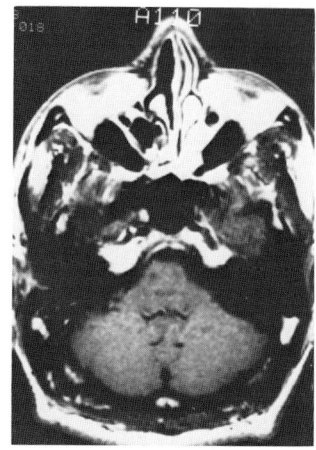

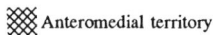 Anteromedial territory   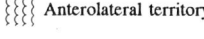 Anterolateral territory   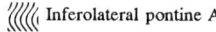 Inferolateral pontine A

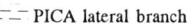 PICA lateral branch   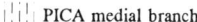 PICA medial branch   AICA

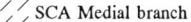 SCA Medial branch

Anatomical key:
1. Pyramidal tract
2. Anterior spinocerebellar tract
3. Medial lemniscus
4. Facial nerve
5. Spinal trigeminal tract and nucleus
6. Nucleus solitarius
7. Facial nerve nucleus
8. Abducens nerve nucleus
9. Central tegmental tract
10. Medial longitudinal fasciculus
11. Vestibulocochlear nerve
12. Ventral cochlear nucleus
13. Dorsal cochlear nucleus
14. Inferior cerebellar peduncle
15. Vestibular nuclei
16. Nucleus prepositus hypoglossi

SECTION 22. Axial scan through caudal pons.

The posterior part of the lateral pons is supplied by the AICA at this level (63). The more anterior and medial structures such as the lateral part of the medial lemniscus, the facial nucleus, and the central tegmental tract are probably outside of AICA territory and are probably supplied by the lateral pontine arteries (70,77). Fisher has reported an infarct affecting this territory (98). The area posterior to this is supplied by perforating branches from the proximal stem of the AICA (63,80). The areas supplied by the AICA include the superior olivary nucleus, the facial nucleus, the lateral lemniscus, and sometimes the lateral part of the abducens nucleus and the central tegmental tract according to Duvernoy (63). Autopsy correlations of AICA territory infarcts show a less restricted distribution (as shown in this figure), which includes the eighth nerve, the inferior cerebellar peduncle, and part of the vestibular nuclei (70,81).

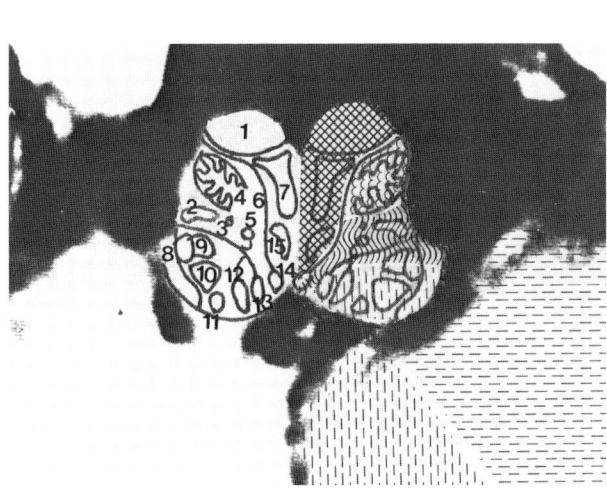
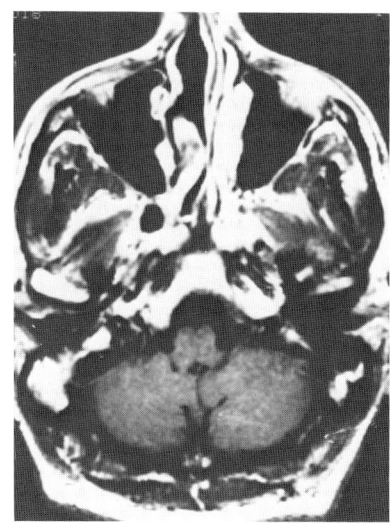

▓ Anteromedial territory   ₍₍₍ Anterolateral (olivary) territory   ⁾⁾⁾⁾ Lateral territory

┊┊ PICA medial branch   ═ PICA lateral branch

Anatomical key:
1. Pyramidal tract
2. Spinothalamic tract
3. Ventral trigeminothalamic tract
4. Inferior olivary nucleus
5. Nucleus ambiguous and vagus nerve
6. Hypoglossal nerve
7. Medial lemniscus
8. Inferior cerebellar peduncle
9. Spinal trigeminal tract and nucleus
10. Nucleus cuneatus
11. Nucleus gracilis
12. Nucleus solitarius
13. Dorsal vagal nucleus
14. Hypoglossal nucleus
15. Medial longitudinal fasciculus

SECTION 23. Axial scan through olivary nucleus.

The anteromedial territory is supplied mostly by branches from the terminal segments of the vertebral artery (63). These supply the hypoglossal nucleus and the medial lemniscus.

The anterolateral territory depicted here is the olivary territory that appears to fit better with the published extent of infarcts in this region (83,85,99). It does not include the pyramids as Duvernoy's anterolateral territory does (63). This territory principally includes the olive, but may include the spinothalamic tract (85).

The arteries of the lateral group usually arise predominantly from the vertebral artery in the lateral medullary fossa and not from the PICA, as is generally believed (63). The relative positions of the spinothalamic tract, the spinal trigeminal tract and nucleus, and the ventral trigeminothalamic tract explain how ipsilateral facial sensory loss may be combined with contralateral hemisensory loss with or without a sensory level (100).

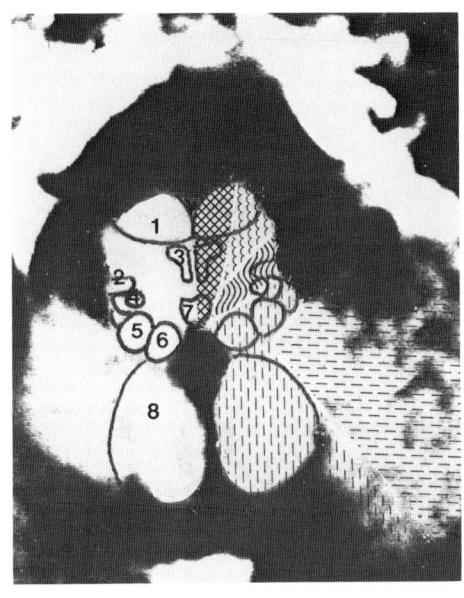 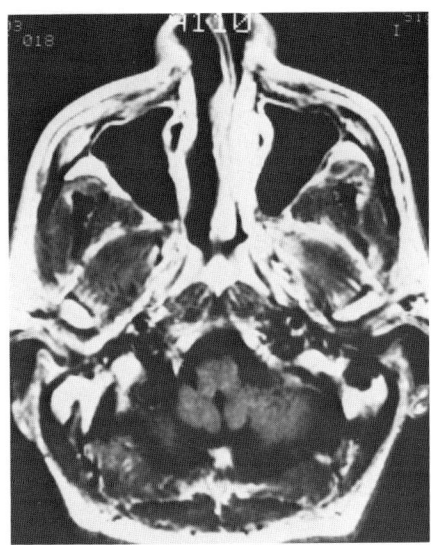

▓ Anteromedial territory ⦃⦃⦃ Anterolateral territory ⁾⁾⁾⁾ Lateral territory

═ PICA Lateral branch   ┆┆┆ PICA Medial branch

Anatomical key:
1. Pyramidal tract
2. Spinocerebellar tract
3. Medial lemniscus
4. Spinal trigeminal tract and nucleus
5. Nucleus cuneatus
6. Nucleus gracilis
7. Solitary nucleus, dorsal nucleus of vagus, and hypoglossal nucleus
8. Cerebellar tonsil

SECTION 24. Axial scan through caudal lemniscal decussation (medulla).

The anterior and anterolateral territories at this level are supplied mostly by the anterior spinal artery (77). The lateral and posterior territories are supplied by the vertebral artery and PICA (63).

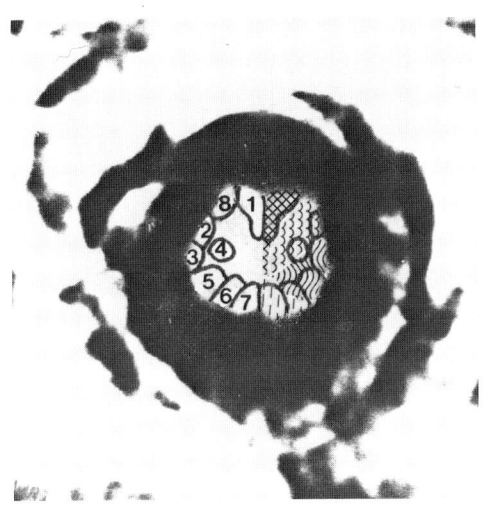 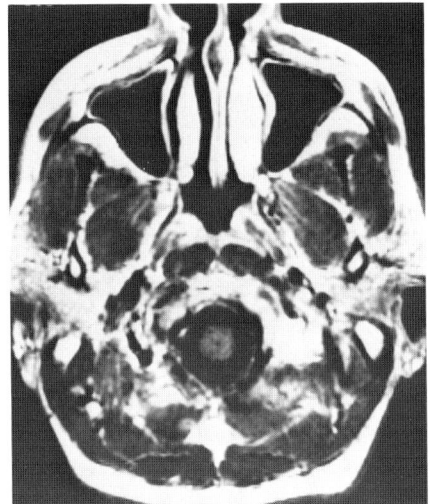

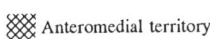 Anteromedial territory   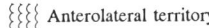 Anterolateral territory   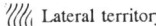 Lateral territory

|||| Posterior territory

Anatomical key:
1. Pyramidal tract
2. Anterior spinocerebellar tract
3. Posterior spinocerebellar tract
4. Lateral corticospinal tract
5. Spinal trigeminal tract
6. Fasciculus cuneatus
7. Fasciculus gracilis.
8. Spinothalamic tract

SECTION 25. Axial scan through pyramidal decussation of medulla.

The territories of supply are similar to those seen in Section 24.

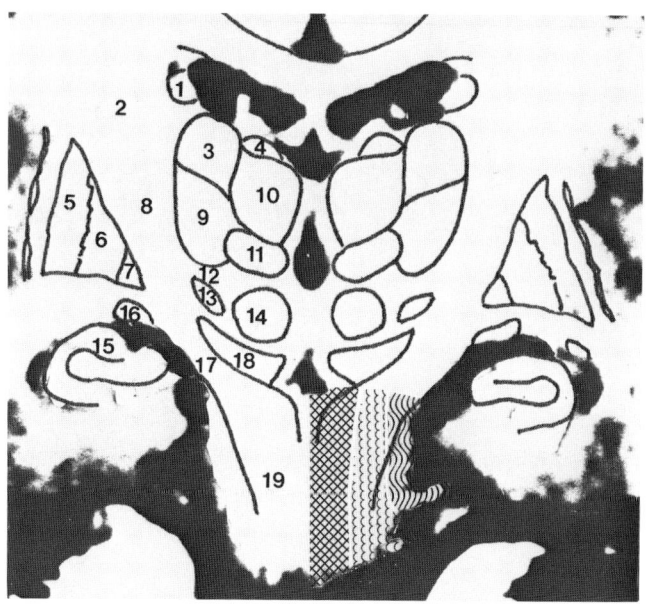
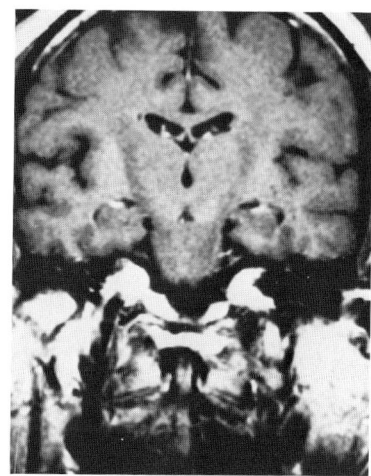

⁄⁄⁄⁄ Lateral pontine territory   ▓▓ Anteromedial pontine territory   ≀≀≀ Anterolateral pontine territory

Anatomical key:
1. Body of caudate nucleus
2. Corona radiata
3. Dorsocaudal nucleus (lateral posterior nucleus)
4. Dorsal superficial nucleus (lateral dorsal nucleus)
5. Putamen
6. Globus pallidus, lateral segment
7. Globus pallidus, medial segment
8. Posterior limb of internal capsule
9. Ventrocaudal nucleus (ventral posterolateral nucleus)
10. Medical nucleus (dorsomedial nucleus)
11. Parafascicular nucleus
12. Zona incerta
13. Subthalamic nucleus
14. Red nucleus
15. Hippocampal formation
16. Optic tract
17. Cerebral peduncle
18. Substantia nigra
19. Pyramidal tract (pons)

SECTION 26. Coronal scan through cerebral peduncles.

The base of the pons is shown supplied by branches from the basilar artery.

SMALL ARTERIAL TERRITORIES

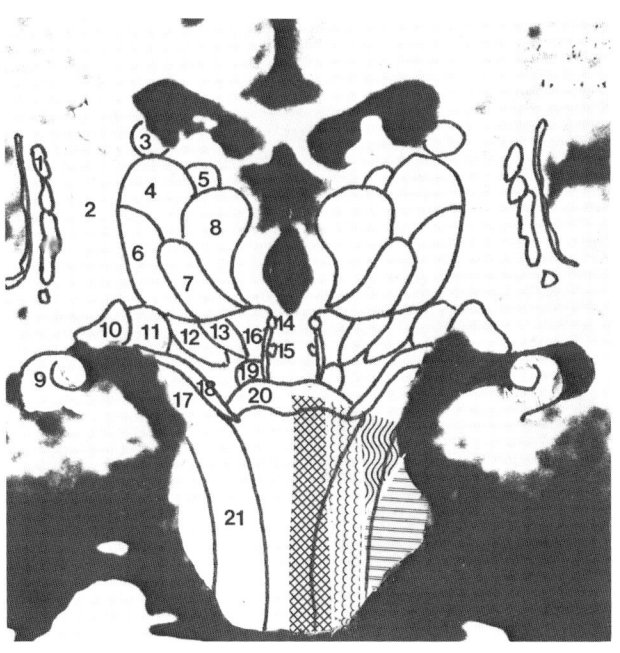 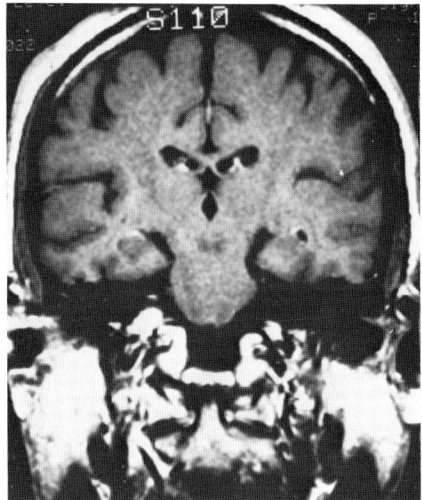

▓ Anteromedial pontine territory   ))) Lateral Pontine territory   ≡ AICA

{{{ Anterolateral pontine territory

Anatomical key:
1. Putamen
2. Posterior limb of internal capsule
3. Body of caudate nucleus
4. Dorsocaudal nucleus (lateral posterior nucleus)
5. Dorsal superficial nucleus (lateral dorsal nucleus)
6. Ventrocaudal nucleus (ventral posterolateral nucleus)
7. Central (centromedian) nucleus and parafascicular nucleus
8. Medial nucleus (dorsomedial nucleus)
9. Hippocampal formation
10. Lateral geniculate body
11. Medial geniculate body
12. Medial lemniscus
13. Superior cerebellar peduncle
14. Nucleus of Darkschewitsch and interstitial nucleus of Cajal
15. Accessory oculomotor nucleus
16. Medial longitudinal fasciculus
17. Cerebral peduncle
18. Substantia nigra
19. Central tegmental tract
20. Decussation of superior cerebellar peduncle
21. Pyramidal tract (pons)

SECTION 27. Coronal scan through decussation of superior cerebellar peduncle.

The territories are similar to those seen in Section 26.

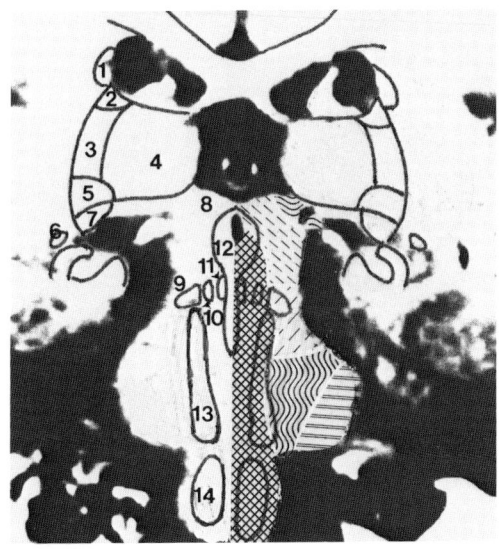 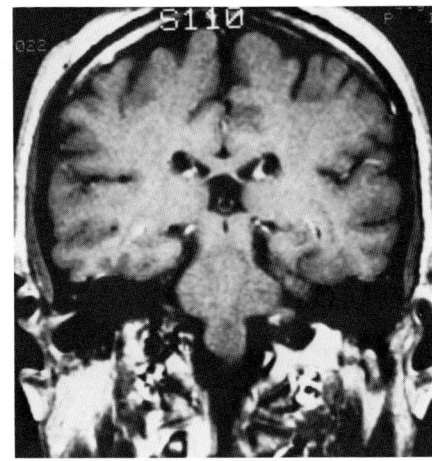

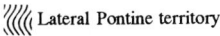 Lateral Pontine territory   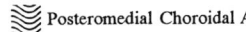 Posteromedial Choroidal A   AICA

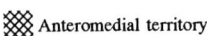 Anteromedial territory   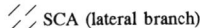 SCA (lateral branch)   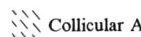 Collicular A

Anatomical key:
1. Body of caudate nucleus
2. Dorsocaudal nucleus (lateral posterior nucleus)
3. Lateral pulvinar nucleus
4. Medial pulvinar nucleus
5. Pulvinar nucleus
6. Tail of caudate nucleus
7. Lateral geniculate body
8. Superior colliculus
9. Superior cerebellar peduncle
10. Central tegmental tract
11. Medial longitudinal fasciculus
12. Periaqueductal gray matter
13. Medial lemniscus
14. Pyramidal tract (medulla)

SECTION 28. Coronal scan through medial lemniscus.

The anteromedial territory supplied by the basilar artery paramedian perforators extends posteriorly to the aqueduct and region of the medial longitudinal fasciculus. The medial lemniscus can be seen extending down in the lateral brainstem territory.

REFERENCES*

1. Marinkovic S, Milisavljevic M, Kovacevic M. Anatomical bases for surgical approach to the initial segment of the anterior cerebral artery. *Surg Radiol Anat* 1986;8:7–18.
2. Rosner SS, Rhoton AL Jr, Ono M, Barry M. Microsurgical anatomy of the anterior perforating arteries. *J Neurosurg* 1984;61:468–485.
3. Perlmutter D, Rhoton AL Jr. Microsurgical anatomy of the anterior cerebral-anterior communicating-recurrent artery complex. *J Neurosurg* 1976;45:259–272.
4. Lazorthes G, Poulhes J, Gaubert J. Les artères et les territoires vasculaires de l'hypothalamus. *Presse Med* 1956;64:1701–1703.

*This reference list is a combination of references from chapters 2 and 3.

5. Ostrowski AZ, Webster JE, Gurdjian ES. The proximal anterior cerebral artery: an anatomic study. *Arch Neurol* 1960;3:661–664.
6. Alexander L. The vascular supply of the strio-pallidum. *Proc Assoc Res Nerv Ment Dis* 1942;21:77–132.
7. Kaplan HA, Ford DH. *The brain vascular system.* Amsterdam: Elsevier; 1966.
8. Dunker RO, Harris AB. Surgical anatomy of the proximal anterior cerebral artery. *J Neurosurg* 1976;44:359–367.
9. Crowell RM, Morawetz RB. The anterior communicating artery has significant branches. *Stroke* 1977;8:272–273.
10. Marinkovic S, Milisavljevic M, Marinkovic A. Branches of the anterior communicating artery. Microsurgical anatomy. *Acta Neurochir* 1990;106:78–85.
11. Vincentelli F, Lehman G, Caruso G, Grisoli F, Rabehanta P, Gouaze A. Extracerebral course of the perforating branches of the anterior communicating artery:

microsurgical anatomical study. *Surg Neurol* 1991;35: 98–104.
12. Phillips S, Sangalang V, Sterns G. Basal forebrain infarction. *Arch Neurol* 1987;44:1134–1138.
13. Heubner O. Zur Topographie der Ernahrungsgebiete der einzelnen Hirnarterien. *Centralbl Med Wiss* 1872; 10:817–821.
14. Lazorthes G, Gaubert J, Poulhes J. La distribution centrale et corticale de l'artère cérébrale antérieure. Etude anatomique et incidences neurochirurgicales. *Neurochirurgie* 1956;2:237–253.
15. Gorczyca W, Mohr G. Microvascular anatomy of Heubner's recurrent artery. *Neurol Res* 1987;9:259–264.
16. Gomes F, Dujovny M, Umansky F, et al. Microsurgical anatomy of the recurrent artery of Heubner. *J Neurosurg* 1984;60:130–139.
17. Umansky F, Gomes FB, Dujovny M, et al. The perforating branches of the middle cerebral artery. *J Neurosurg* 1985;62:261–268.
18. Kaplan HA. The lateral perforating branches of the anterior and middle cerebral arteries. *J Neurosurg* 1965;23:305–310.
19. Gibo H, Lenkey C, Rhoton AL Jr. Microsurgical anatomy of the supraclinoid portion of the internal carotid artery. *J Neurosurg* 1981;55:560–574.
20. Marinkovic SV, Milisavljevic MM, Marinkovic ZD. Microanatomy and possible clinical significance of anastomoses among hypothalamic arteries. *Stroke* 1989; 20:1341–1352.
21. Marinkovic S, Milisavljevic M, Marinkovic ZD. The perforating branches of the internal carotid artery: the microsurgical anatomy of their extracerebral segments. *Neurosurgery* 1990;26:472–479.
22. Lazorthes G, Gouaze A, Salamon G. Les artères centrales du cerveau. In: *Vascularisation et circulation de l'encéphale*. Paris: Masson; 1976:154–182.
23. Marinkovic SV, Kovacevic MS, Marinkovic JM. Perforating branches of the middle cerebral artery. *J Neurosurg* 1985;63:266–271.
24. Vincentelli F, Caruso G, Andriamamonjy C, et al. Etude micro-anatomique des branches collatérales perforantes de l'artère cérébrale moyenne. *Neurochirurgie* 1990;36:3–15.
25. Shellshear JI. The basal arteries of the forebrain and their functional significance. *J Anat* 1920;55:27–35.
26. Ghika JA, Bogousslavsky J, Regli F. Deep perforators from the carotid system. *Arch Neurol* 1990;47:1097–1100.
27. Marinkovic SV, Milisavljevic MM, Kovacevic MS, Stevic ZD. Perforating branches of the middle cerebral artery. *Stroke* 1985;16:1022–1029.
28. Herman LH, Ostrowski AZ, Gurdjian ES. Perforating branches of the middle cerebral artery. *Arch Neurol* 1963;1:32–34.
29. Manelfe C, Clanet M, Gigaud M, Bonafé A, Guiraud B, Rascol A. Internal capsule: normal anatomy and ischemic changes demonstrated by computed tomography. *AJNR* 1981;2:149–155.
30. Beevor CE. On the distribution of the different arteries supplying the human brain. *Philos Trans R Soc Lond [Biol]* 1909;200:1–55.
31. De Reuck J. La limite du territoire profond de l'artère Sylvienne chez l'homme. *Acta Anat* 1969;74:30–35.
32. Percheron G. Les artères du thalamus humain. Les artères choroidiennes. *Rev Neurol (Paris)* 1977;133:547–558.
33. Duret H. Recherches anatomiques sur la circulation de l'encéphale. *Arch Physiol Norm Pathol* 1874;1:60–91.
34. Abbie AA. The anatomy of capsular vascular disease. *Aust Med J* 1937;2:564–568.
35. Herman LH, Fernando OU, Gurdjian ES. The anterior choroidal artery: an anatomical study of its area of distribution. *Anat Rec* 1966;154:95–102.
36. Carpenter MB, Noback CR, Moss ML. The anterior choroidal artery. *Arch Neurol Psych* 1954;71:714–722.
37. Saeki N, Rhoton AL Jr. Microsurgical anatomy of the upper basilar artery and the posterior circle of Willis. *J Neurosurg* 1977;46:563–578.
38. Hussein S, Renella RR, Dietz H. Microsurgical anatomy of the anterior choroidal artery. *Acta Neurochir* 1988;92:19–28.
39. Abbie AA. The blood supply of the lateral geniculate body with a note on the morphology of the choroidal arteries. *J Anat* 1933;67:491–521.
40. Rhoton AL Jr, Fujii K, Fradd B. Microsurgical anatomy of the anterior choroidal artery. *Surg Neurol* 1979;12:171–187.
41. Schlesinger B. *The upper brainstem in the human. Its nuclear configuration and vascular supply*. Berlin: Springer-Verlag; 1976.
42. Abbie AA. The clinical significance of the anterior choroidal artery. *Brain* 1933;56:233–246.
43. Mohr JP, Steinke W, Timsit SG, Sacco RL, Tatemichi TK. The anterior choroidal artery does not supply the corona radiata and lateral ventricular wall. *Stroke* 1991;22:1502–1507.
44. Beevor CE. the cerebral arterial supply. *Brain* 1908; 30:403–425.
45. Khan NM. *The blood supply of the midbrain in man and monkey* [PhD Thesis]. London: University of London, 1969.
46. Foix C, Chavany H, Hillemand P, Schiff-Wertheimer M. Oblitération de l'artère choroidienne antérieure. Ramollissement de son territoire cérébral. Hémiplégie, hémianesthésie, hémianopsie. *Bull Soc Ophthalmol* 1925;27:221–223.
47. Buge A, Escourolle R, Hauw JJ, Rancurel G, Gray F, Tempier P. Syndrome pseudobulbaire aigu par infarctus bilatéral. Limite du territoire des artères choroidiennes antérieures. *Rev Neurol (Paris)* 1979;135:313–318.
48. Poppi U. Sindrome talamo-capsulare per rammolimento nel territorio dell'arteria coroidea anteriore. *Riv Patol Nerv Ment* 1928;33:505–542.
49. Van Buren JM, Borke RC. *Variations and connection of the human thalamus. Vol 1. The nuclei and cerebral connections of the human thalamus*. Berlin: Springer; 1972.
50. Percheron G. Les artères du thalamus humain. I. Artère et territoire thalamiques polaires de l'artère communicante postérieure. *Rev Neurol (Paris)* 1976;132: 297–307.
51. Vincentelli F, Caruso G, Grisoli F, Rabehanta P, Andriamamonjy C, Gouaze A. Microsurgical anatomy of the cisternal course of the perforating branches of the posterior communicating artery. *Neurosurgery* 1990; 26:824–831.
52. Pedroza A, Dujovny M, Ausman JI, et al. Microvascular anatomy of the interpeduncular fossa. *J Neurosurg* 1986;64:484–493.
53. Marinkovic S, Milisavljevic M, Kovacevic M. Interpeduncular perforating branches of the posterior cerebral artery. *Surg Neurol* 1986;26:349–359.
54. Castaigne P, Lhermitte F, Buge A, Escourolle R, Hauw JJ, Lyon-Caen O. Paramedian thalamic and midbrain infarcts: clinical and neuropathological study. *Ann Neurol* 1981;10:127–148.
55. Takahashi S, Goto K, Fukasawa H, Kawata Y, Uemura K, Yaguchi K. Computed tomography of cerebral infarction along the distribution of the basal perforating arteries. Part II: thalamic arterial group. *Radiology* 1985;155:119–130.
56. Zeal AA, Rhoton AL Jr. Microsurgical anatomy of the posterior cerebral artery. *J Neurosurg* 1978;48:534–559.
57. Milisavljevic M, Marinkovic S, Marinkovic Z, Malobabic S. Anatomic basis for surgical approach to the

distal segment of the posterior cerebral artery. *Surg Radiol Anat* 1988;10:259-266.
58. Milisavljevic MM, Marinkovic SV, Gibo H, Puskas LF. The thalamogeniculate perforators of the posterior cerebral artery: the microsurgical anatomy. *Neurosurgery* 1991;28:523-530.
59. Marinkovic SV, Milisavljevic MM, Kovacevic MS. Anastomoses among the thalamoperforating branches of the posterior cerebral artery. *Arch Neurol* 1986; 43:811-814.
60. Milisavljevic M, Marinkovic S, Lolic-Draganic V, Djordjevic L. Anastomoses in the territory of the posterior cerebral arteries. *Acta Anat* 1986;127:221-225.
61. Percheron G. Les artères du thalamus humain. II. Artères et territoires thalamiques paramedians de l'artère basilaire communicante. *Rev Neurol (Paris)* 1976;132: 309-324.
62. Pierrot-Deseilligny C, Chain F, Gray F, Serdaru M, Escourolle R, Lhermitte F. Parinaud's syndrome. *Brain* 1982;105:667—696.
63. Duvernoy HM. *Human brainstem vessels*. Berlin: Springer-Verlag; 1978.
64. Percheron G. Les artères du thalamus humain. Les artères choroidiennes. *Rev Neurol (Paris)* 1977;133:533-545.
65. Plets C, De Reuck J, Vander Eecken H, Van Den Bergh R. The vascularization of the human thalamus. *Acta Neurol Belg* 1970;70:687-770.
66. Devic M, Michel F, Lenglet JP. Nystagmus retractorius, paralysie de la verticalité, aréflexie pupillaire et anomalie de la posture du regard par ramollissement dans la territoire de la choroidienne postérieure. *Rev Neurol (Paris)* 1964;110:399-404.
67. Alezais, D'Astros L. La circulation artérielle du pédoncule cérébral. *J Anat Physiol* 1892;28:519-528.
68. Marinkovic SV, Milisavljevic MM, Vuckovic VD. Microvascular anatomy of the uncus and the parahippocampal gyrus. *Neurosurgery* 1991;29:805-814.
69. Milisavljevic M, Marinkovic S, Lolic-Draganic V, Kovacevic M. Oculomotor, trochlear, and abducens nerves penetrated by cerebral vessels. *Arch Neurol* 1986;43:58-61.
70. Amarenco P, Hauw JJ. Anatomie des artères cérébelleuses. *Rev Neurol (Paris)* 1989;145:267-276.
71. Foix C, Hillemand P. Les artères de l'axe encéphalique jusqu'au diencéphale inclusivement. *Rev Neurol (Paris)* 1925;32:705-739.
72. Gillilan LA. The correlation of the blood supply to the human brain stem with clinical brain stem lesions. *J Neuropathol Exp Neurol* 1964;23:78-108.
73. Stephens RB, Stilwell DL. *Arteries of the human brain*. Springfield, IL: Charles C. Thomas; 1969.
74. Davison C, Goodhart SP, Savitsky N. The syndrome of the superior cerebellar artery. *Arch Neurol Psychol* 1935;33:1143-1174.
75. Amarenco P, Hauw JJ. Cerebellar infarction in the territory of the superior cerebellar artery. *Neurology* 1990;40:1383-1390.
76. Stopford JSB. The arteries of the pons and medulla oblongata. *J Anat Physiol* 1916;50:131-164.
77. Stopford JSB. The arteries of the pons and medulla oblongata: part II. *J Anat Physiol* 1916;51:255-280.
78. Fisher CM, Tapia J. Lateral medullary infarction extending to the lower pons. *J Neurol Neurosurg Psychiatry* 1987;50:620-624.
79. Lazorthes G. *Vascularisation et circulation cérébrales*. Paris: Masson; 1961.
80. Atkinson WJ. The anterior inferior cerebellar artery. *J Neurol Neurosurg Psychiatry* 1949;12:137-151.
81. Amarenco P. The spectrum of cerebellar infarctions. *Neurology* 1991;41:973-979.
82. Duret H. Artères nourricières du bulbe rachidien. *Arch Physiol Norm Pathol* 1873;5:97-113.
83. Hauw JJ, Der Agopian P, Trelles L, Escourolle R. Les infarctus bulbaires. *J Neurol Sci* 1976;28:83-102.
84. Böhne C. Uber die arterielle Blutversorgung der Medulla oblongata. *Z Anat Entwickl-Gesch* 1927;84:760-776.
85. DeSmet Y, Brucher JM, Gonsette RE. L'infarctus du territoire olivaire du bulbe. *Rev Neurol (Paris)* 1984; 140:559-566.
86. Hiller F. The vascular syndromes of the basilar and vertebral arteries and their branches. *J Nerv Ment Dis* 1952;116:988-1016.
87. Escourolle R, Hauw JJ, Der Agopian P, Trelles L. Les infarctus bulbaires. *J Neurol Sci* 1976;28:103-113.
88. Goodhart SP, Davison C. Syndrome of the posterior inferior and anterior inferior cerebellar arteries and their branches. *Arch Neurol Psychol* 1936;35:501-524.
89. Foix C, Hillemand P, Schalit. Irrigation du bulbe. *C R Soc Biol (Paris)* 1925;92:33-35.
90. DeArmond SJ, Fusco MM, Dewey MM. *Structure of the human brain. A photographic atlas*. 2nd ed. New York: Oxford University Press; 1976.
91. Nieuwenhuys R, Voogd J, van Huijsen C. *The human central nervous system. A synopsis and atlas*. Berlin: Springer-Verlag; 1981.
92. Fix JD. *Atlas of the human brain and spinal cord*. Rockville, MD: Aspen; 1987.
93. Damasio HA. A computed tomographic guide to the identification of cerebral vascular territories. *Arch Neurol* 1983;40:138-142.
94. Takahashi S, Goto K, Fukasawa H, Kawata Y, Uemura K, Suzuki K. Computed tomography of cerebral infarction along the distribution of the basal perforating arteries. Part 1: striate arterial group. *Radiology* 1985;155:107-118.
95. Savoiardo M, Bracchi M, Passerini A, Visciani A. The vascular territories in the cerebellum and brainstem: CT and MR study. *AJNR* 1987;8:199-209.
96. Frisen L, Holmegaard L, Rosencrantz M. Sectorial optic atrophy and homonymous, horizontal sectoranopia: a lateral choroidal artery syndrome? *J Neurol Neurosurg Psychiatry* 1978;41:374-380.
97. Frisen L. Quadruple sectoranopia and sectorial optic atrophy: a syndrome of the distal anterior choroidal artery. *J Neurol Neurosurg Psychiatry* 1979;42:590-594.
98. Fisher CM. Lacunar infarct of the tegmentum of the lower lateral pons. *Arch Neurol* 1989;46:566-567.
99. Jagiella WM, Sung JH. Bilateral infarction of the medullary pyramids in humans. *Neurology* 1989;39:21-24.
100. Matsumoto S, Okuda B, Imai T, Kameyama M. A sensory level on the trunk in lower lateral brainstem lesions. *Neurology* 1988;38:1515-1519.

4

Computed Tomography and Magnetic Resonance of Subcortical Ischemic Lesions

Patrick M. Pullicino and *Reza Pordell

*Department of Neurology, State University of New York at Buffalo, Buffalo General Hospital, Buffalo, New York 14203; and *Division of Neuroradiology, Department of Radiology, State University of New York at Buffalo, Buffalo General Hospital, Buffalo, New York 14203*

TERMINOLOGY

In this chapter the term lacunar infarct will be restricted to pathologically proven ischemic lesions that appear to be caused by occlusion of a single penetrating artery (1). The term lacune will be used for any small cystic space due to a vascular cause, including enlarged perivascular spaces. The term small deep infarct will be used for small subcortical presumed infarcts seen on magnetic resonance (MR) or computed tomography (CT) of less than about 15 mm in diameter. The term presumed lacunar infarction will be used for a small deep infarct that corresponds with the clinical presentation of one of the four main lacunar syndromes (pure motor, pure sensory, and sensorimotor stroke, and the different types of ataxic hemiparesis). Small deep infarcts corresponding to clinical signs that are compatible with a small focal lesion site in a patient with hypertension or diabetes and no other obvious etiology for an infarct (in particular, cardiac or carotid disease) are also classified as presumed lacunar infarcts (1).

CT AND MR APPEARANCE OF PATHOLOGICALLY PROVEN INFARCTS

CT of Pathologically Proven Lacunar Infarcts

The axial CT appearance of autopsy-proven lacunar infarcts that are more than several weeks old is that of well-circumscribed, small circular, oval, oblong, or slit-like areas of low attenuation in the territories of the basal perforating arteries (2–10). The low attenuation may be wedge-shaped or drop-shaped if the infarct is adjacent to a ventricular surface (3). Lacunar infarcts are often quite elongated in the axis of the supplying arteriole (4). The infarct is thus often seen in cross-section on more than one sequential axial scan (3). The cross-sectional dimensions of chronic lacunar infarcts that are well demarcated on CT appear to be a true reflection of the cross-sectional dimensions of the infarct at autopsy (2–7), although no systematic study of this has been performed. Most lacunes less than 2 mm in diameter cannot be detected by CT

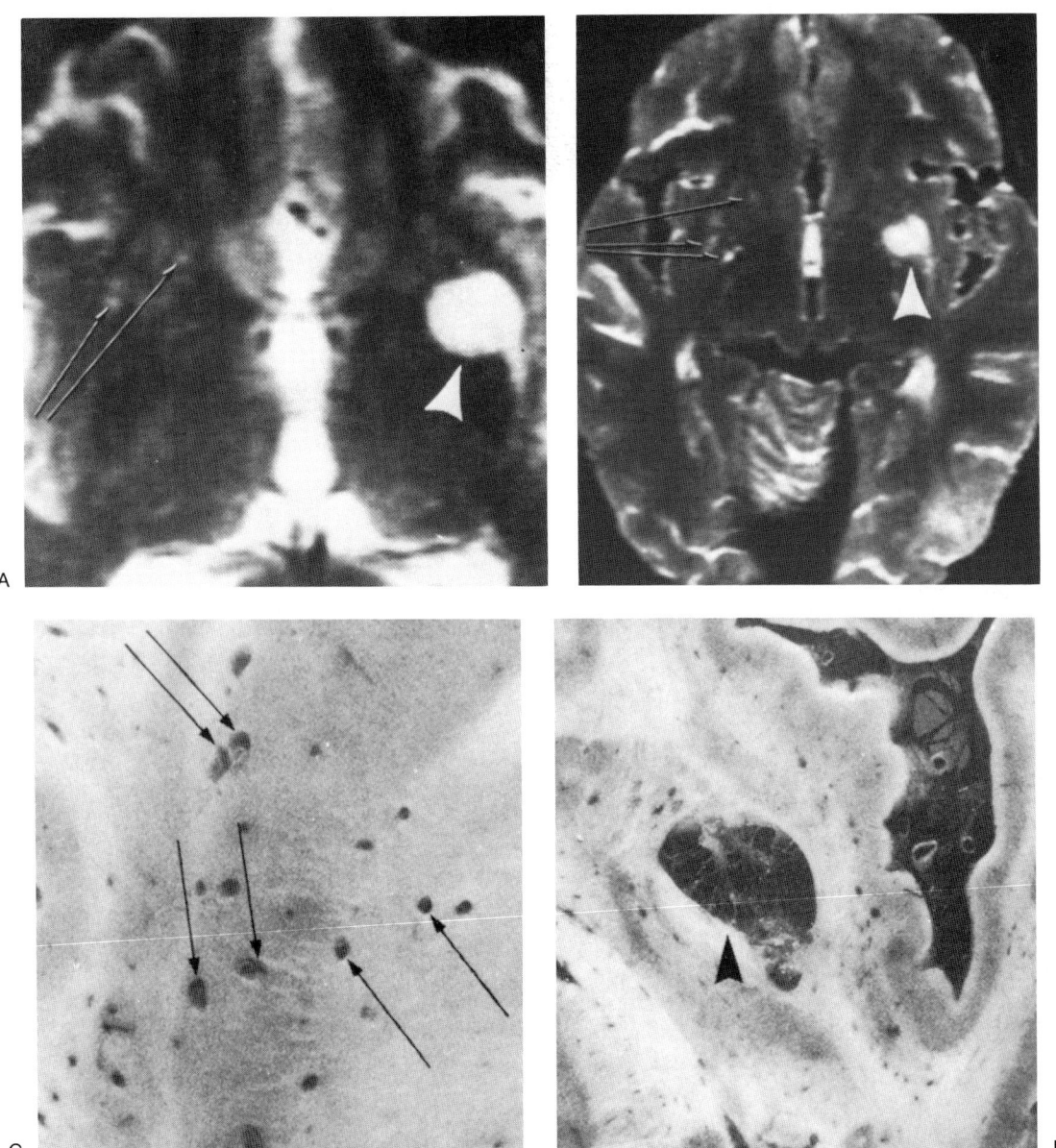

FIG. 1. Pathological correlation of dilated Virchow-Robin spaces and lacune. (**A**) *In vivo* T2-weighted MR scan showing small punctate lesions isointense with cerebrospinal fluid (arrows) and larger round hyperintense lesions in the contralateral inferior putamen (arrowhead). (**B**) Postmortem T2-weighted MR scan showing the same lesions. (**C**) Gross pathology shows the punctate lesions to be dilated Virchow-Robin spaces. (**D**) A round cavitated lesion was the pathological counterpart of the larger MR lesion. The wall of this lesion was found to have reactive astrocytosis on histopathology, indicative of a lacunar infarct. From ref. 10, with permission.

(11,12). Using a second-generation scanner, Toghi et al. reported that only 36 of 112 (32%) small infarcts found at autopsy were detected by CT. Conversely, these authors found that 153 of 189 (81%) small areas of reduced attenuation on CT were not associated with an abnormality at autopsy (13).

MR of Pathologically Proven Lacunar Infarcts

Braffman et al. (10) illustrated two different autopsy-proven lacunar infarcts. The first was a small, slitlike lesion in the left caudate nucleus and anterior limb of the internal capsule measuring 2 mm by 8 mm that was hyperintense on T2-weighted images, but had a brighter signal and was more clearly seen on the more heavily weighted T2 sequences than on proton density images. The second was a 14 mm by 13 mm round lesion in the inferior putamen that was hypointense on T1-weighted images, isointense with white matter on intermediate T2 images, and hyperintense only on heavily T2-weighted images (Fig. 1).

Lacunar infarcts may not be detected by MR: Besson (14) illustrated a pontine lacune shown at autopsy but not by *in vivo* MR. He suggested that the lesion was missed because of a combination of partial volume and slice thickness effects. Salgado et al. (15) illustrated an autopsy specimen showing a thalamic infarct about 3 mm by 2 mm that was not detected by *in vivo* MR.

Pathologically Proven Lacunar Infarcts on Postmortem MR

Revész et al. illustrated a brain slice showing a lacunar infarct in the temporo-occipital white matter that appeared as a small area of hypersignal on a T2 postmortem MR (the limitations of postmortem MR are discussed below). On the MR image, it was difficult to distinguish the infarct from a larger irregular area of hypersignal due to intense gliosis (16). DeWitt et al. performed postmortem MR in a patient with a 2-day-old small deep infarct. The infarct, which was proven at autopsy, was seen as an oval hypointense area on T1 images and as a hyperintense area on T2 images (17). Jungreis et al. illustrated a brain slice showing an elongated lacunar infarct in the outer putamen (18). This infarct was clearly seen on postmortem MR but it appeared much smaller on the T1 images than on the T2 images. Two of Marshall et al.'s six abnormal brains showed lacunar infarcts that appeared as areas of hypersignal on T2 images (19).

CT AND MR OF PRESUMED LACUNAR INFARCTS AND SMALL DEEP INFARCTS

CT

Nelson et al. found that 18 (49%) of 37 patients presenting with a lacunar syndrome had a compatible presumed lacunar infarct (8). Selgado et al. found that 7 of 12 patients (58%) who presented with lacunar syndromes had a compatible presumed lacunar infarct on CT (15). Kappelle et al. detected a higher percentage (76%) of presumed lacunar infarcts when only probable supratentorial lacunar infarcts were included. These authors suggested performing supplementary 3-mm cuts to look for small infarcts not shown on routine CT scans (20).

Miyashita et al. noted that old small cerebral hemorrhages were indistinguishable from old small deep infarcts (21). Since patients with small intracerebral hemorrhages often present with a lacunar syndrome (see Chapter 10), this study emphasizes the difficulty of making a diagnosis of lacunar infarction from a small deep infarct seen on CT.

MR

MR is significantly superior to CT in the detection of small deep infarcts (22,23), particularly in the brainstem (24,25). Seventy-four percent to 89% of patients presenting with lacunar syndromes have presumed lacunar infarcts on MR consistent with the clinical deficit (15,22,26,27). Hommel et al. found that 89% of patients with a lacunar syndrome had a compatible presumed lacunar infarct on MR (26), but this figure increased to 95% if only the four classic lacunar syndromes were included. The mean volume of presumed lacunar infarcts responsible for lacunar syndromes was 0.8 ml (SD = 0.92; maximum volume 4.4 ml) (26). There was a significant difference between the mean volumes of the presumed lacunar infarcts associated with the four different classical lacunar syndromes: sensorimotor stroke (1.7 ml), pure motor hemiparesis (1.2 ml), ataxic hemiparesis (0.6 ml), and pure sensory stroke (0.2 ml) (26).

Brown et al. described the MR appearance of presumed lacunar infarcts together with small deep infarcts. The typical appearance was a focal area of hypointensity on T1-weighted images and a focal area of hyperintensity on T2-weighted images (28). Infarcts were better seen on T2 images than on T1 images, and especially on strongly weighted T2 images (28). Some presumed lacunar infarcts had an atypical appearance on proton density images, with a hyperintense perimeter (possibly due to gliosis) surrounding a more hypointense center (28).

Hemorrhagic Infarction

Nabatame et al. have noted areas of hyperintensity on noncontrast T1-weighted scans in two patients with recent small deep infarcts involving the thalamus. The first showed an area of hypointensity surrounded by a rim of hyperintensity on T2 images and a poorly defined hypointensity on T1 images, 10 days after the onset of the stroke. A CT scan performed at the same time showed a low-attenuation area compatible with an infarct with no areas of high attenuation. A repeat MR 3 weeks later showed a predominantly hyperintense area on T2 images with only a small residual central hypointensity. The lesion was now hyperintense on T1 images. The authors suggested that the T1 hyperintensity was due to hemorrhagic changes at the periphery of the infarct (29). The signal characteristics of these infarcts appear to correspond with Brown et al.'s "atypical" infarcts (see above) (28).

Challa and Moody (30) reported the pathological findings of a cystic hemorrhagic lacunar infarct of the pons that occurred 52 days earlier. An MR scan performed during the acute stage showed that the infarct was isointense with hyperintense areas on a T1 image and uniformly hyperintense on a T2 image.

Old small hemorrhagic infarcts can be distinguished from old small hemorrhages by the fact that they appear as an area of hyperintensity with central hypointensity on T2 images. Old small hemorrhages are predominantly hypointense on T2 images, but may have a small central hyperintensity (21).

Change in Imaging Characteristics of Small Deep Infarcts with Time

Small deep infarcts change in size, particularly within the first ten days of a stroke (4). Small deep infarcts have been shown to increase in size between scans performed in the first few days after a stroke and 2 to 3 weeks later (31). This increase in size may be due to edema (32) and mass effect may be seen on scans of larger deep infarcts between days 2 and 6 (33). The extent of abnormal T2 hyperintensity on MR in acute small deep infarcts, particularly of the pons, may be more extensive than the clinical findings suggest (34,35). Peri-infarct edema has been suggested as the cause of this discrepancy (35). Following this early increase, there is a subsequent decrease in the size of an infarct to the eventual dimensions of the cystic cavity it produces (31,36). After several months to years, small deep infarcts tend to become more clearly demarcated on CT, but occasionally may become undetectable, possibly because the infarct has become too small for the resolution of the scanner (31). Longstanding small deep infarcts are brighter than acute small deep infarcts on proton density images (28). Positron emission tomography showed a focal area of hypoperfusion and hypometabolism in the striatum in a patient with transient pure motor hemiparesis in whom the CT and MR were normal (37).

Hommel et al. found that an infarct whose volume was 0.7 ml 10 days after a stroke was 0.36 ml 14 months later (26). Donnan et al. found that the size of a lacunar infarct at autopsy was half the estimated size of the infarct when measured 7 weeks after the causative stroke (9).

Small deep infarcts may be seen on CT as early as 17 hours after a stroke (31), but they are often not seen on CT during the first 24 hours. Scans remain negative in 28 to 48% (8,9,28) of patients with a clinical lacunar syndrome. A small deep infarct may take days or weeks to appear: 79% of small deep infarcts detected by CT are seen by 10 days and 92% by a month of the onset of symptoms (9). On CT a small deep infarct that is seen initially may transiently become isodense in the second week after the ictus, due to "fogging effect" but this is less common than in larger infarcts (31,38).

MR of Acute Presumed Lacunar Infarcts and Small Deep Infarcts

Acute presumed lacunar infarcts (within 1 week of the stroke) are generally only seen on T2 MR images (28,39). Deep infarcts are not reliably seen on MR until 8 hours after the stroke, and are best seen on strongly weighted T2 images within the first 24 hours after a stroke (40).

Hommel et al. found that in patients with a lacunar syndrome, the MR is more likely to show a relevant infarct before the first 2 weeks after a stroke (98% before versus 80% after 2 weeks) (26). Rothrock et al. found that 92% of patients with lacunar syndromes scanned within 5 days of a stroke showed an appropriate presumed lacunar infarct, whereas only 67% of patients scanned between 5 days and 30 days after the stroke and 62% scanned after 30 days had an appropriate infarct (22).

MR may be normal in small subcortical or brainstem infarcts, and Alberts et al. (41) reported a normal MR at 24 hours after a stroke in a patient later found to have an internal capsule small deep infarct and a normal MR at 12 weeks after a stroke in a patient who previously had been found to have a small deep infarct in the pons.

Enhancement Characteristics of Small Deep Infarcts (CT and MR)

Thirteen percent to 40% of small deep infarcts seen on CT enhance following intravenous contrast, which is less frequently than large infarcts (65%) (9,42). Enhancement is maximal during the second and third weeks after a stroke, but may be seen as early as day 2 and as late as day 26 after a small deep infarct (31). CT usually shows enhancement of involved or adjacent deep gray matter structures, such as the caudate nucleus, rather than of the white matter (31).

On MR, enhancement of small deep infarcts can be seen on the second day after a stroke (33); dynamic contrast-enhanced MR imaging may even show abnormalities immediately after a stroke, although this technique is not reliable with infarcts smaller than 20 mm in diameter (43). Enhancement develops earlier in small deep infarcts than in cortical infarcts, where it usually begins after 7 days, but enhancement is usually seen later than the appearance of the T2 signal abnormality (44). An average of 67% of small deep infarcts enhance during the first week and this increases to 100% by the second week (33,39). From the third week the percentage of infarcts that enhance decreases, and enhancement is not seen after 3 months (33). Enhancement appears as a faint rim in the first week (Fig. 2), but by the second week the enhancement pattern becomes more dense and progresses toward the center of the infarct, by which time most presumed lacunar infarcts enhance (44). Miyashita et al. found that contrast injection may help to distinguish a recent small deep infarct from longstanding infarcts in patients with multiple small deep infarcts (39).

Arterial enhancement, which is seen during the first few days after a cortical infarct, may be seen in the vertebral or basilar arteries with moderately sized brainstem infarctions (33,44). Meningeal enhancement, which is also seen with cortical infarcts, is not seen in association with small deep infarcts (33).

DIFFERENTIATION OF PATHOGENESIS OF SUBCORTICAL ISCHEMIC LESIONS BY IMAGING

The imaging characteristics of small deep ischemic lesions may sometimes give an indication of the underlying pathogenesis. This is particularly true of subcortical ischemia caused by hypoperfusion, which tends to occur in the characteristic locations of watershed zones between subcortical arterial territories or in "terminal" arterial zones.

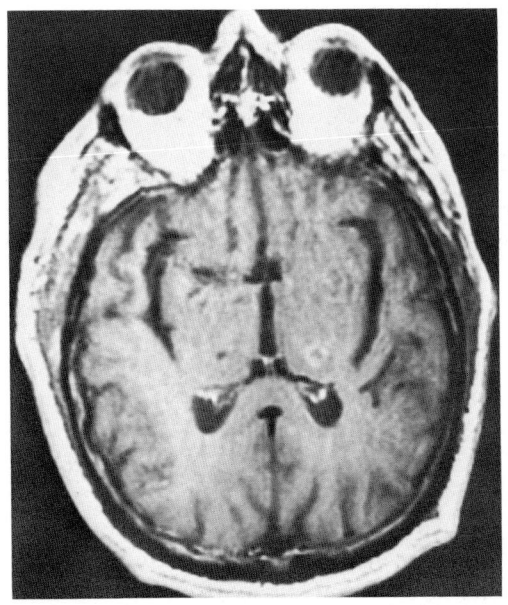 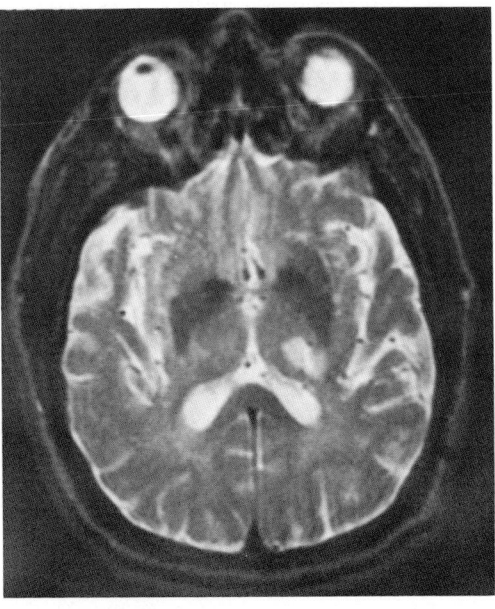

FIG. 2. (**A**) Small deep thalamic infarct shown on T2-weighted MR. (**B**) On T2-weighted images, the infarct shows faint peripheral enhancement following intravenous gadolinium. Note that the area of signal change on the T2 images exceeds the area of enhancement on the T1 image. From ref. 44, with permission.

Low-Flow Infarcts and Terminal Zone Infarcts

Low-flow infarcts are characteristically situated either in the white matter of the centrum semiovale or at the periphery of the putamen or caudate nucleus and they may be bilateral (45–47). These infarcts are associated with ipsilateral tight internal carotid stenosis or occlusion (Fig. 3) and may be associated with reduced cerebral blood flow reactivity in the ipsilateral hemisphere. Low-flow infarcts are often situated in the watershed zone between the basal perforator and cortical perforator territory. Zulch, however, has shown that infarcts at the outer angle of the lateral ventricle may be situated within the territory of the terminal ramifications of the lenticulostriate arteries or Heubner's artery, and are more properly called terminal zone infarcts than watershed infarcts (48). Like watershed infarcts, terminal zone infarcts appear to have a hemodynamic origin. Waterston et al. described 10 patients with tight carotid stenosis or carotid occlusion, some of whom had reduced cerebrovascular reactivity to carbon dioxide. CT showed small deep infarcts in the centrum semiovale or the head of the caudate nucleus and anterior limb of the internal capsule (45). Infarction was bilateral in two cases. Weiler et al. illustrated the site of infarction seen on MR in 17 cases of low-flow infarction (Fig. 4).

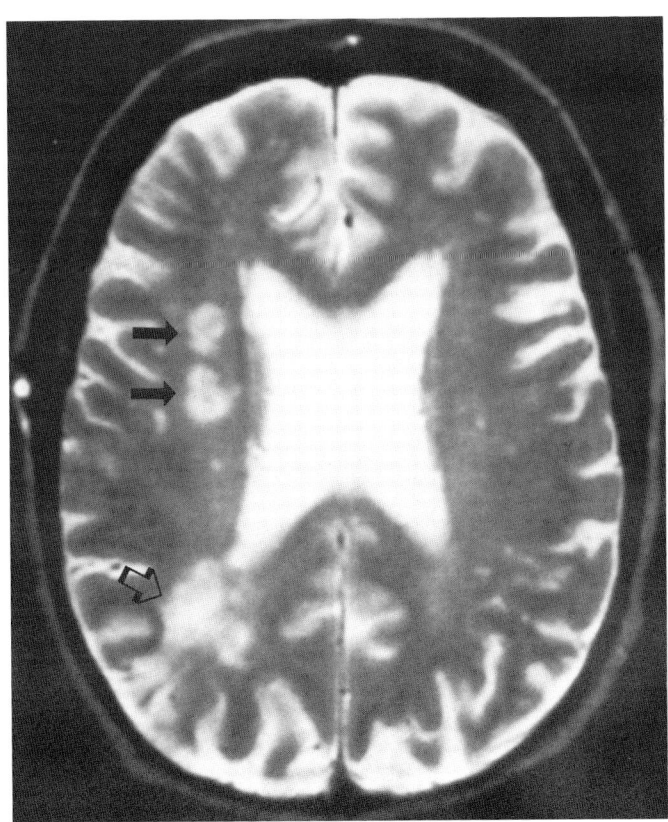

FIG. 3. T2-weighted image showing two low-flow infarcts (black arrows) and a watershed infarct (open arrow) in a patient with an ipsilateral carotid occlusion.

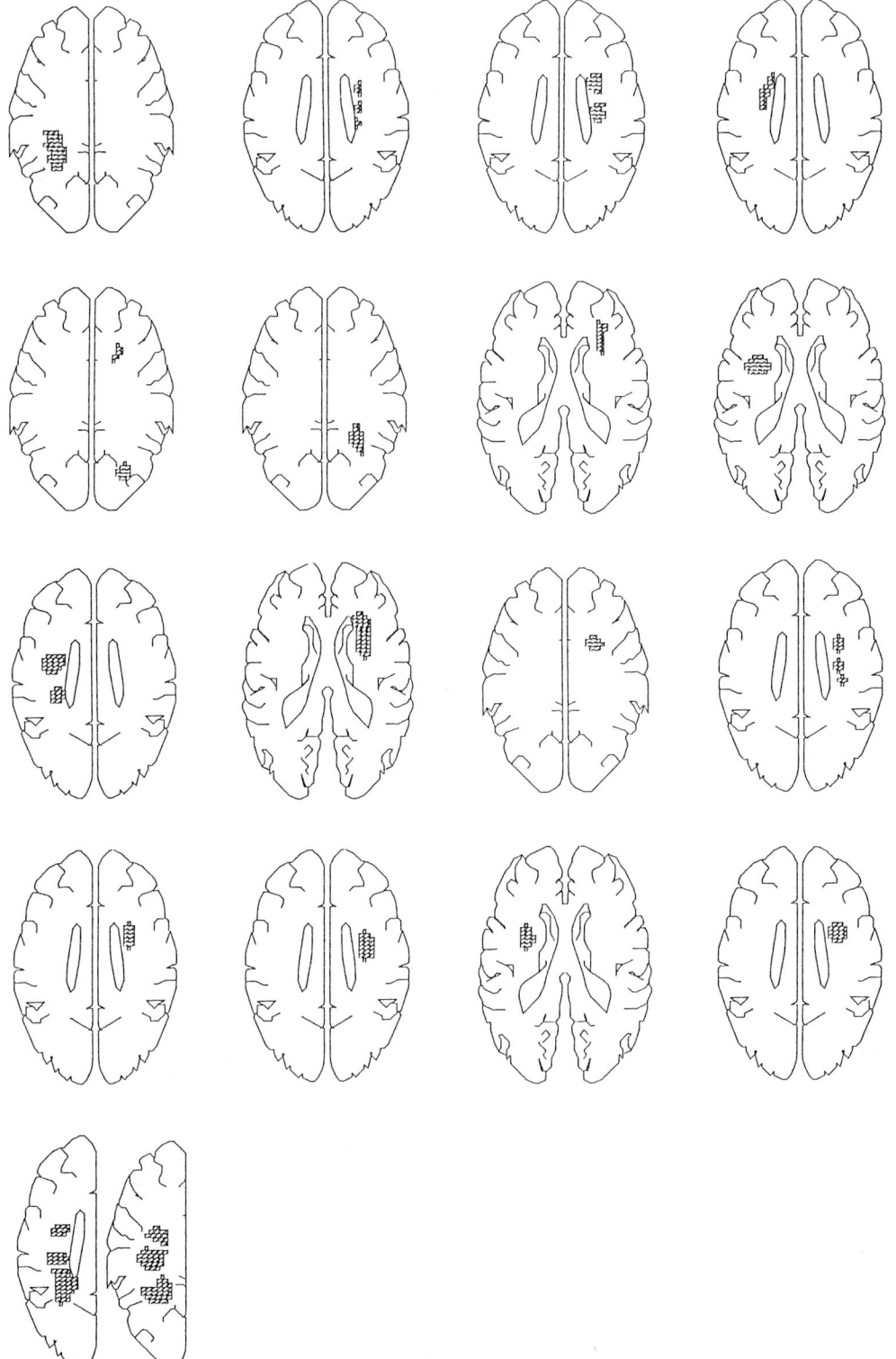

FIG. 4. Diagram showing the site of infarction in 17 patients with low-flow infarcts. From ref. 46, with permission.

All had severe carotid artery occlusive disease and impaired cerebrovascular reactivity. The infarcts were small and situated in the corona radiata or centrum semiovale (46). Yamauchi et al. described a confluent area of hypersignal on T2 images in the mid-centrum semiovale in five patients with unilateral carotid occlusive disease (47). They found that all patients with this confluent hypersignal had evidence of hemodynamic compromise on positron emission tomography, and concluded that the presence of confluent hypersignal in the deep white matter of the mid-centrum semiovale was indicative of hemodynamic compromise in patients with carotid occlusive disease.

Internal Borderzone Infarcts

Angeloni et al. (49) reported seven patients with internal borderzone infarction and illustrated the CT of one of these patients. These infarcts were associated with distal pial middle cerebral artery branch occlusions and were thought to be due to vascular compromise at the interface between cortical branches of the middle cerebral and the lenticulostriate arteries. They were situated in the subinsular region, extending anteriorly and superiorly to the margins of the lateral ventricles (Fig. 5).

Linear Subinsular Infarction

Cobb et al. (50) reported a series of 22 patients with curvilinear subinsular areas of decreased attenuation on CT. These authors described four patterns of lesions: Pattern 1 was that of a curvilinear lucency limited to the lateral striatum and not crossing the white matter boundaries of the anterior or posterior limb of the internal capsule. This pattern was seen in 13 patients,

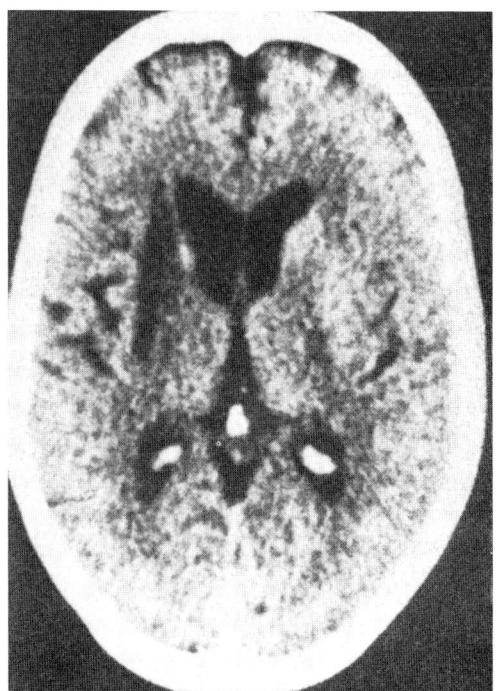
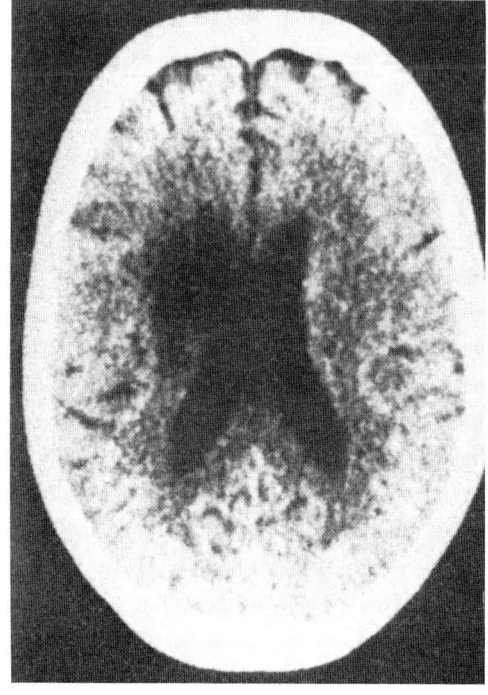

FIG. 5. Extensive internal borderzone infarct in a patient with occlusion of the middle cerebral artery distal to the origin of the temporal pial branches. From ref. 49, with permission.

all of whom had a history of stroke or strokelike symptoms, and Cobb et al. thought that the cause was a previous lateral striatal hemorrhage. Pattern 3 was seen in six elderly patients, and the subinsular lucency was continuous with a frontal periventricular lucency. This pattern was thought to be a manifestation of subcortical arteriosclerotic encephalopathy, but two of these patients had pattern 1 lesions as well. Pattern 2 was a transient lucency seen in young patients with altered mental status and pattern 4 was thought to be an infarction in the lateral lenticulostriate territory.

Pullicino et al. found linear subinsular hyperintensities in 7 of 49 MR scans (14%) of patients over 60 years of age (51). These subinsular lesions appeared to correspond with Cobb et al.'s patterns 1 and 3, but there was no MR evidence of previous hemorrhage, suggesting that previous lateral striatal hemorrhage is an uncommon cause for these lesions. The hyperintensities were narrower than the internal borderzone infarct illustrated by Angeloni et al., and there was no history of middle cerebral artery occlusion in these patients. Patients with subinsular hyperintensities were older and had a higher frequency of subcortical arteriosclerotic encephalopathy than controls, and 57% had vascular risk factors. Postmortem histology and MR in a case with subinsular lesions on CT (Fig. 6) showed cavitary infarction, and postmortem microangiography showed that the infarcts were in the watershed zone between cortical and basal penetrating arteries.

Embolism

Yadav et al. (52) found that 55 of 72 patients (76%) who had focal MR hyperintensities that were situated at the corticomedullary junction or in the cortex had clinical evidence of either cardiogenic or artery-to-artery embolism. No pathological correlation was given, however.

The only report of pathologically proven lacunar infarcts caused by embolism is that

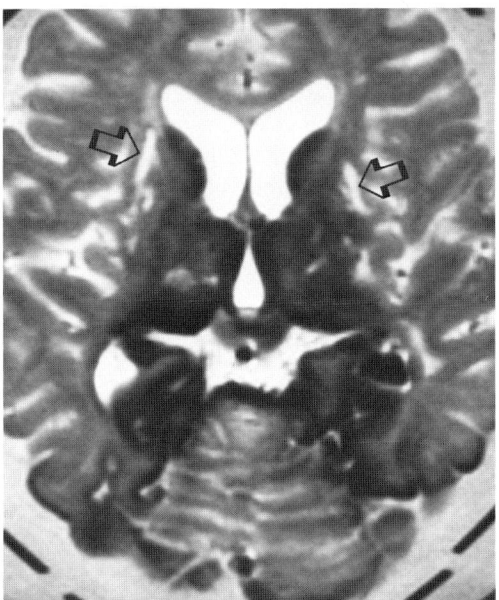

FIG. 6. Postmortem MR showing bilateral linear subinsular hyperintensities (arrows) shown to be due to infarction in a watershed distribution (see text).

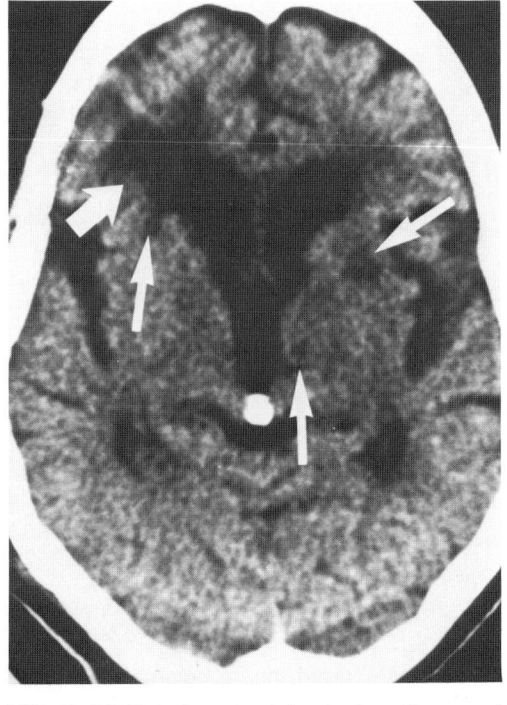

FIG. 7. Multiple lacunar infarcts (small arrows) of embolic origin. From ref. 53, with permission.

of Laloux and Brucher (53). These authors illustrated a CT showing three small deep infarcts that were not distinguished by their location or size from the CT appearance of nonembolic lacunar infarcts (Fig. 7). At autopsy, multiple small arteries including a narrowed artery adjacent to a lacune were occluded by cholesterol crystals. An aortic dissection with large amounts of cholesterol crystals was also found at autopsy.

POSTMORTEM MR

Validity of Postmortem MR Images

Unlike CT, MR images of reasonable quality can be obtained by scanning a brain postmortem (54). Using an early generation 0.15-tesla scanner, Nagara et al. found that both the T1 and T2 relaxation times of gray and of white matter were reduced in brains that had been fixed for over 2 years compared to *in vivo* scans in normals (54). Relatively few studies, however, have compared *in vivo* and postmortem MR of the same brain. Using an early generation MR scanner, Pykett et al. (55) compared *in vivo* CT, MR, and postmortem cranial MR (before removal of the brain) with the brain slices at autopsy. These authors showed that infarcts were clearly seen on postmortem MR. Whilst brain anatomy was well seen on the postmortem MR, the extracerebral spaces appeared more prominent than on the *in vivo* MR, although the authors did not make any systematic comparisons (55). Awad et al. compared the MR of fresh (unfixed but after removal from the cranium) with the MR of fixed brains (56). They noted that MR lesions were identical in the fresh and fixed states, and the overall quality of the image did not seem to be impaired by fixation. Their illustrations, however, appear to show a reduction of ventricular size in the fixed brain. Marshall et al. compared an *in vivo* MR to the MR of a formalin-fixed brain. Although hyperintensities present antemortem were seen postmortem, the shape of the brain was clearly distorted postmortem (19). Braffman et al. performed MR *in vivo* and after fixation postmortem in two cases (10). They found gray matter to be hyperintense relative to white matter on T1 images, which is different from *in vivo* MR. Fazekas et al. compared *in vivo* MR with MR of fixed postmortem brains and found that there was less contrast between focal abnormalities and normal white matter on the postmortem MR scans. The detectability of small lesions was impaired, and small hyperintensities were sometimes not seen or only seen on heavily weighted T2 images. There appeared to be a better distinction between gray and white matter structures on postmortem MR (57).

Although postmortem MR gives good anatomical images, there appear to be significant alterations in dimensions of lesions, in ventricular size, and in the visibility of small hyperintensities (57). There may also be an alteration of the signal characteristics of normal structures.

Size of Vascular Lesions on Postmortem MR

Several reports have appeared correlating postmortem MR with vascular lesions at autopsy (10,16,18,19,55–60). Most MR scans were performed on fixed autopsy brains, although DeWitt et al. performed postmortem MR on the cranium prior to brain removal (17). These authors found that the area of hyperintensity on MR may overestimate the size of a chronic infarct because Wallerian degeneration adjacent to the infarct had similar signal characteristics to the infarct. Using postmortem MR, Marshall et al. found that a white matter infarct may appear up to three times its length due to extensive associated isomorphic gliosis, which gave a similar hypersignal on T2 images (19). Postmortem MR is useful in localizing small hyperintensities, which represent small ischemic lesions that may otherwise be missed at autopsy (61). Hyperintensities on postmortem MR, however, do not always correspond with detectable pathological abnormalities (60).

MR APPEARANCE OF DIFFERENT AUTOPSY-CONFIRMED VASCULAR LESIONS

White Matter Infarcts

Braffman et al. found that 6 of 15 (40%) small focal white matter hyperintensities (WMHIs) noted on postmortem MR were infarcts with varying amounts of cavitation. All of these six hyperintensities were less than 10 mm in diameter. Two of the 15 hyperintensities (13%) were either minute infarcts or gliosis (60).

Marshall et al. correlated focal T2 hyperintensities in the white matter found in three out of six abnormal postmortem MRs (19). Brain number 1 in his series had both multiple discrete small hyperintensities as well as more confluent lesions. These were all found to be intermediate or old infarcts with surrounding isomorphic gliosis. In brain 2, the MR scan showed a linear 3-cm hyperintensity that was found to be a cavitary infarct 1 cm in length with an associated area of isomorphic gliosis 2 cm in length. Brain 3 had a discrete 5-mm hyperintense lesion that was found to be a small cavitary infarct with surrounding gliosis.

Noncystic Small Deep Infarcts

Braffman et al. (10) reported the pathological correlation of small T2 hyperintense lesions seen on MR of postmortem fixed brains in 36 cases and *in vivo* MR in three cases. They divided these lesions on the basis of pathological findings into cystic and noncystic "lacunar" infarcts. These two lesions could be differentiated on *in vivo* MR scans: the noncystic infarcts were hyperintense on proton density images, whereas the cystic infarcts were hypointense. This difference was not seen on the postmortem scans. The locations of several of the noncystic "lacunar" infarcts corresponded with known watershed areas (upper outer lateral ventricular margin, dentate nuclei) suggesting that the pathogenesis of some of these may be different from that of typical lacunar infarcts.

Perivascular Demyelination

Perivascular demyelination has been found to be the cause of focal white WMHIs in elderly individuals (27). Fazekas et al. (57) found that 10 of 14 (71%) hyperintensities in which a lesion was identified pathologically were due to perivascular pathology. This was periarteriolar demyelination in six (Fig. 8), periarterial fibrosis in one, perivenous demyelination in two, and perivenous edema in one.

Small Artery Ectasia

Small artery ectasia was one of the vascular abnormalities Awad et al. found in areas of MR hypersignal intensity (56).

Normal Perivascular Spaces

Thirty-five percent of routine MR scans performed with a high-field scanner showed two or three tiny foci of cerebrospinal fluid (CSF) intensity in the inferior lateral putamen, lateral to the anterior commissure (62) (Fig. 1A). These foci probably represent large perivascular (Virchow-Robin) spaces around the lateral lenticulostriate arteries. Heier et al. found that if these foci are under 2 mm, they are not age related and probably represent normal anatomy (62). Less commonly (15% of routine MR scans), similar foci of CSF intensity are seen in the high-convexity gray matter extending into the centra semiovalia (62) (Fig. 9). When these spaces are less than 2 mm in diameter they are also probably normal (62).

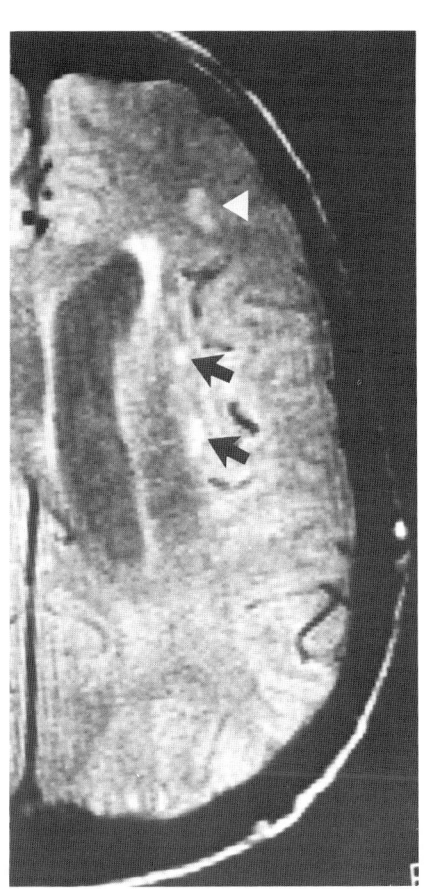 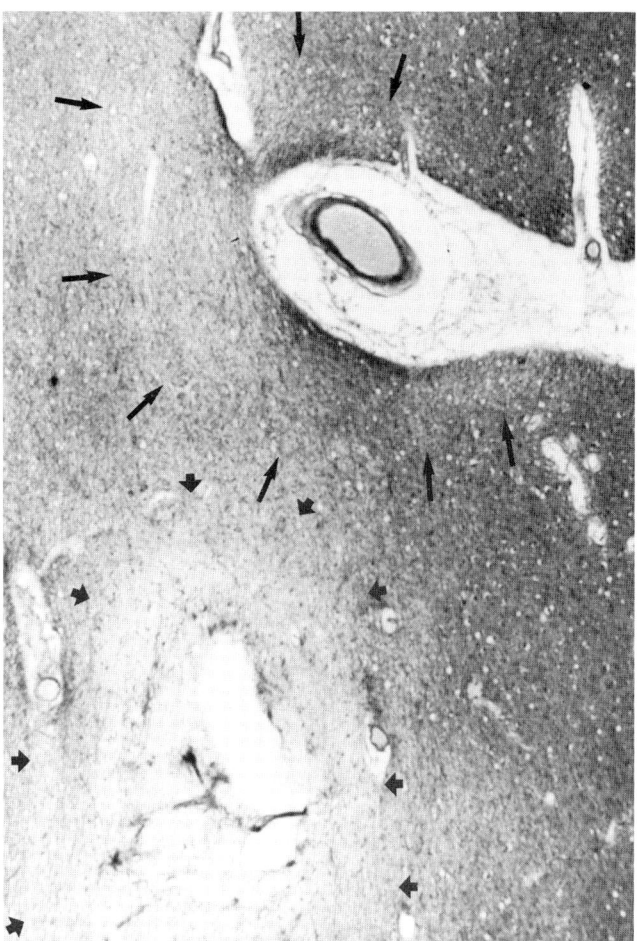

FIG. 8. (A) Focal hyperintensities on proton-density–weighted *in vivo* MR (black arrows), shown on histology **(B)** to be due to perivascular demyelination. This shows as a halo of decreased myelin staining surrounding an artery (upper ring of long arrows) and a vein (lower ring of short arrows). From ref. 57, with permission.

Jungreis et al. found that 59% of axial MR scans showed areas of CSF signal intensity in the medial temporal lobes or corpus striatum that could be attributed to normal perivascular spaces (18). Fifty percent of patients had multiple (two or three) small hyperintensities, but in eight patients the areas were larger than 5 mm. The most common shape of these lesions was round or oval, but they could be tubular in shape if scanned in the long axis of the artery. Jungreis et al. did not show any pathological confirmation that these lesions were normal perivascular spaces, however.

Dilated Perivascular Spaces

Braffman et al. showed the ante- and postmortem MR scans of a patient with multiple very small round or linear lesions situated in the lateral inferior putamen, just above the anterior perforated substance. These lesions were isointense with CSF on

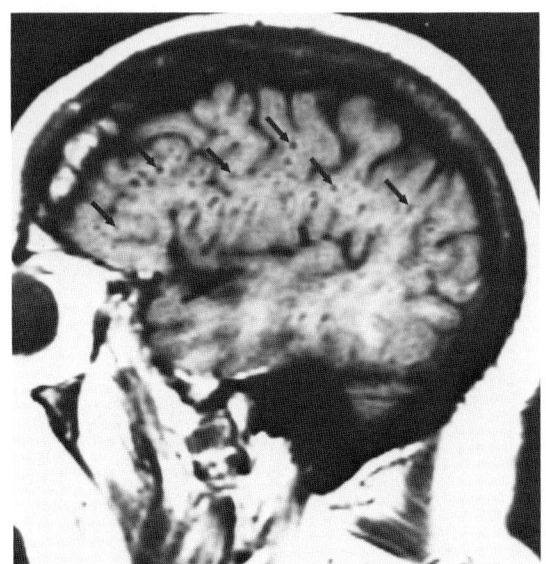 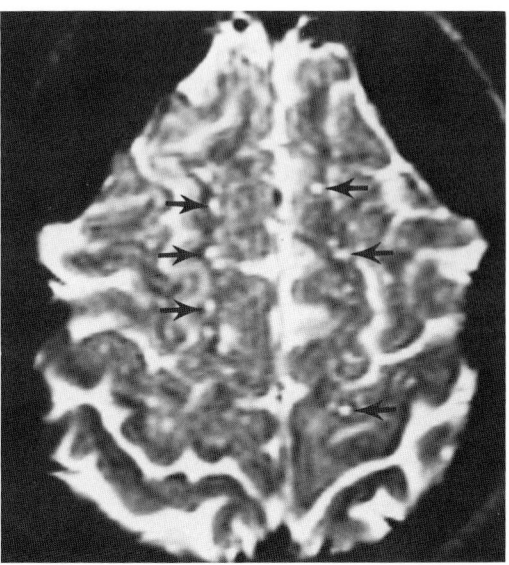

FIG. 9. (**A**) Multiple focal areas of hypointensity over the cerebral convexities on T1-weighted MR due to enlarged perivascular spaces. (**B**) Multiple punctate hyperintensities are seen on T2-weighted images in the same patient.

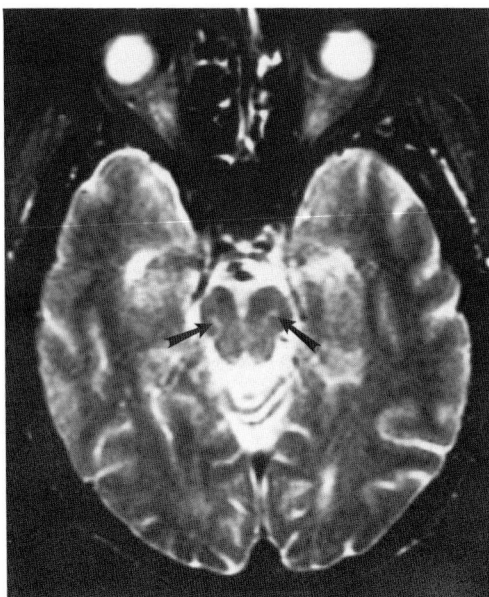

FIG. 10. Symmetrical hyperintensities in the midbrain due to enlarged perivascular spaces.

both T1 and T2 images. Histology showed multiple small dilated perivascular spaces compatible with *état criblé* (Fig. 1) (10).

Heier et al. found that when presumed Virchow-Robin spaces in the inferior basal ganglia or high-convexity foci were 2 mm or greater in diameter there was a significant correlation with age, hypertension, dementia, and focal WMHIs (62). Logistic regression analysis, however, showed that age was the only significant risk factor for these foci.

Elster and Richardson reported punctate or linear hyperintensities on T2 images in the inferior midbrain near the junction of the substantia nigra and the cerebral peduncle (63). Twenty percent of 157 serial MR scans had this finding, which correlated with the site of penetrating branches of the collicular or accessory collicular arteries. Enlargement of the perivascular spaces around these arteries was thought to account for these hyperintensities (Fig. 10).

Awad et al. compared the histology from areas of confluent white matter hyperintensity seen on postmortem MR with areas from the same brains without hyperintensities. They found that sclerosis and ectasia of small arteries and enlarged perivascular spaces were more common and normal myelin staining was less common in the areas showing confluent WMHIs on MR (56).

Giant Perivascular Space

Poirier et al. illustrated a CT that showed a focal round area of reduced attenuation in the midbrain, which was found to be a giant perivascular space at autopsy (64).

DIFFERENTIAL DIAGNOSIS OF WHITE MATTER HYPERINTENSITIES

MR is very sensitive at detecting small deep infarcts and other white matter lesions. This high sensitivity often makes interpretation of MR images difficult, because of the nonspecific appearance of a wide variety of both ischemic and nonischemic lesions. WMHIs are usually divided into four groups (Fig. 11): ventricular caps, periventricular rims, focal or punctate WMHIs, and confluent WMHIs or patches (65). All of these different types of WMHIs can be caused by penetrating artery disease (see Chapter 11) and a pathology like that seen in subcortical arteriosclerotic encephalopathy (Binswanger's disease) is one of the most common underlying causes of WMHIs (18,60).

Rims have been found to be characterized pathologically by subependymal gliosis and loss of the ependymal lining (65). Thin rims may be a feature of normal aging (66) but thick rims are suggestive of underlying small artery disease (66). Other differentials are given in Table 1.

Small, localized caps are a normal finding (66–68). The usual histopathological counterpart of caps has been found to be myelin pallor and dilated perivascular spaces (56,65). Enlarged caps may be caused by several conditions (see Table 1).

Focal WMHIs are well circumscribed lesions in the white matter, ranging in size from tiny lesions about a millimeter in

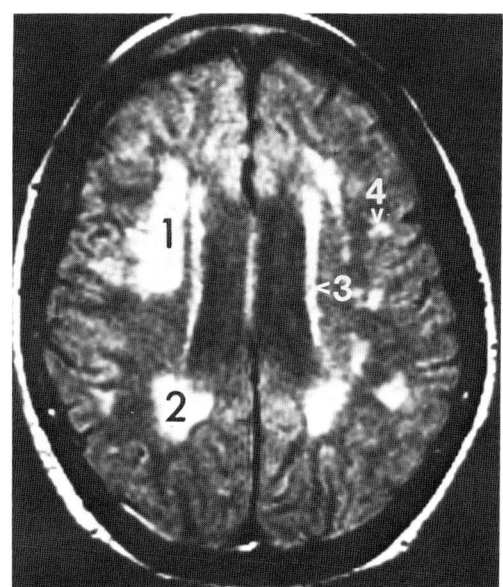

FIG. 11. Proton density MR scan showing (**1**) confluent WMHI, (**2**) cap, (**3**) rim, and (**4**) focal WMHI.

TABLE 1. *Differential diagnosis of periventricular white matter hyperintensities*

Caps
  Normal finding if small and localized (66–68)
  Subcortical arteriosclerotic encephalopathy (67)
  Multiple sclerosis (67,78)
  Wallerian degeneration adjacent to an infarct (67,79)
  Etat criblé (56)
  Sarcoidosis (80)
  Anoxic encephalopathy (81)
  Epstein-Barr virus (mononucleosis) (82)
  Behçet's disease (78)
  Globoid cell leukodystrophy (83)
  Adrenomyeloneuropathy (84)
Rims
  Normal aging if thin (66)
  Secondary to small artery vascular disease if thick (66)
  Multiple sclerosis (thick) (67)
  Communicating hydrocephalus (85)

diameter to a diameter of about a centimeter. Focal WMHIs may be caused by small infarcts (19,60), focal gliosis (60), focal demyelination (60), dilated perivascular spaces, and perivascular gliosis (65) or perivascular demyelination (57). There is a wide differential diagnosis of focal or punctate WMHIs (Table 2). The site and the size of the WMHIs may help in the differential diagnosis. Multiple very small WMHIs in the high-convexity gray matter or in the inferior lateral putamen are likely to be dilated perivascular spaces (62) (Figs. 1 and 9). The white matter adjacent to the upper outer angle of the lateral ventricle is a characteristic site for low-flow infarcts (46) (Figs. 3 and 4), but also for multiple sclerosis plaques. Multiple focal WMHIs may appear to coalesce to form confluent patches.

Confluent WMHI ranges from small irregular patches to extensive involvement of the whole white matter. Confluent WMHI may be continuous with caps over the ventricles. WMHI patches have been found to be associated with myelin pallor and dilated perivascular spaces at autopsy (65), and the most common underlying pathology associated with extensive confluent WMHI is that of subcortical arteriosclerotic encephalopathy (Binswanger's disease) (69). The differential diagnosis of confluent WMHI is given in Table 3.

TABLE 2. *Differential diagnosis of small focal hyperintensities*

White matter infarcts (19,60)
Focal demyelination (60)
Focal areas of gliosis (60)
Dilated perivascular spaces and perivascular gliosis or demyelination (57,65)
"Brain cyst" (60)
Systemic lupus erythematosus (78,86,94)
Hypertensive encephalopathy (95)
Moyamoya disease (92)
Chicken pox encephalitis (78)
Toxoplasmosis (89)
Adrenomyeloneuropathy (84)
Sjogren's syndrome (88)
Sarcoidosis (80)
Isolated CNS angiitis (96)

TABLE 3. *Differential diagnosis of confluent irregular white matter lesions*

Subcortical arteriosclerotic encephalopathy (16,67)
White matter infarcts with surrounding isomorphic gliosis (19)
SLE (86,87)
Acute disseminated encephalomyelitis (85)
Acute hemorrhagic leukoencephalopathy (85)
Epstein-Barr virus (mononucleosis) (82)
Sjogren's syndrome (88)
Sarcoidosis (80)
Anoxic encephalopathy and carbon monoxide poisoning (81,85)
HIV encephalitis (89)
Progressive multifocal leukoencephalopathy (89)
Radiation injury (90)
High-dose methotrexate (91)
Moyamoya disease (92)
Metachromatic leukodystrophy (78)
Dominant adult-onset leukodystrophy (93)
Adrenomyeloneuropathy (84)

MEASUREMENT OF SMALL DEEP INFARCTS

Reliability of Assessment of Small Deep Infarcts

The interpretation of pictographic data entailed in the diagnosis of a small infarct is dependent on the past experience and expectancy of the observer (70). For senior neurologists there is substantial interobserver agreement (kappa coefficient greater than 0.6) in identifying either a normal CT scan or a small deep infarct (70). However, there does not seem to be any difference between neurologists and neuroradiologists in interpretation of CT scans (71). The interobserver agreement is not so good (kappa = 0.45) when some of the raters are still in training (72). The diagnosis of a small deep infarct may be biased by the accompanying clinical information if the infarct is very small (71). Bonke et al. advised that if the presence of a small deep infarct on CT is thought to be equivocal, then the scan should be interpreted as such without looking at the clinical information (71).

Using MR, Hommel et al. found good statistical agreement between a neurologist and a radiologist in deciding on the location of small deep lesions (kappa coefficient 0.65) and also in differentiating between small deep infarcts, nonlacunar infarcts, and enlarged perivascular spaces (kappa = 0.7) (26). Yetkin et al. found excellent intraobserver variability in deciding on the presence of focal hyperintensities, but showed poor interobserver reliability (kappa < 0.35) in deciding on the number of small (< 5 mm) or large (> 5 mm) hyperintensities on a scan (73). Interobserver reliability was slightly better, but still remained only fair (kappa = 0.53 to 0.73) when the two observers first reached a consensus on the interpretation of the scans. These authors concluded that in order to compare the frequency of focal hyperintensities, observer variability must be controlled by using proper control subjects.

Van Swieten et al. (74) reported a three-point scale for grading periventricular white matter lesions on CT or MR. They found a good level of interobserver agreement for this scale for both CT (weighted kappa coefficient 0.63) and for MR (weighted kappa coefficient 0.78). On CT the interobserver agreement for degree of radiolucency was the same as that for anatomical extent of the periventricular lesions.

METHODS OF MEASUREMENT OF INFARCTS

1. Method of Nelson et al.: The longest dimension of the infarct and the greatest dimension at right angle to this (both corrected for the size of the hard copy) are multiplied, and the product is multiplied by the thickness and number of slices showing the infarct. This result represents the volume of a cuboid containing the lesion. Since lacunar infarcts approximate more to a spherical shape, the above result is divided by two to approximate a spheroid (8).

2. Method of Brott et al. (75): These authors traced the area of low attenuation on each CT slice, and the area was summed for the slices showing the infarct. The volume was derived from the area and the slice thickness.

3. Viewing console, computer assisted method of measuring infarct area and area of white matter lesions as used by Liu et al. (76).

4. Method of Okada et al.: These authors express the area of the infarct as a percentage of the total ipsilateral hemisphere area (77).

REFERENCES

1. Bogousslavsky J. The plurality of subcortical infarction. *Stroke* 1992;23:629–631.
2. Caplan LR, DeWitt LD, Pessin MS, Gorelick PB, Adelman LS. Lateral thalamic infarcts. *Arch Neurol* 1988;45:959–964.
3. Graff-Radford NR, Schelper RL, Ilinsky IA, Damasio H. Computed tomographic and postmortem study of a nonhemorrhagic thalamic infarction. *Arch Neurol* 1985;42:761–763.
4. Pullicino P, Nelson RF, Kendall BE, Marshall J. Small deep infarcts diagnosed on computed tomography. *Neurology* 1980;30:1090–1096.
5. Lepore FE, Gulli V, Miller DC. Neuro-ophthalmological findings with neuropathological correlation in bilateral thalamic-mesencephalic infarction. *J Clin Neuro Ophthalmol* 1985;5:224–228.
6. Hochman MS, Sowers JJ, Bruce-Gregorios J. Syndrome of the mesencephalic artery: report of a case with CT and necropsy findings. *J Neurol Neurosurg Psychiatry* 1985;48:1179–1181.
7. Collard M, Saint-Val C, Mohr M, Kiesmann M. Paralysie isolé du nerf moteur oculaire commun par infarctus de ses fibres fasciculaires. *Rev Neurol (Paris)* 1990;146:128–132.
8. Nelson RF, Pullicino P, Kendall BE, Marshall J. Computed tomography in patients presenting with lacunar syndromes. *Stroke* 1980;11:256–261.
9. Donnan GA, Tress BM, Bladin PF. A prospective study of lacunar infarction using computerized tomography. *Neurology* 1982;32:49–56.
10. Braffman BH, Zimmerman RA, Trojanowski JQ, Gonatas NK, Hickey WF, Schlaepfer WW. Brain MR: pathologic correlation with gross and histopathology. I. Lacunar infarction and Virchow-Robin spaces. *AJR* 1988;151:551–558.
11. Alcala H, Gado M, Torack RM. The effect of size, histologic elements, and water content on the visualisation of cerebral infarcts. A computerized cranial tomographic study. *Arch Neurol* 1978;35:1–7.
12. Weisberg LA. Lacunar infarcts. Clinical and computed tomographic correlations. *Arch Neurol* 1982;39:37–40.
13. Toghi H, Mochizuki H, Yamanouchi H, et al. A comparison between the computed tomogram

and the neuropathological findings in cerebrovascular disease. *J Neurol* 1981;224:211–220.
14. Besson G. *Les infarctus lacunaires. Evaluation clinique et par l'imagerie par resonance magnetique* [MD thesis]. Grenoble, France: University of Grenoble, 1989.
15. Salgado ED, Weinstein M, Furlan AJ, et al. Proton magnetic resonance imaging in ischemic cerebrovascular disease. *Ann Neurol* 1986;20:502–507.
16. Revész T, Hawkins CP, du Boulay EPGH, Barnard RO, McDonald WI. Pathological findings correlated with magnetic resonance imaging in subcortical arteriosclerotic encephalopathy (Binswanger's disease). *J Neurol Neurosurg Psychiatry* 1989;52:1337–1344.
17. DeWitt LD, Kistler JP, Miller DC, Richardson EP Jr, Buonanno FS. NMR-neuropathologic correlation in stroke. *Stroke* 1987;18:342–351.
18. Jungreis CA, Kanal E, Hirsch WL, Martinez AJ, Moossy J. Normal perivascular spaces mimicking lacunar infarction: MR imaging. *Radiology* 1988;169:101–104.
19. Marshall VG, Bradley WG Jr, Marshall CE, Bhoopat T, Rhodes RH. Deep white matter infarction: correlation of MR imaging and histopathologic findings. *Radiology* 1988;167:517–522.
20. Kappelle LJ, Ramos LMP, Van Gijn J. The role of computed tomography in patients with lacunar stroke in the carotid territory. *Neuroradiology* 1989;31:316–319.
21. Miyashita K, Naritomi H, Nakamura M, Kazui S, Sawada T. Old cerebral hemorrhage in cases of multiple lacunar infarction found by magnetic resonance imaging. *Cerebrovasc Dis* 1991;1:321–326.
22. Rothrock JF, Lyden PD, Hesselink JR, Brown JJ, Healy ME. Brain magnetic resonance imaging in the evaluation of lacunar stroke. *Stroke* 1987;18:781–786.
23. Arboix A, Marti-Vilalta JL, Pujol J, Sanz M. Lacunar cerebral infarct and nuclear magnetic resonance. A review of sixty cases. *Eur Neurol* 1990;30:47–51.
24. Bogousslavsky J, Fox AJ, Barnett HJM, Hachinski VC, Vinitski S, Carey LS. Clinico-topographic correlation of small vertebrobasilar infarct using magnetic resonance imaging. *Stroke* 1986;17:929–938.
25. Kistler JP, Buonanno FS, DeWitt LD, Davis KR, Brady TJ, Fisher CM. Vertebral-basilar posterior cerebral territory stroke—delineation by proton nuclear magnetic resonance imaging. *Stroke* 1984;15:417–426.
26. Hommel M, Besson G, Le Bas JF, et al. Prospective study of lacunar infarction using magnetic resonance imaging. *Stroke* 1990;21:546–554.
27. Fazekas F, Schmidt R, Kleinert R, et al. Follow up of MRI white matter lesions and histopathologic correlation. *J Neurol* 1990;237:147(abst).
28. Brown JJ, Hesselink JR, Rothrock JF. MR and CT of lacunar infarcts. *AJR* 1988;151:367–372.
29. Nabatame H, Fujimoto N, Nakamura K, et al. High intensity areas on noncontrast T1-weighted MR images in cerebral infarction. *J Comput Assist Tomogr* 1990;14:521–526.
30. Challa VR, Moody DM. The value of magnetic resonance imaging in the detection of type II hemorrhagic lacunes. *Stroke* 1989;20:822–825.
31. Launay M, N'Diaye M, Bories J. X-ray computed tomography (CT) study of small, deep and recent infarcts (SDRIs) of the cerebral hemispheres in adults. *Neuroradiology* 1985;27:494–508.
32. Virapongse C, Mancuso A, Quisling R. Human brain infarcts: Gd-CTPA-enhanced MR imaging. *Radiology* 1986;161:785–794.
33. Elster AD. MR contrast enhancement in brainstem and deep cerebral infarction. *AJNR* 1991;12:1127–1132.
34. Biller J, Adams HP Jr, Dunn V, Simmons Z, Jacoby CG. Dichotomy between clinical findings and MR abnormalities in pontine infarction. *J Comput Assist Tomogr* 1986;10:379–385.
35. Durif F, Hommel M, Bennani W, et al. Magnetic resonance imaging in ischaemic accidents of the brain stem. *J Neuroradiol* 1989;16:25–37.
36. Fisher CM. Lacunes: small deep cerebral infarcts. *Neurology* 1965;15:774–784.
37. Heiss WD, Herholz K, Bocher-Schwarz HG, et al. PET, CT and MR imaging in cerebrovascular disease. *J Comput Assist Tomogr* 1986;10:903–911.
38. Skrivner EB, Olsen TS. Repeated computed tomography in lacunar infarcts of the brain. *Acta Radiol [Diagn] (Stockh)* 1989;30:1–6.
39. Miyashita K, Naritomi H, Sawada T, et al. Identification of recent lacunar lesions in cases of multiple small infarctions by magnetic resonance imaging. *Stroke* 1988;19:834–839.
40. Yuh WTC, Crain MR, Loes DJ, Greene GM, Ryals TJ, Sato Y. MR imaging of cerebral ischemia. Findings in the first 24 hours. *AJNR* 1991;12:621–629.
41. Alberts MJ, Faulstich ME, Gray L. Stroke with negative brain magnetic resonance imaging. *Stroke* 1992;23:663–667.
42. Pullicino P, Kendall BE. Contrast enhancement in ischaemic lesions. I. Relationship to prognosis. *Neuroradiology* 1980;19:235–239.
43. Warach S, Li W, Ronthal M, Edelman RR. Acute cerebral ischemia: evaluation with dynamic contrast-enhanced MR imaging and MR angiography. *Radiology* 1992;182:41–47.
44. Crain MR, Yuh WTC, Greene GM, et al. Cerebral ischemia: evaluation with contrast-enhanced MR imaging. *AJNR* 1991;12:631–639.
45. Waterston JA, Brown MM, Butler P, Swash M. Small deep cerebral infarcts associated with occlusive internal carotid artery disease. *Arch Neurol* 1990;47:953–957.
46. Weiller C, Ringelstein EB, Reiche W, Buell U. Clinical and hemodynamic aspects of low-flow infarcts. *Stroke* 1991;22:1117–1123.
47. Yamauchi H, Fukuyama H, Yamaguchi S, Miyoshi T, Kimura J, Konishi J. High-intensity

area in deep white matter indicating hemodynamic compromise in internal carotid artery occlusive disorders. *Arch Neurol* 1991;48:1067–1071.
48. Zülch K-J. *The cerebral infarct. Pathology, pathogenesis and computed tomography.* Berlin: Springer-Verlag; 1985.
49. Angeloni U, Bozzao L, Fantozzi L, Bastianello S, Kushner M, Fieschi C. Internal borderzone infarction following acute middle cerebral artery occlusion. *Neurology* 1990;40:1196–1198.
50. Cobb SR, Mehringer CM, Itabashi HH, Pribram H. CT of subinsular infarction and ischemia. *AJNR* 1987;8:221–227.
51. Pullicino P, Miller LL, Munschauer FE, Ostrow PT. Linear subinsular MR hyperintensities. *Ann Neurol* 1992;32:267(abst).
52. Yadav JS, Kinkel PR, Klee D, Bates V, Calcano J, Kinkel WR. Small cerebral embolic infarctions: evaluation by magnetic resonance imaging. *Neurology* 1989;39:160 (abst).
53. Laloux P, Brucher JM. Lacunar infarctions due to cholesterol emboli. *Stroke* 1991;22:1440–1444.
54. Nagara H, Inoue T, Koga T, Kitaguchi T, Tateishi J, Goto I. Formalin fixed brains are useful for magnetic resonance imaging (MRI) study. *J Neurol Sci* 1987;81:67–77.
55. Pykett IL, Buonanno FS, Brady TJ, Kistler P. True three-dimensional nuclear magnetic resonance neuro-imaging in ischemic stroke: correlation of NMR, x-ray CT and pathology. *Stroke* 1983;14:173–177.
56. Awad IA, Johnson PC, Spetzler RF, Hodak JA. Incidental subcortical lesions identified on magnetic resonance imaging in the elderly. II. Postmortem pathological correlations. *Stroke* 1986;17:1090–1097.
57. Fazekas F, Kleinert R, Offenbacher H, et al. The morphologic correlate of incidental punctate white matter hyperintensities on MR images. *AJR* 1991;157:1317–1323.
58. Grafton ST, Sumi SM, Stimac GK, Alvord EC Jr, Shaw CM, Nochlin D. Comparison of postmortem magnetic resonance imaging and neuropathologic findings in the cerebral white matter. *Arch Neurol* 1991;48:293–298.
59. Van Swieten JC, Van den Hout JHW, Van Ketel BA, Hijdra A, Wokke JHJ, Van Gijn J. Periventricular lesions in the white matter on magnetic resonance imaging in the elderly. A morphometric correlation with arteriolosclerosis and dilated perivascular spaces. *Brain* 1991;114:761–774.
60. Braffman BH, Zimmerman RA, Trojanowski JQ, Gonatas NK, Hickey WF, Schlaepfer WW. Brain MR: pathologic correlation with gross and histopathology. 2. Hyperintense white-matter foci in the elderly. *AJR* 1988;151:559–566.
61. Miller LL, Pullicino P, Ostrow LW, Ostrow PT. Small deep infarcts demonstrated by post-mortem angiography and magnetic resonanace imaging. *J Neuropathol Exp Neurol* 1992;51:343 (abst).

62. Heier LA, Bauer CJ, Schwartz L, Zimmerman RD, Morgello S, Deck MDF. Large Virchow-Robin spaces: MR-clinical correlation. *AJNR* 1989;10:929–936.
63. Elster AD, Richardson DN. Focal high signal on MR scans of the midbrain caused by enlarged perivascular spaces: MR-pathologic correlation. *AJNR* 1991;11:1119–1122.
64. Poirier J, Barbizet J, Gaston A, Meyrignac C. Démence thalamique. Lacunes expansives du territoire thalamo-mésencéphalique paramédian. Hydrocéphalie par sténose de l'aqueduc de Sylvius. *Rev Neurol* 1983;139:349–358.
65. Chimowitz MI, Estes ML, Furlan AJ, Awad IA. Further observations on the pathology of subcortical lesions identified on magnetic resonance imaging. *Arch Neurol* 1992;49:747–752.
66. Kertesz A, Black SE, Tokar G, Benke T, Carr T, Nicholson L. Periventricular and subcortical hyperintensities on magnetic resonance imaging "rims, caps and unidentified bright objects." *Arch Neurol* 1988;45:404–408.
67. Leifer D, Buonanno FS, Richardson EP Jr. Clinicopathologic correlations of cranial magnetic resonance imaging of periventricular white matter. *Neurology* 1990;40:911–918.
68. Sze G, De Armond SJ, Brant-Zawadzki M, Davis RL, Norman D, Newton TH. Foci of MRI signal (pseudo lesions) anterior to the frontal horns: histologic correlations of a normal finding. *AJNR* 1986;7:381–387.
69. Van Swieten JC. *Periventricular leuko-encephalopathy: vascular dementia revisited* [Thesis]. Utrecht, The Netherlands: University of Utrecht, 1992.
70. Shinar D, Gross CR, Hier DB, et al. Interobserver reliability in the interpretation of computed tomography scans of stroke patients. *Arch Neurol* 1987;44:149–155.
71. Bonke B, Kwakernaak A, Van den Berg M, Koudstaal PJ. Bias in the assessment of computed tomography scans for lacunar infarction. *Cerebrovasc Dis* 1992;2:107–110.
72. Schneider R, Kluge R, Willmes K. Interrater agreement for CT scans of patients with lacunar infarcts and leuko-araiosis. *Acta Neurol Scand* 1991;84:527–530.
73. Yetkin FZ, Haughton VM, Fischer ME, et al. High-signal foci on MR images of the brain: observer variability in their quantification. *AJR* 1992;159:185–188.
74. Van Swieten JC, Hijdra A, Koudstaal PJ, Van Gijn J. Grading of white matter lesions on CT and MRI: a simple scale. *J Neurol Neurosurg Psychiatry* 1990;53:1080–1083.
75. Brott T, Marler JR, Olinger CP, et al. Measurements of acute cerebral infarction: lesion size by computed tomography. *Stroke* 1989;20:871–875.
76. Liu CK, Miller BL, Cummings JL, et al. A quantitative MRI study of vascular dementia. *Neurology* 1992;42:138–143.
77. Okada Y, Yamaguchi T, Minematsu K, et al. Hemorrhagic transformation in cerebral embolism. *Stroke* 1989;20:598–603.

78. Ormerod IEC, Miller DH, McDonald WI, et al. The role of NMR imaging in the assessment of multiple sclerosis and isolated neurological lesions. *Brain* 1987;110:1579–1616.
79. Lu JQ, Zhu YH, Han ZY. Periventricular hyperintensity. *Neurology* 1992;42:1256.
80. Miller DH, Kendall BE, Barter S, et al. Magnetic resonance imaging in central nervous system sarcoidosis. *Neurology* 1988;38:378–383.
81. Sawada H, Udaka F, Seriu N, Shindou K, Kameyama M, Tsujimura M. MRI demonstration of cortical laminar necrosis and delayed white matter injury in anoxic encephalopathy. *Neuroradiology* 1990;32:319–321.
82. Tolly TL, Wells RG, Sty JR. MR features of fleeting CNS lesions associated with Epstein-Barr virus infection. *J Comput Assist Tomogr* 1989;13:665–668.
83. Verdru P, Lammens M, Dom R, Van Elsen A, Carton H. Globoid cell leukodystrophy: a family with both late-infantile and adult type. *Neurology* 1991;41:1382–1384.
84. Aubourg P, Adamsbaum C, Lavallard-Rousseau MC, et al. Brain MRI and electrophysiologic abnormalities in preclinical and clinical adrenomyeloneuropathy. *Neurology* 1992;42:85–91.
85. Soila KP. MRI of demyelinating and other white matter diseases. In: Pomeranz SJ, ed. *Craniospinal magnetic resonance imaging*. Philadelphia: WB Saunders; 1989:459–488.
86. Bell CL, Partington C, Robbins M, Graziano F, Turski P, Kornguth S. Magnetic resonance imaging of central nervous system lesions in patients with lupus erythematosus. *Arthritis Rheum* 1991;34:432–441.
87. Aisen AM, Gabrielsen TO, McCune WJ. MR imaging of systemic lupus erythematosus involving the brain. *AJR* 1985;144:1027–1031.
88. Alexander EL, Beall SS, Gordon B, et al. Magnetic resonance imaging of cerebral lesions in patients with the Sjogren syndrome. *Ann Intern Med* 1988;108:815–823.
89. Jarvik JG, Hesselink JR, Kennedy C, et al. Acquired immunodeficiency syndrome. Magnetic resonance patterns of brain involvement with pathologic correlation. *Arch Neurol* 1988;45:731–736.
90. DeAngelis LM, Delattre JY, Posner JB. Radiation-induced dementia in patients cured of brain metastases. *Neurology* 1989;39:789–796.
91. Lien HH, Blomlie V, Saeter G, Solheim O, Fossa SD. Osteogenic sarcoma: MR signal abnormalities of the brain in asymptomatic patients treated with high-dose methotrexate. *Radiology* 1991;179:547–550.
92. Bruno A, Yuh WTC, Biller J, Adams HP Jr, Cornell SH. Magnetic resonance imaging in young adults with cerebral infarction due to Moyamoya. *Arch Neurol* 1988;45:303–306.
93. Schwankhaus JD, Patronas N, Dorwart R, Eldridge R, Schlesinger S, McFarland H. Computed tomography and magnetic resonance imaging in adult-onset leukodystrophy. *Arch Neurol* 1988;45:1004–1008.
94. Vermess M, Bernstein RM, Bydder GM, Steiner RE, Young IR, Hughes GRV. Nuclear magnetic resonance (NMR) imaging of the brain in systemic lupus erythematosus. *J Comput Assist Tomogr* 1983;7:461–467.
95. Hauser RA, Lacey M, Knight MR. Hypertensive encephalopathy. Magnetic resonance imaging demonstration of reversible cortical and white matter lesions. *Arch Neurol* 1988;45:1078–1083.
96. Kattah JC, Cupps TR, Di Chiro G, Manz HJ. An unusual case of central nervous system vasculitis. *J Neurol* 1987;234:344–347.

5

Pathology of Small Artery Disease

Peter T. Ostrow and Lucia L. Miller

Department of Pathology, State University of New York at Buffalo, Buffalo General Hospital, Buffalo, New York 14203

This chapter will review the changes that occur in small arteries in several disease processes, and the consequences of those vascular changes on the brain parenchyma. A central theme will be that these changes are orderly and comprehensible. The vessels and the brain have a limited repertoire of responses to injury; most of the lesions encountered represent a continuum of alterations, and are much less heterogeneous than suggested by the profusion of names they have been called in the literature.

GENERAL OVERVIEW OF SMALL ARTERY DISEASE

Small arteries and arterioles throughout the body undergo arteriosclerotic changes with aging. These include hyaline deposits in their walls and intimal atheroma formation. The wall becomes rigid and the lumen becomes narrow, impeding blood flow. If flow is reduced below a critical level, tissue supplied by the artery is injured. This is an extremely simple concept, but it is important to keep in mind that vascular disorders produce ischemic damage in the brain by narrowing the arteries, usually through some modification of the basic process of arteriosclerosis. For example, hypertension and diabetes will exacerbate/accelerate the process of arterial narrowing, making ischemic consequences more likely to occur, and at a younger age. Tissue damage is most often associated with local stenosis that has become severe or has developed rapidly, but systemic hemodynamic factors are also important. Reduction of blood flow or of oxygen delivery, due to systemic hypotension or hypoxemia secondary to respiratory disease, may produce damage in the territories of arteries that are only moderately narrowed.

Another simple but fundamental principle is that the topography of brain lesions is determined by the type and distribution of vascular pathology. The arterial changes are not uniformly distributed, so focal lesions will be seen in the territories of those most severely affected. Complete occlusion of a single small artery may produce necrosis in its territory of supply, while gradual narrowing of many small arteries may damage the tissue in the border zones between their territories to varying degrees. Once again, this is an intuitively obvious concept that, if kept in mind, will help explain some of the minute distinctions among types of lesions reported in the literature. We must also bear in mind that the selective vulnerability to hypoxia/ischemia of different cell types in the nervous system (neurons > oligodendroglia > astrocytes) will also influence the occurrence and location of lesions, as will proximal vessel disease, cardiovascular status, and respiratory function. If all these contributing factors are regarded appropriately as modifying influences on a basic, rather stereotyped process, then the spectrum of abnormalities a pathologist must interpret becomes manageable, perhaps even user-friendly.

GENERAL OVERVIEW OF TISSUE CHANGES FOLLOWING HYPOXIA/ISCHEMIA

An infarct is a localized area of tissue necrosis that follows a severe, prolonged interruption of blood flow (Fig. 1). All the cellular elements (neurons, glia, blood vessels, nerve fibers) are destroyed, and the necrotic tissue is removed by a standard inflammatory response. This includes early appearance of polymorphonuclear leukocytes, followed by macrophages, then ingrowth of delicate capillaries that represent the brain's analogue of granulation tissue. In the rest of the body, fibroblasts also grow into the lesion and produce a collagenous scar. That does not happen in the brain; instead, reactive astrocytes proliferate at the margin, and the end result is a cavity, notably smaller than the original volume of infarcted brain, traversed by a delicate meshwork of capillaries and surrounded by a zone of fibrillary gliosis (Fig. 2). This process is dependably stereotyped, regardless of the location or size of the infarct.

Many hypoxic/ischemic episodes are insufficiently prolonged or severe to produce true infarction, but may damage some vulnerable tissue elements. Neurons may be dispatched, either singly or in small clusters, while the rest of the tissue remains intact. The dead cells become eosinophilic, then shrink and disappear over several days. There is no inflammatory response, only occasional mild gliosis in the adjacent tissue. Hippocampal pyramidal cells and cerebellar Purkinje cells are exceptionally sensitive to mild or brief hypoxic insults (Fig. 3).

Hypoxic/ischemic injuries produce many combinations of neuronal and glial damage that are intermediate between the extremes of infarction and focal neuronal loss. They result in varying degrees of loss of myelin and axons, reactive astrocytosis, and tissue rarefaction that falls short of cavitation. These lesions produce a variety of clinical syndromes and appearances on computed tomography (CT) and magnetic resonance (MR) images, and have engendered new descriptive terms such as incomplete infarction (1) and leukoaraiosis (2, 3), as well as various interpretations of what constitutes "subcortical arteriosclerotic encephalopathy/ Binswanger's disease" (4, 5), and the lacunar state (6, 7).

ANATOMY OF THE MICROCIRCULATION AND ITS PATHOGENETIC IMPLICATIONS

The origin and distribution of perforating arteries to the deep cerebral gray matter and arteries to the brainstem are detailed in Chapters 2 and 3. Blood flow through these arteries may be impeded in several ways:

1. The lumen of individual arteries may become narrowed by atherosclerosis. Complete occlusion of one of these vessels produces the "classic" lacunar infarct as described by Fisher (8) (Figs. 4, 5).
2. The ostium of a branch point may become stenotic due to the atherogenic effects of local turbulence. This is particularly likely if the branch is at a sharp angle, which is typically seen in the deep penetrators (Fig. 6).
3. The parent artery from which the perforating branches arise may become similarly narrowed, lowering blood flow to the territory of many branches simultaneously. Superimposed acute occlusion of the parent artery produces large deep infarcts, with or without a cortical component (9) (Fig. 7).

These changes are not mutually exclusive; they usually occur together in various combinations. They produce cumulative re-

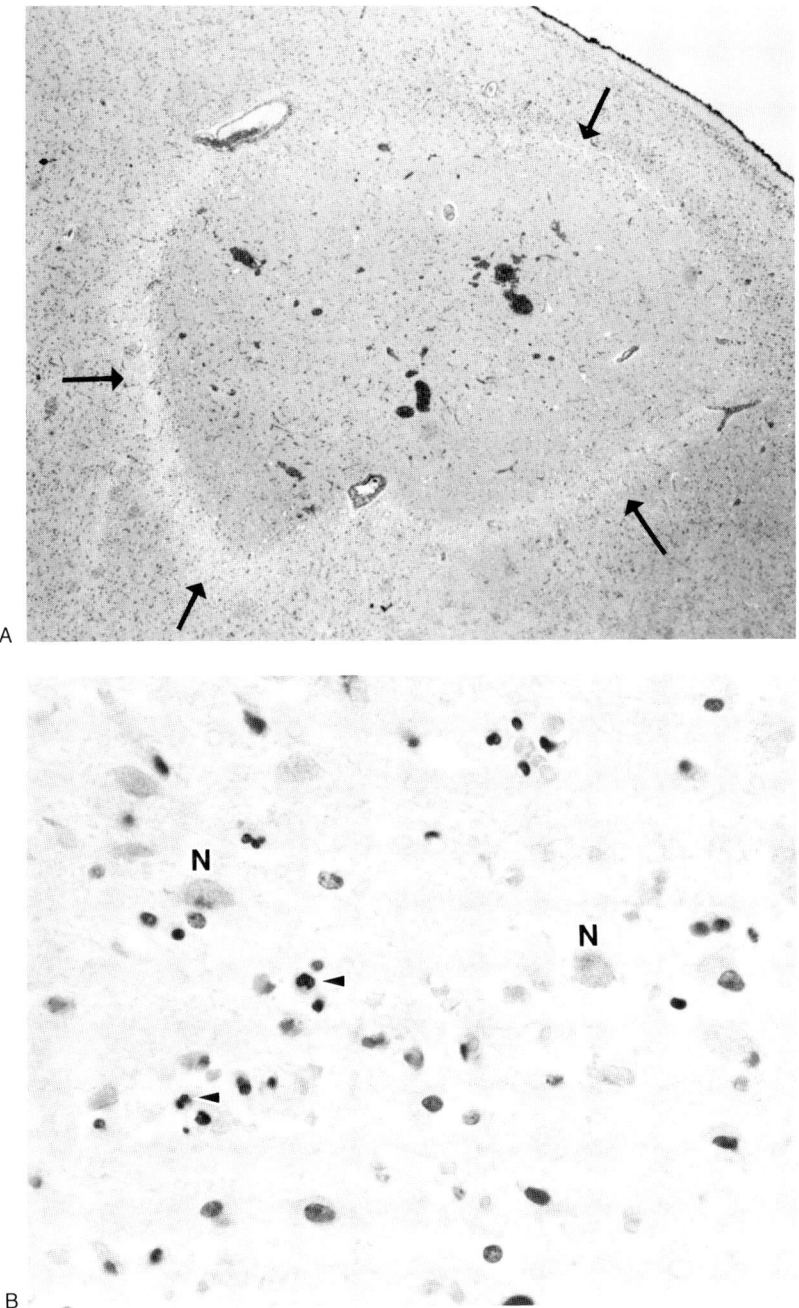

FIG. 1. Acute small deep infarct in caudate. **A:** Low power photomicrograph. *Arrows* point to edema at margin. **B:** High power photomicrograph of center of infarcted zone. Note ischemic neurons (N) and early infiltration by polymorphonuclear leukocytes (*arrows*).

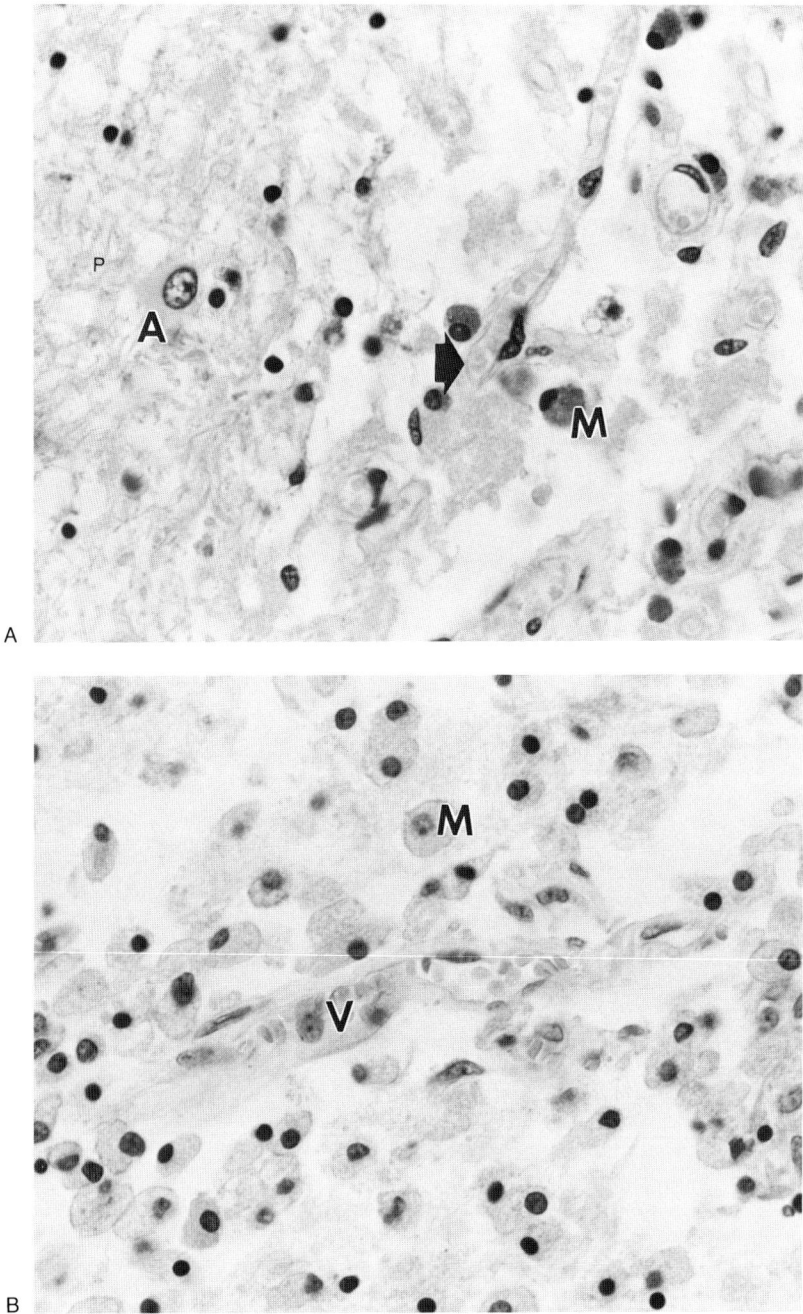

FIG. 2. Resolution of infarct. **A:** 7–10 days. Macrophages (M) accumulating; vessels growing in from margin (*arrow*); tissue fragmented; reactive astrocytes at margin **A**. **B:** 21 days. Loose network of delicate vessels (V) with macrophages (M).

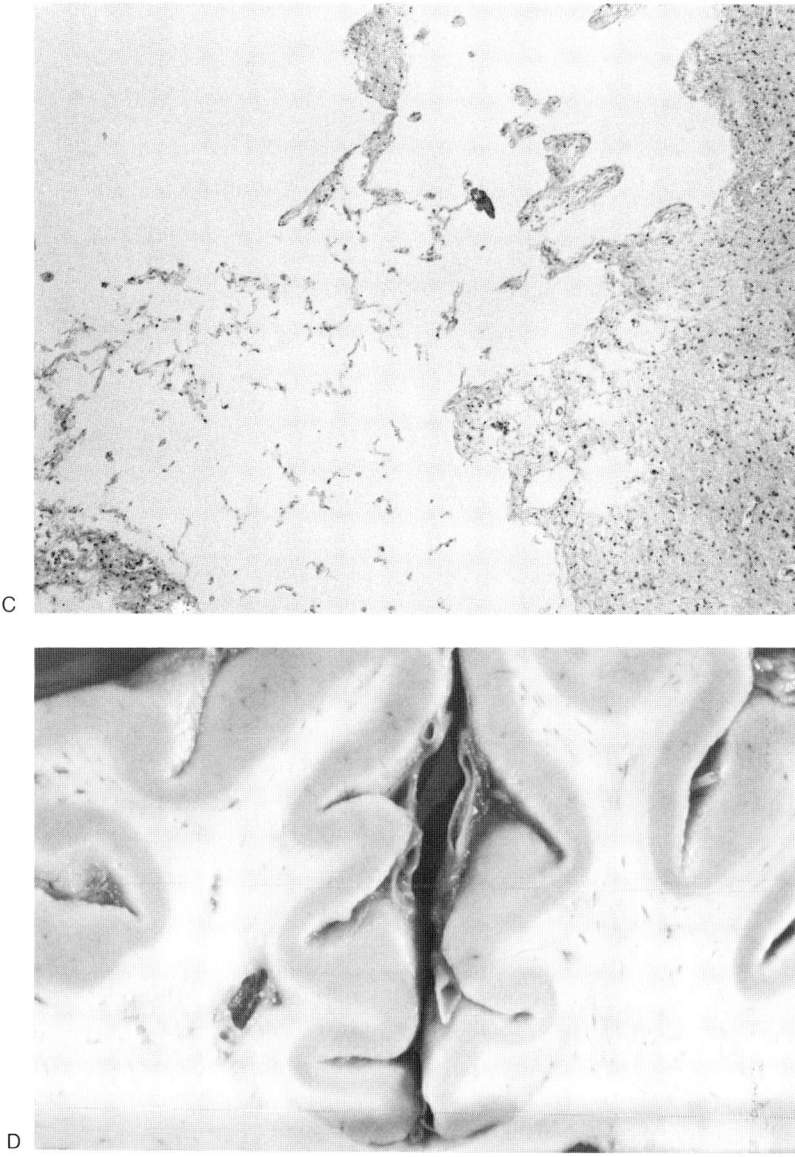

FIG. 2. *Continued*. **C:** 6 months. Cavity traversed by delicate meshwork of vessels with occasional residual macrophages. Gliotic margin. **D:** Gross photograph of cavitated infarct.

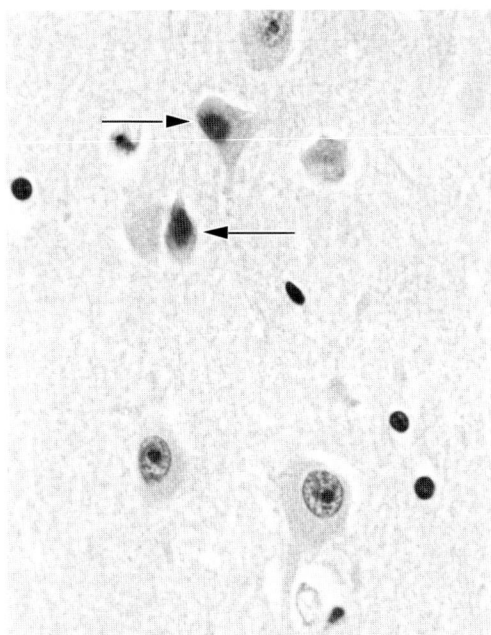

FIG. 3. Photomicrograph of hippocampus of patient who experienced brief cardiac arrest and resuscitation 1 day prior to death. Note cytoplasmic shrinkage and pyknosis of nuclei in some neurons, while others appear normal.

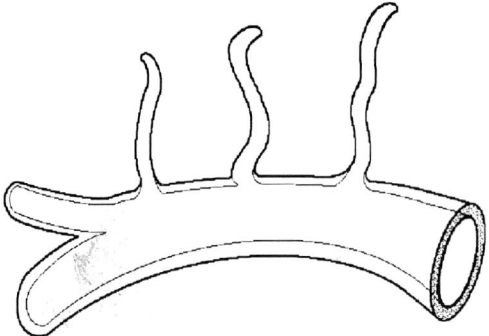

FIG. 4. Schematic diagram of origin of deep perforating branches from a parent artery.

ductions in flow, so that distal territories become highly vulnerable to superimposed proximal disease that falls short of total occlusion, or to systemic hypoxemia or hypotension (10). The prodigious diversity of these vascular lesions and of the underlying conditions and superimposed acute events that influence them easily explains the ungainly multitude of clinical syndromes attributed to small deep lesions.

After giving off their deep perforators, the main cerebral arteries continue as leptomeningeal arteries and ramify over the surface of the brain. Their adjacent distal territories form anastomotic border zones through which collateral circulation may flow. Individual pial arteries give off penetrating branches that extend into the cortex and white matter (Fig. 8). These comprise short and medium length cortical penetrators, which supply a rich cortical capillary network, long cortical penetrators, which supply the deep cortex and the subcortical U fibers, and white matter ("medullary") penetrators, which supply the gyral white matter and centrum semiovale, and terminate in border zones with deep perforators, notably in the periventricular regions and beneath the insula. The territories supplied by the pial penetrators may be damaged, either singly or in various combinations:

1. Narrowing or occlusion of a cortical penetrator produces a small area of necrosis. This ultimately results in a tiny collapsed cavity. The focal loss of cortical volume is seen as irregular narrowing of the cortical ribbon and minute pitting of the surface (Fig. 9). When this affects the territories of many nearby superficial penetrators, we describe the appearance as "granular atrophy."

2. A similar process in the white matter penetrators may lead to focal necrosis in their territories or, since these arteries have very few collaterals, may result in border zone hypoxia/ischemia in the white matter. This, in simplest terms, is the pathogenetic mechanism of "subcortical arteriosclerotic encephalopathy/ Binswanger's disease."

3. Systemic hypoxemia or hypotension may produce necrosis, either as an infarct in a border zone (11), or as "laminar necrosis," in which a linear zone of vulnerable

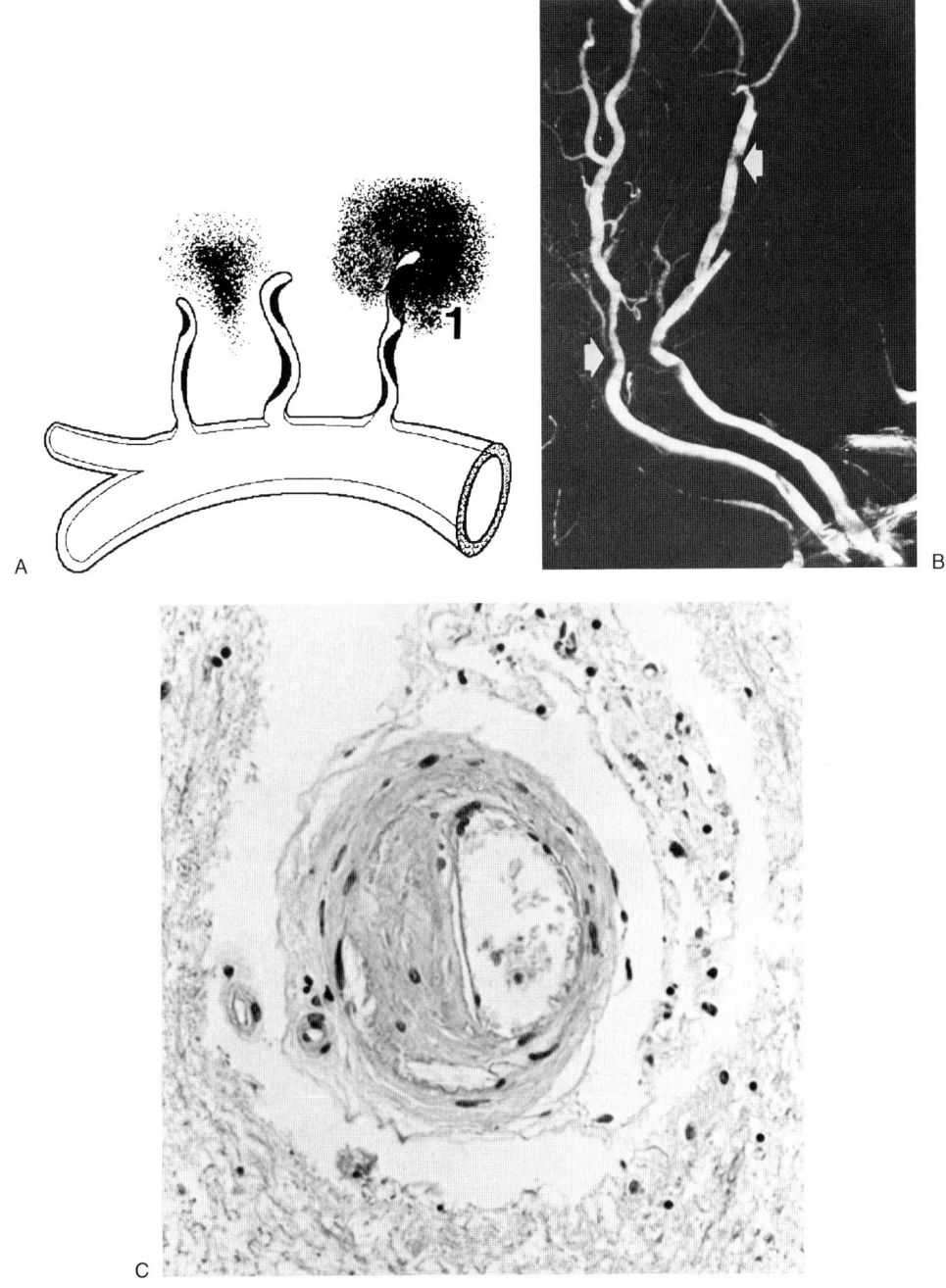

FIG. 5. A: Narrowing of perforating branches by microatheroma formation. Total occlusion of one branch (1) leads to infarction (stippled area) in its distal territory. The border zone between two adjacent narrowed vessels is vulnerable to systemic hypotension or hypoxemia. **B:** Post mortem microangiogram of perforating arteries with focal stenoses (*arrows*). **C:** Photomicrograph of microatheroma in a perforating vessel. Note eccentric narrowing of lumen.

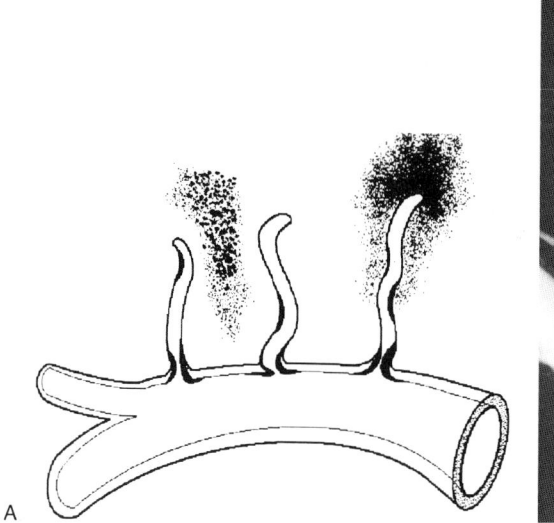
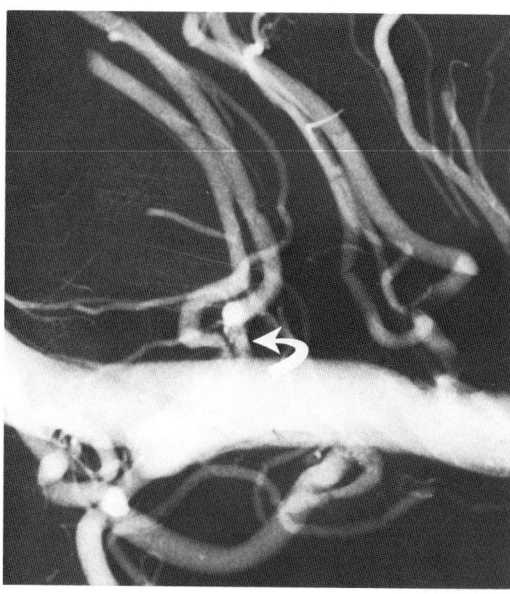

FIG. 6. A: Perforating branches with narrowing at ostia. Severe narrowing may produce infarction in the territory of a single branch, while border zone lesions may occur between arteries with moderate stenoses. **B:** Microangiogram of branch points showing narrowing of the ostia. *Arrow* points to focal narrowing of dye column in stenotic proximal portion of deep perforators.

tissue (perhaps related to specific length of the penetrators) is destroyed.

Again, these are not mutually exclusive, and are usually found in some combination. Of course, occlusive proximal vessel disease exacerbates their effects, and increases the likelihood of further hemodynamic consequences.

FACTORS THAT INFLUENCE THE DEVELOPMENT OF SMALL VESSEL LESIONS

Hypertension

Almost every cerebrovascular disorder—infarct, hemorrhage, Binswanger's disease—is more common and more severe in people whose blood pressure is too high (12–14). Yet these disorders do occur in normotensives, and similar vascular lesions are seen in normotensives. Hypertension, then, may be regarded as an aggravating and accelerating influence on degenerative vascular disease.

Throughout the body, hypertension has similar effects upon the "resistance vessels," small arteries and arterioles that are believed to regulate flow by maintaining tone. These effects consist of thickening of the muscular media and proliferation of the intima, with net reduction in the size of the lumen and increased resistance to flow. In arterioles, the medial thickening may include hyaline deposition, "hyaline arteriolosclerosis" (Fig. 10) thought to be due to insudation of plasma constituents into the wall. In more severe cases of hypertension, there may be necrotizing lesions such as fibrinoid necrosis or arteriolitis, which may weaken the vessel walls leading to local dilatation and extravasation. As arterial narrowing becomes severe, it leads to a dangerous decline in perfusion of the capillary bed, which can result in ischemia and infarction. On the bright side, however, the luminal narrowing probably has the salu-

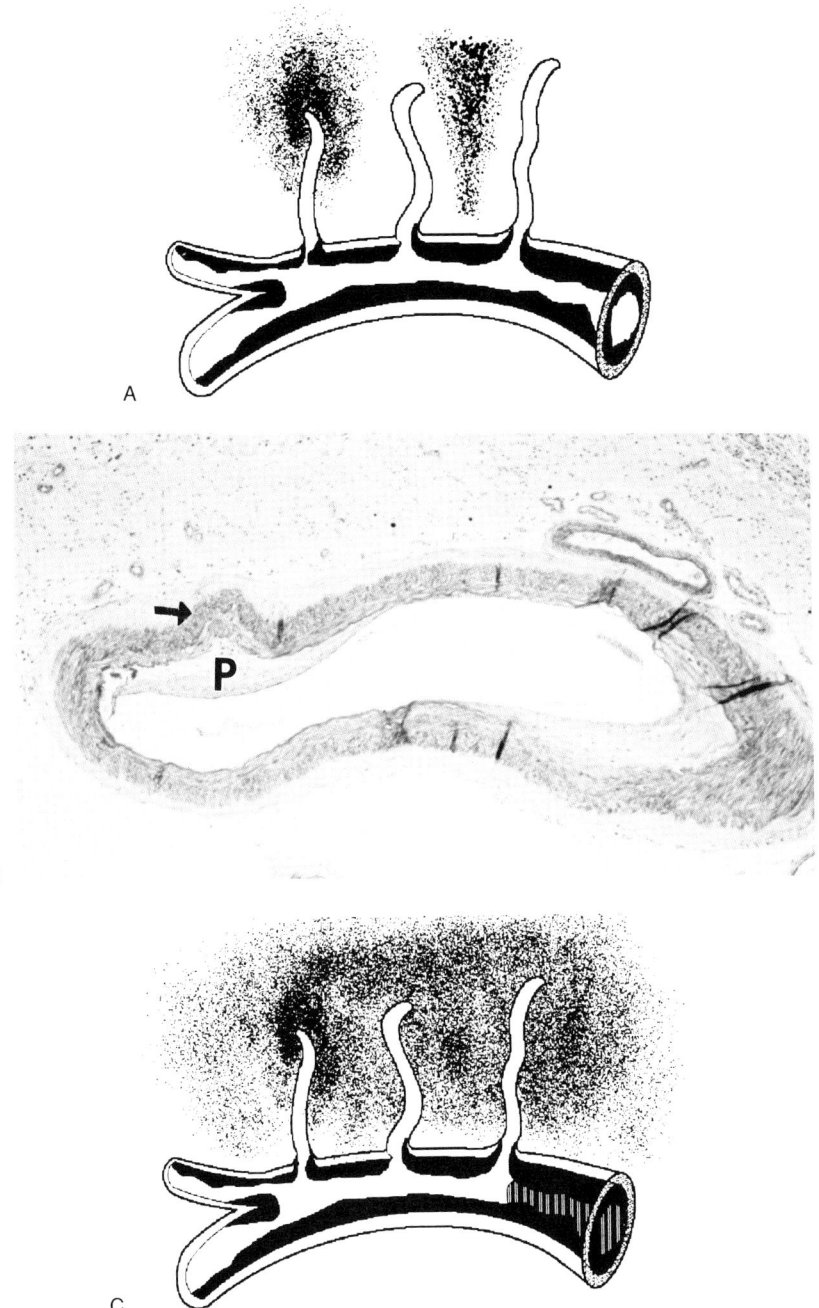

FIG. 7. A: Atherosclerotic narrowing of a parent artery. Plaques encroach upon branch points; as in the other examples, this may produce either distal infarction or border zone hypoperfusion. **B:** Atherosclerotic plaque (P) in artery occluding branch point (*arrow*). **C:** Proximal thrombus or embolus in atherosclerotic artery leads to large infarct in the territory of several perforators.

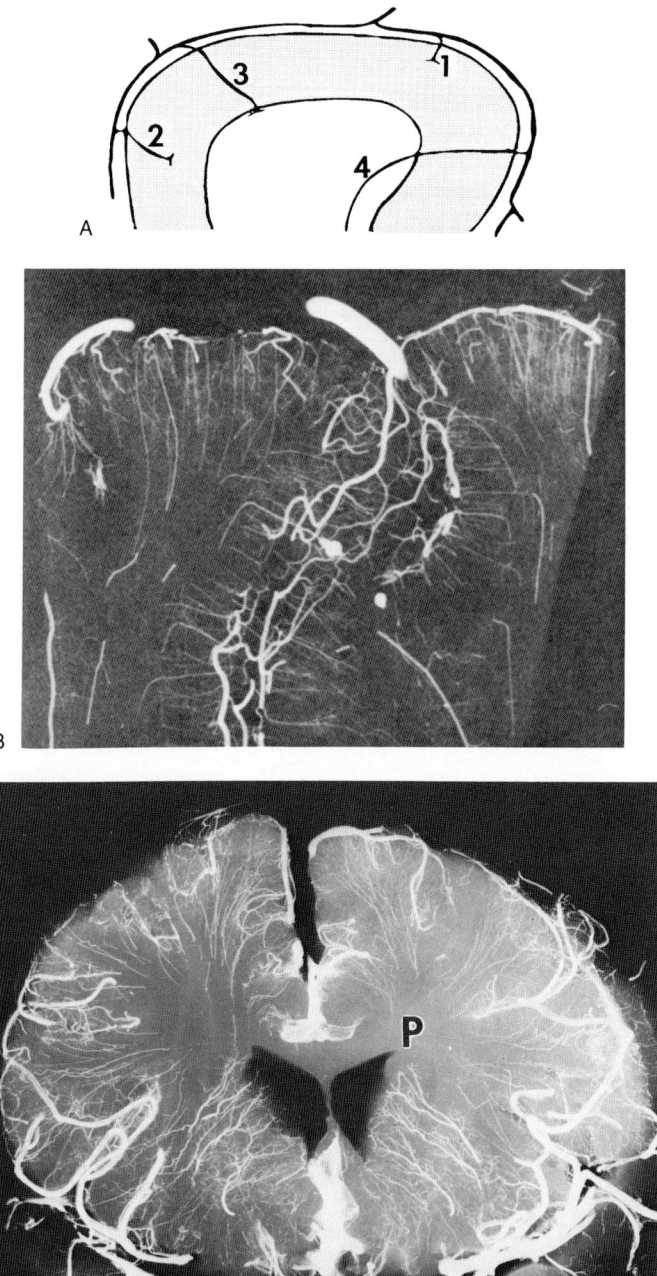

FIG. 8. A: Schematic drawing of a gyrus with a pial artery giving off (1) short, (2) medium, and (3) long cortical penetrators and (4) a white matter penetrator. **B:** Microangiogram of the arterial supply to 2 adjacent gyri. **C:** Angiogram of blood supply to hemisphere. Note border zones in periventricular (P) regions.

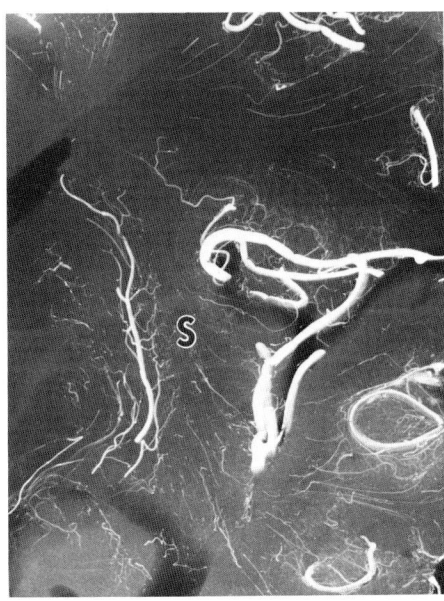

FIG. 8. *Continued.* **D:** Angiogram showing border zone (S) in subinsular region.

tary effect of protecting the capillary bed from pressures that would otherwise produce hemorrhage.

All these are routine, general pathologic findings in hypertension, seen in many organs. Does the brain have any unique lesions attributable to hypertension?

One candidate is the arterial lesion described by Fisher (8) as responsible for lacunes. He coined the term "segmental arterial disorganization" to denote a set of appearances that included "mural destruction, focal expansion of the vessel, thrombotic occlusion, hemorrhagic extravasation, and fibrinoid deposit." Fisher later included the term under the rubric of "lipohyalinosis", which he pointed out encompassed the previous designations "fibrinoid necrosis, hyaline arterionecrosis, atherosclerosis of small arteries, hyaline fatty change, plasmatic vascular destruction, hyalinosis, angionecrosis and fibrinoid arteritis" that had been used by others (15). Thus, the process of lipohyalinosis includes a continuum of alterations, from the earliest thickening of the vessel wall to progressive narrowing, poststenotic dilatation, thrombosis, fibrinoid necrosis, etc. Fisher identified true occlusive lesions in the vast majority of arteries associated with lacunes, with obliteration of the lumen by fibrous connective tissue, fibrinoid material, or apparent old organized thrombus. Many of these vessels also exhibited focal enlargements, "suggesting the formation of a microaneurysm presumably as a result of weakening of the wall." He did not claim these were aneurysms, since the arteries were occluded and there was no evidence that their lumens ever had been dilated. He proposed that the occlusions were responsible for the lacunar infarcts that were seen distal to these lesions. However, the infarcts he studied were old, and the destructive and occlusive components Fisher described may have represented *post hoc* changes that develop after an infarct occurs. Lipohyalinosis is probably a close cousin of the hypertensive lesions seen elsewhere in the body, rather than a hypertensive lesion unique to the brain.

Another possibly unique lesion is the miliary (Charcot-Bouchard) aneurysm, thought to be responsible for hypertensive

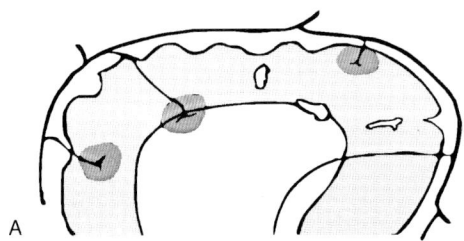

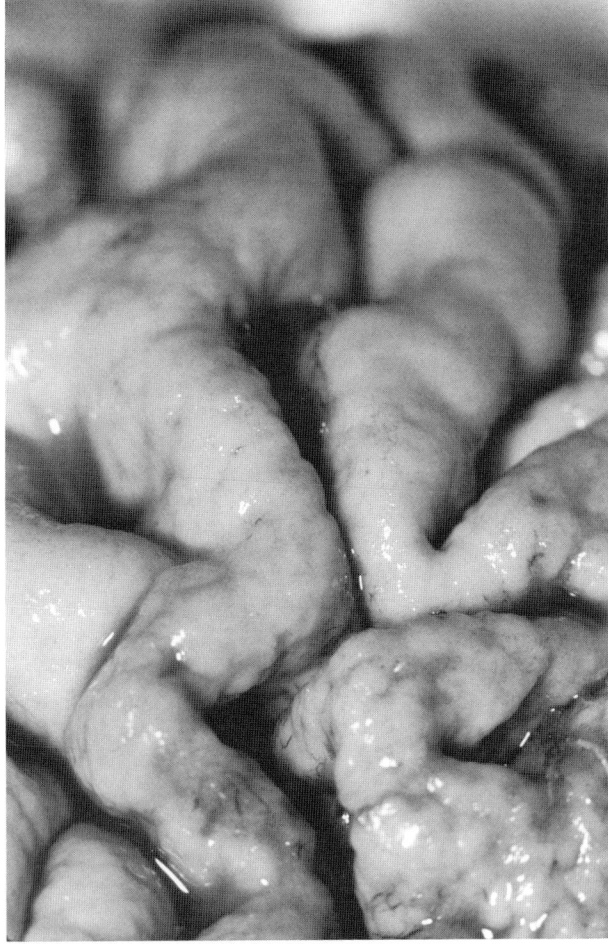

FIG. 9. A: Necrosis (*dark gray*) in the territories of individual pial penetrators leads to minute foci of cavitation (empty spaces). This results in irregular gyral shrinkage and surface indentation, producing the pattern known as granular atrophy. **B:** Surface of brain showing granular atrophy.

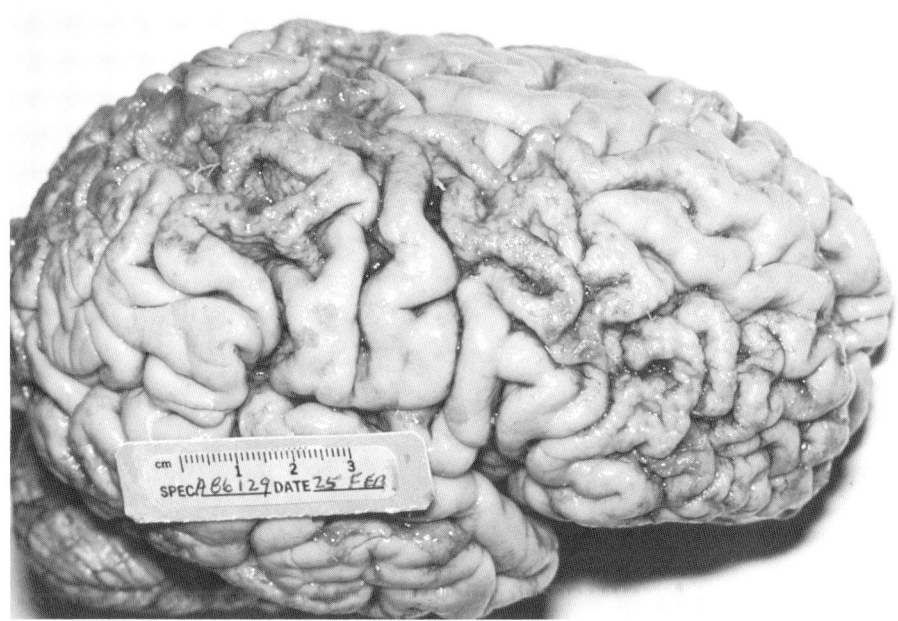

FIG. 9. Continued. **C:** Same brain as (**B**), showing that the granular atrophy is distributed in the arterial border zones.

intracerebral hemorrhage. Strong circumstantial evidence for that relationship was provided by Cole and Yates (16), who performed postmortem angiography on 100 brains from hypertensives and 100 brains from age-matched normotensive controls. Microaneurysms were found in 46 of the hypertensives and seven of the normotensives. In the hypertensives, aneurysms occurred as early as age 44, while the youngest normotensive patient with aneurysms was 66. Patients with aneurysms had a minimum of nine each, and the frequency of location of the aneurysms (deep gray > gray-white junction > pons > cerebellum) was comparable to the frequency of location of hypertensive hemorrhages. Microaneurysms have been reported by others in both autopsy (15, 17) and surgical (18) material, and it has been proposed that the aneurysms arise from the weakened walls of vessels with lipohyalinosis (19). If true, this points toward a convenient unifying concept, in that the lesions that presumably underlie both infarcts and hemorrhages arise from the same pathogenetic mechanism.

However, a recent report by Challa et al. (20) disputed the significance and prevalence of Charcot-Bouchard aneurysms. They used a histochemical stain that labelled the alkaline phosphatase of endothelial cells with a radiodense lead sulfide precipitate. Microradiographs of 500- or 1000-μm thick celloidin sections from brains of 35 hypertensive and 20 normotensive patients yielded elegant images of the arteriolar lumens. There were no aneurysms; instead, the vessels contained many tight coils and twists. The authors pointed out that previous investigators who identified microaneurysms by injection techniques might have been misled by artifacts. If the lumen of a tight coil is filled with contrast medium, an x-ray of the overlapping

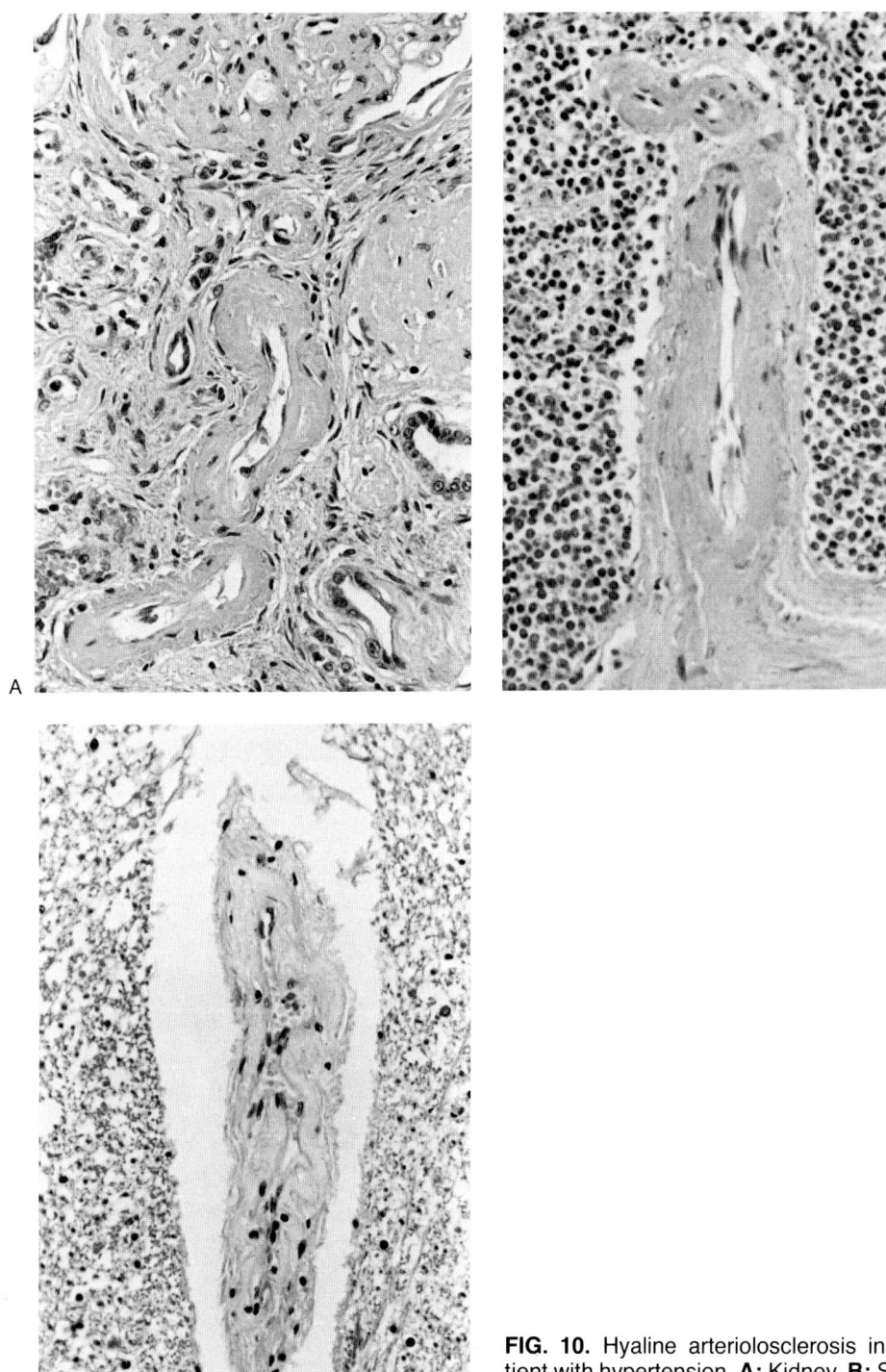

FIG. 10. Hyaline arteriolosclerosis in a patient with hypertension. **A:** Kidney. **B:** Spleen. **C:** Brain.

loop could be misinterpreted as showing a solid structure that would be called an aneurysm. Also, the pressure of the injection itself might suffice to produce localized bulges in the very thin-walled vessels. They noted that most pathologists have difficulty identifying Charcot-Bouchard aneurysms in histologic material, compared to the frequency of aneurysms reported in injection studies. Our experience agrees with this report. We have used a low viscosity lead/gelatin mixture injected at low pressure in 20 brains from hypertensive patients and have found several tightly coiled and tortuous vessels, but no microaneurysms (Fig. 11).

Coiling and tortuosity are not surprising findings, since hypertension lengthens the arteries. Hughes (21) referred to this process as "unfolding," and noted that it leads to displacement and kinking of branch points. Flow through tortuous or kinked vessels generates considerable turbulence, which engenders intimal thickening and fosters atheroma formation, especially at branch points (22). Again, this is not unique to the brain, and it occurs to a lesser extent in normotensive people with aging, but it represents a significant mechanism by which hypertension impedes flow through small cerebral arteries.

Diabetes

Diabetes mellitus produces well-known microvascular pathology. Hyaline arteriolosclerosis, the most common lesion, is more frequent and more severe in diabetics than in nondiabetics, but is also associated with hypertension. A more specific change in diabetes is thickening of capillary basement membranes (23), which leads to noteworthy lesions in the kidney and the retina. Microangiopathy has also been implicated in the pathogenesis of diabetic neuropathy, and one may speculate on its possible effects on cerebral perfusion.

Diabetes has been reported to be associated with both lacunar and nonlacunar infarction (see Chapter 12). Aronson (24) studied a series of 5,479 consecutive adult autopsies, which included 677 diabetics, and noted that diabetes was associated with an increased frequency of small deep infarcts. He noted that the exacerbating effect of diabetes seemed to be greater in the posterior fossa, with diabetics exhibiting a threefold increase in the incidence of pontine lacunes. Aronson also noted that both intracerebral hemorrhages and fibrinoid necrosis of small arteries were less common in diabetics than in nondiabetics, and that among patients who suffered fatal intracerebral hemorrhages, the average age of diabetics was considerably higher than that of nondiabetics. He speculated that diabetic microangiopathy might induce a structural change that deters the subsequent effects of hypertension (fibrinoid necrosis) upon the same arteries.

Amyloid Angiopathy

Cerebral amyloid angiopathy (CAA) is characterized by the deposition of amyloid protein in the adventitia and outer media of leptomeningeal vessels, small arteries, and arterioles of the outer cerebral cortex (Fig. 12). Vessels of the cerebellum are affected to a lesser degree. Deep white matter penetrators and vessels supplying the deep gray matter are usually spared. A striking association between CAA and Alzheimer's disease (AD) (25) led to the suggestion that the vascular amyloid might play a pathogenetic role in the formation of AD plaque amyloid, but this has been disputed (26). Amyloid angiopathy is strongly related to aging; it is virtually never seen in persons younger than 60 years of age and increases in incidence with increasing age (27). It has also been seen in patients with a variety of conditions, including hemorrhage, infarction, vasculitides, and leukoencephalopathy (28).

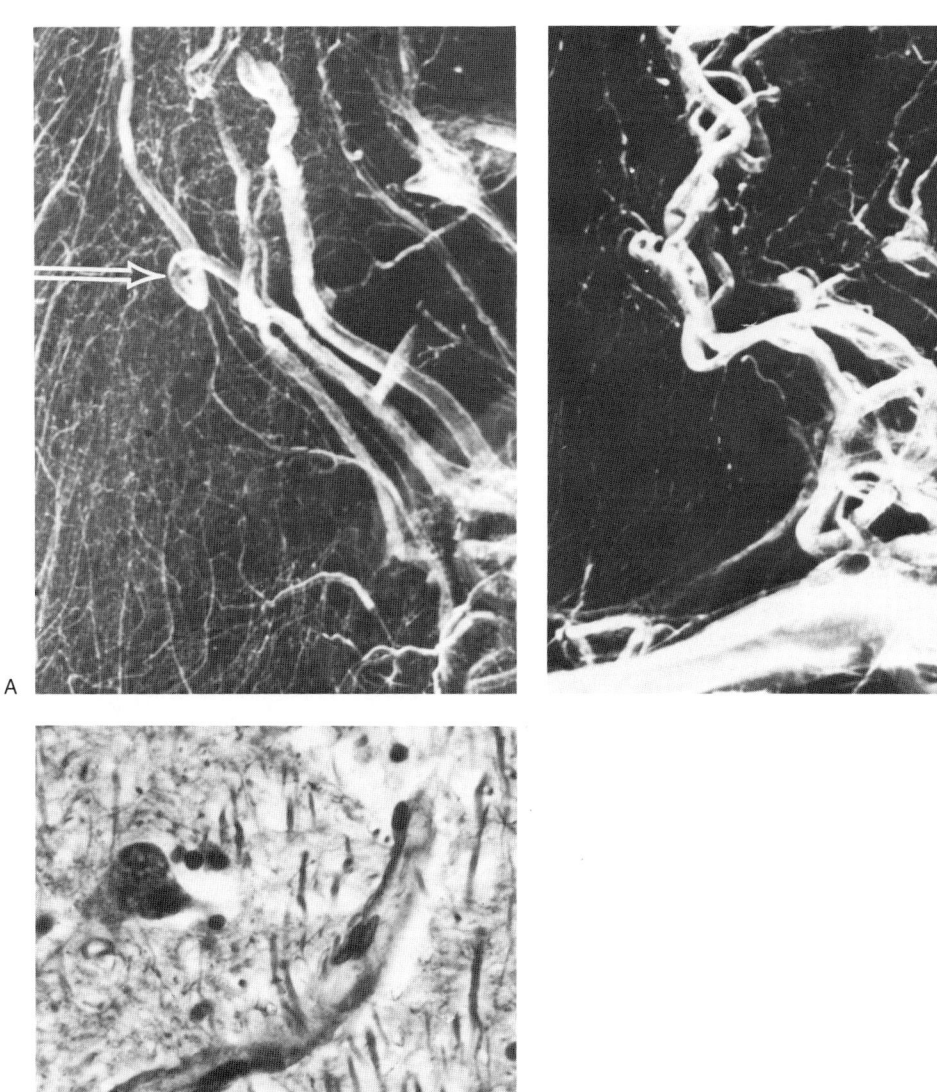

FIG. 11. **A** and **B:** Post-mortem angiograms of brain from a hypertensive patient. **A:** tight loop in deep basal perforator (*arrow*). **B:** tortuous small arteries. **C:** Photomicrograph of a coiled arteriole.

Both sporadic and familial forms of CAA have become recognized as causes of spontaneous intracerebral hemorrhage. The sporadic form tends to occur in elderly individuals, many of whom also have some combination of hypertension and diabetes, so that its relative pathogenetic importance may be difficult to discern. However, when Vinters (28) reviewed 20 previous reports comprising 107 cases of CAA with hemorrhage, he noted that, with rare exception, the hemorrhages occurred in the cortex and subcortical white matter. This superficial location was frequently associated with spread to the subarachnoid space. Thus, the hemorrhages seen in CAA exhibit the same geographic distribution as the angiopathy. This contrasts starkly with the lo-

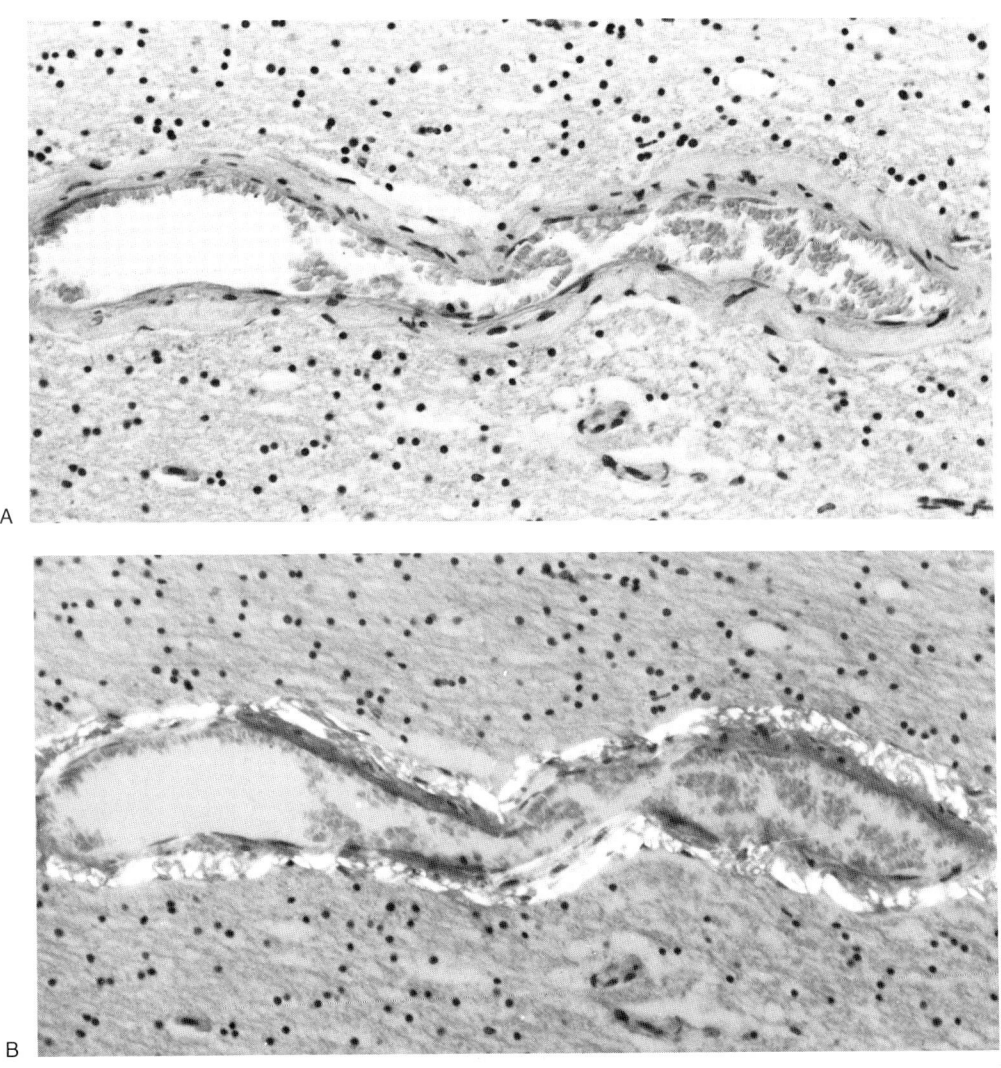

FIG. 12. Amyloid angiopathy in superficial artery. **A:** Congo red stain for amyloid. The vessel wall appears thickened similar to hyaline arteriosclerosis. **B:** Same section viewed with polarized light. Amyloid is seen in the outer aspects of the wall.

cation of typical hypertensive intracerebral hemorrhages, which most commonly occur in the deep gray matter and are more likely to rupture into the lateral ventricles. Some hemorrhages followed relatively minor head trauma, suggesting that the amyloid-laden superficial vessels are brittle or fragile.

The familial variants, known as hereditary cerebral hemorrhage with amyloidosis, tend to affect younger individuals. They also demonstrate geographic correspondence between the hemorrhages and the affected vessels, and are not related to hypertension or Alzheimer's disease, reinforcing the intuitive assumption that amyloid deposition weakens the vessel wall.

Amyloid angiopathy also narrows the lumen, thus impeding blood flow in a manner similar to hypertensive or diabetic changes. Accordingly, these lesions may result in various forms of hypoxic/ischemic injury, including small infarcts and leukoencephalopathy (29).

Vasculitides and Miscellaneous Conditions

Vasculitis, autoimmune disorders, and infectious agents may afflict the small cerebral vessels. They all involve some form of injury to the arterial wall, followed by a characteristically modified inflammatory response and repair process. Like arteriosclerosis, vasculitis may produce obstruction or dilatation of the artery and lead to similar ischemic or hemorrhagic consequences.

The vasculitides are of unknown etiology and have overlapping clinical syndromes as well as similarities in their histopathology. They tend to affect vessels of particular size and location. Two conditions that have a predilection for small arteries are polyarteritis nodosa (PAN) and granulomatous angiitis of the nervous system (GANS). Clinically, PAN is a systemic disease and can be differentiated from GANS by involvement of other organs, especially the kidney, heart, liver, and gastrointestinal tract (30). Lesions are commonly seen at all stages of organization. Small arteries and arterioles undergo segmental fibrinoid necrosis, which may involve the full thickness of the wall. There is a dense neutrophilic infiltrate in and around the vessel wall. This often results in small aneurysm formation (31), and there may also be thrombosis of the lumen. Healing involves fibroblast proliferation, which may extend into the periphery, producing the characteristic nodularity. GANS is by definition a primary central nervous system (CNS) vasculitis, segmentally affecting meningeal vessels, small parenchymal arteries and arterioles, and veins (32). Branch points of vessels are preferred sites. The lesions have a predominantly mononuclear cell infiltrate; multinucleated giant cells may be present, but are not necessary for the diagnosis (33). Again, the net result will be some combination of focal obstruction and dilatation.

Among the rheumatologic disorders, systemic lupus erythematosis (SLE) shows great predilection for clinical CNS involvement. The pathologic findings often seem disproportionately sparse with respect to the symptoms. When vasculitis is present, it affects very small vessels (< 100 μm in diameter), producing focal fibrinoid necrosis and/or eccentric thickening of the wall, with a surrounding lymphocytic infiltrate. Occasionally, the existence of such a lesion may be inferred from the discovery of a small "ring hemorrhage" in the perivascular space, which is presumptive evidence of focal damage and extravasation at a site proximal or distal to the section examined. Although active vasculitis is uncommon, the brain frequently exhibits multiple small infarcts (34). An autopsy study of 50 cases suggested that brain lesions may be due to emboli from either valvular vegetations or mural thrombi (35). However, the functional abnormalities may not occur solely on a hemodynamic basis. Immunologic studies have identified immune complexes in the cerebrospinal fluid (CSF) of SLE patients with active CNS disease. Antineuronal antibodies that cross-react with lymphocytes are present in the CSF and serum in active CNS lupus (36,37). These findings indicate the possibility of direct autoimmune damage to the nervous system in SLE.

A substantial proportion of patients with SLE and about 2% of the general population produce an anticardiolipin antibody, which is one of many antiphospholipid antibodies (38). Persons with this antibody may exhibit the anticardiolipin syndrome, which is characterized by recurrent spontaneous abortions, thrombocytopenia, arterial and venous thromboses, livedo reticularis, Coomb's positivity, false-positive VDRL, and cardiac and neurologic manifestations (39). Among 80 patients with the syndrome, 25 had neurologic symptoms, 16 of these had cerebral infarcts. CT scan showed the majority of the lesions to be small and cortical (40). We have examined two patients with this syndrome at autopsy. One had superior sagittal sinus thrombosis followed by posterior cerebral artery thrombosis with a large occipital lobe infarct, as well as multiple microscopic foci of ischemia in the cortex and centrum semiovale. Our other patient, who had been on long-term anticoagulant therapy, had multiple bilateral subdural hematomas and a small superficial cerebellar hematoma.

Vasculitis also has been seen following drug abuse, particularly of amphetamines, either alone or in combination with other drugs (41), and more recently in cocaine abuse (42). Amphetamines produce a necrotizing arteritis resembling PAN, while cocaine causes small artery lesions characterized by endothelial swelling and intramural and perivascular lymphocytic infiltration without necrosis. This was seen in a biopsy sample from a patient who presented 10 days earlier with multifocal signs and symptoms and several lesions identified by MR imaging in the basal ganglia and deep white matter.

SPECIFIC BRAIN LESIONS ASSOCIATED WITH SMALL ARTERY DISEASE

While the individual vasculopathies have some distinguishing clinical and/or pathologic features, their resultant effects on blood flow through the afflicted vessels and on the tissues they supply are hearteningly similar. Thus, the pathology of the brain lesions is qualitatively rather limited. In spite of this, or perhaps because of it, a bewildering lexicon of terms has been created, with the apparent aim of separating lesions according to quantitative criteria (i.e., severity of ischemic episode, size, location, etc.), or as distinct clinicopathologic entities. These have some utility, in that they foster a disciplined approach to functional anatomy. However, to the neuropathologist who faces the daunting task of finding the elusive lesions that "must be there" to correspond to a patient's signs and symptoms, or to the clinician who, when presented with an unexpected discovery, can only say, "It must have been asymptomatic," the current and emerging jargon seems overly doctrinaire. Modern imaging techniques compound this dilemma when they recognize subtle "new" lesions that cry out for clinical and pathologic explication. Thus, the first chapter of this book concludes with the statement that ". . . it is likely that many small deep infarcts seen on imaging are not what neuropathologists call lacunes."

Let us examine some of these terms in the context of basic principles of pathology.

Necrosis: Small Deep Infarcts Versus Lacunes

Figure 13A illustrates irregular trabeculated cavities produced by the organization

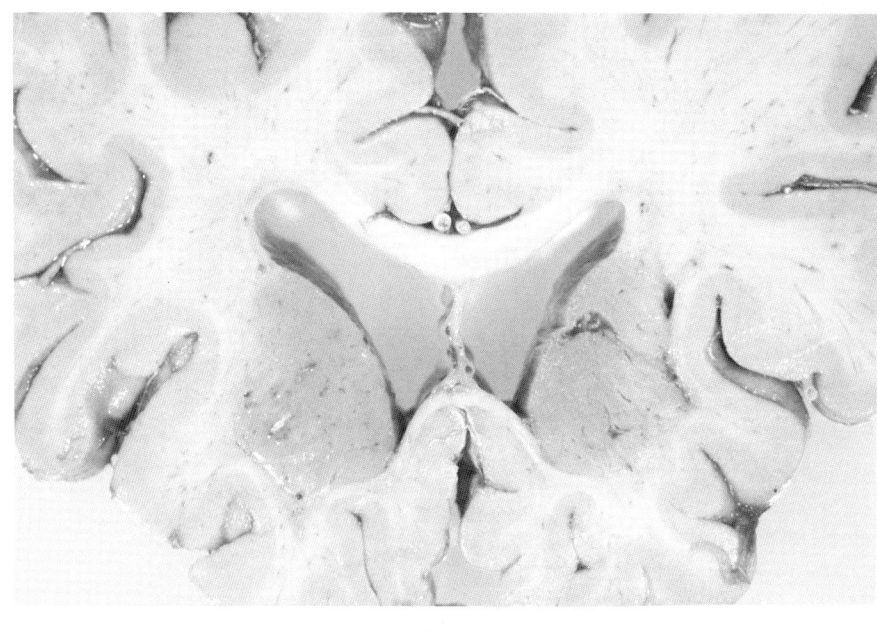

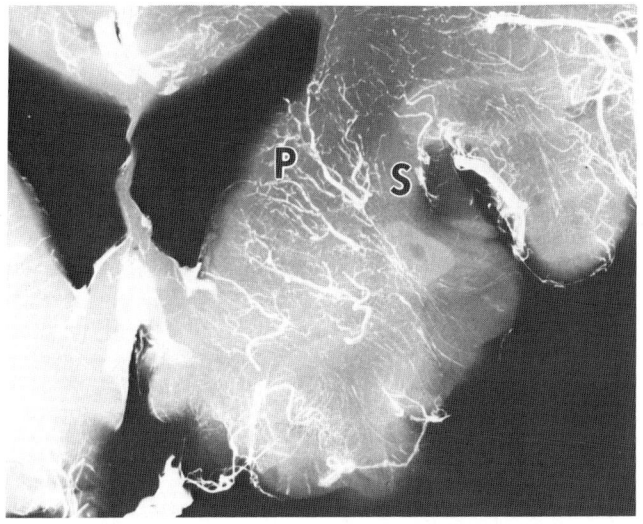

FIG. 13. Small deep infarcts **A:** Coronal brain slice with small cavities in the caudate and beneath the insula. **B:** Angiogram of slice in **A,** showing that the area of the caudate infarct is in the territory of a perforating artery (P), while the subinsular lesions are in a border zone (S) between deep and pial circulations.

of small infarcts. Are they lacunes? The current popular use of the term "lacune" can be traced to Fisher's 1965 article (43), in which the title, "Lacunes: Small Deep Cerebral Infarcts," seems to equate the two entities. Later, however, Fisher examined serial sections and noted that most lacunes were associated with a totally occluded branch of a penetrating artery (8). Thus, the term lacune became restricted, and is now generally used to denote small deep infarcts that are in (or are assumed to be in) the territory of a single occluded penetrator artery (6,7,44). Is that appropriate?

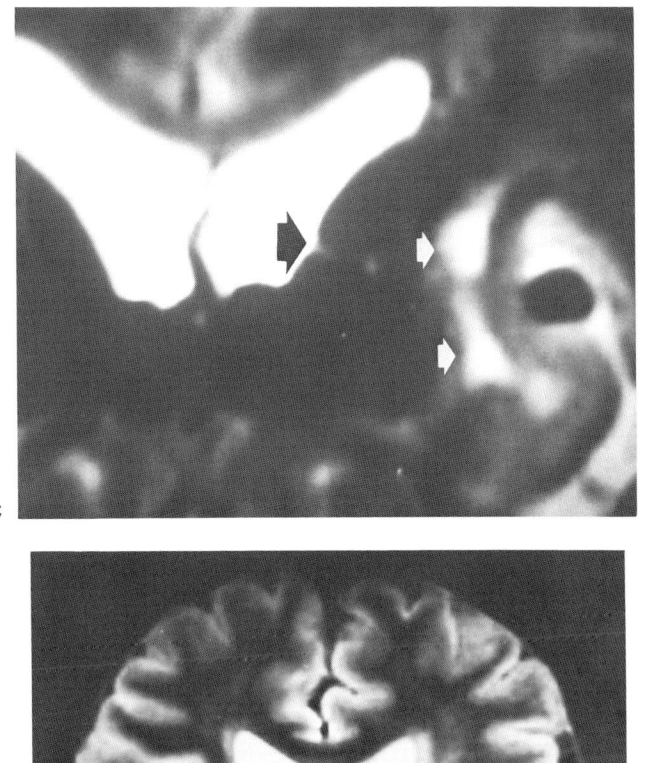

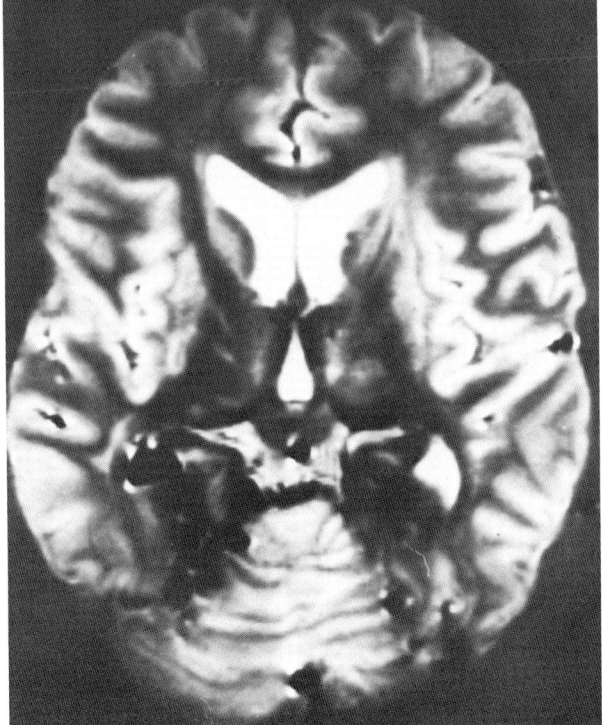

FIG. 13. *Continued.* **C:** Coronal MR image of slice in **A**, showing hyperintensities in cavitated areas (arrows). **D:** Axial MR image showing linear nature of the subinsular lesion.

Figures 5–7 illustrate schematically how small deep infarcts may be produced by various commonly encountered processes. Total occlusion is not necessary, and ischemic necrosis may occur in border zones, rather than in single artery territories. Furthermore, a cavitary lesion produced by ischemic necrosis in a single artery territory is histologically indistinguishable from one that occurs in a border zone. Why not call all of them (or none of them) lacunes? Figures 13B, C, and D illustrate the postmortem MR images and angiograms of the brain in Figure 13A, and demonstrate that one of the lesions may be regarded as occupying the territory of a single vessel, while the others are clearly in a border zone. When a small deep infarct is identified *in vivo* by imaging, it is impossible to be certain whether it is in the territory of a single vessel. Small deep infarcts are seldom fatal, and even at autopsy, most "lacunes" are not thoroughly investigated, so that the claim that "involvement of the territory of one single penetrator defines lacunar infarction pathologically" (44) is largely unsubstantiated.

Regarding vascular occlusion as the cause of lacunes, Fisher, in his painstaking observations of serial sections, was unable to identify occlusive lesions in many instances. He noted that some arteries that ran to the region of infarcts were normal, and inferred that they must once have been occluded by emboli "because emboli generally undergo lysis" (45). This argument seems rather circular, and the finding of a "normal" artery does not exclude other causes of transient hypoperfusion or hypoxemia. Challa et al. used their thick section/alkaline phosphatase technique to study the vascular lesions associated with lacunes in 15 hypertensive patients (46). They found variable narrowing of arteries due to intimal hyperplasia or atherosclerosis in the vast majority, rather than the occlusions described by Fisher. They also noted that a striking proportion (39%) of lacunes occurred in the white matter, and suggested that the natural history of lacunes might have changed since Fisher's earliest reports. Dozono et al. (13) reviewed 532 autopsy cases with lacunes, and noted that the white matter, particularly of the frontal lobe, was the most frequent site. They studied large coronal sections from 200 patients with lacunes in the deep white matter. Occlusions were rare, and the number and distribution of lacunes was related to hyaline arteriolosclerosis in the medullary arteries, rather than to necrotizing lesions or lipohyalinosis.

The meaning of the term lacune has been further clouded by attempts to broaden it to include other cavities found in the brain and lesions seen on imaging studies. Old small hemorrhages and dilated perivascular spaces (Fig. 14) have been called type II and type III lacunes, respectively, by Poirier et al. (47) in a classification system described in Chapter 1, but neither of these is produced by ischemic necrosis. Hemosiderin-laden macrophages indicative of minor extravasation are often seen in old infarct cavities, but a hematoma organizes differently, usually producing a relatively smooth-walled cavity that is not traversed by delicate vessels. Dilated perivascular spaces have been the subject of wild speculation about their origin (see Chapter 6). They appear utterly unrelated, except as coincidence, to small deep infarcts. The variety of conditions included under the term lacunar syndrome has also dramatically increased. Fisher has reviewed over 70 clinical presentations (48) that may be attributed to lacunar infarction, but Bogousslavsky regarded the vast majority as "not specific at all for lacunar infarction" (44).

We confront a situation in which the term lacune either indiscriminately encompasses far too much, without rigorous definition, or is too restricted, admitting some small deep infarcts but not others. Why use a classification system in which, after reading

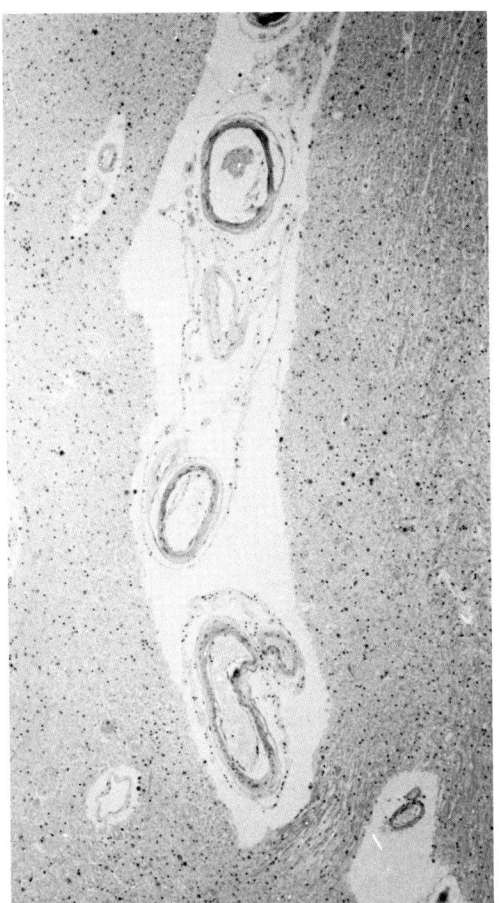

FIG. 14. Dilated perivascular spaces. This appearance has been referred to as "état criblé", or the "cribriform state."

Neuropathologists call small deep cavitated infarcts lacunes, and will probably continue to do so, if only for the economy of verbiage. They are regarded as the result of ischemic necrosis, but it is impractical to determine whether every lacune discovered at autopsy resulted from occlusion of a single artery or hypoperfusion of a border zone. Indeed, many lacunes are missed on routine dissection, since the average diameter of a lacune is smaller than the usual thickness of the brain slice at autopsy. For example, Challa et al. acknowledged that about three fourths of the lacunes in their study were not seen grossly, but were found incidentally in the microscopic sections (46). Accordingly, postmortem MR images have become useful guides to brain dissection, and their importance is likely to increase. When combined with postmortem angiography, they help identify deep ischemic lesions and elucidate their distribution and vascular supply (50). Thus, linear MR hyperintensities in the subinsular region were found to be due to confluent cavities in the border zone between cortical and basal penetrating arteries (51) (Fig. 13D).

that a lesion is a type IIIb lacune, you must then pause to recall whether that means it is a "real" lacune? Why use "lacunar" to mean small, when, as Landau points out (49), lacunes themselves have been described as small, medium, large, and giant? In fact, the reported size of a real lacune (i.e., a small deep infarct) is always conditional. When acute, they are swollen, appearing larger than the actual area of damage; when organized, the cavity occupies only a small fraction of the original volume of destroyed tissue.

Hypoxic/Ischemic Noninfarcts: Subcortical Arteriosclerotic Encephalopathy/Binswanger's Disease; Leukoaraiosis

Since there is a continuum of severity in small vessel disease, and since gradual narrowing along the arteries leads to a cumulative decrement in perfusion which becomes critical in distal territories, the occurrence of ischemic lesions that fall short of infarction is not surprising. Such lesions in the white matter have long been recognized as the hallmarks of Binswanger's disease or "subcortical arteriosclerotic encephalopathy" (see Chapter 11). The tissue changes characteristically include variable loss of axons and myelin,

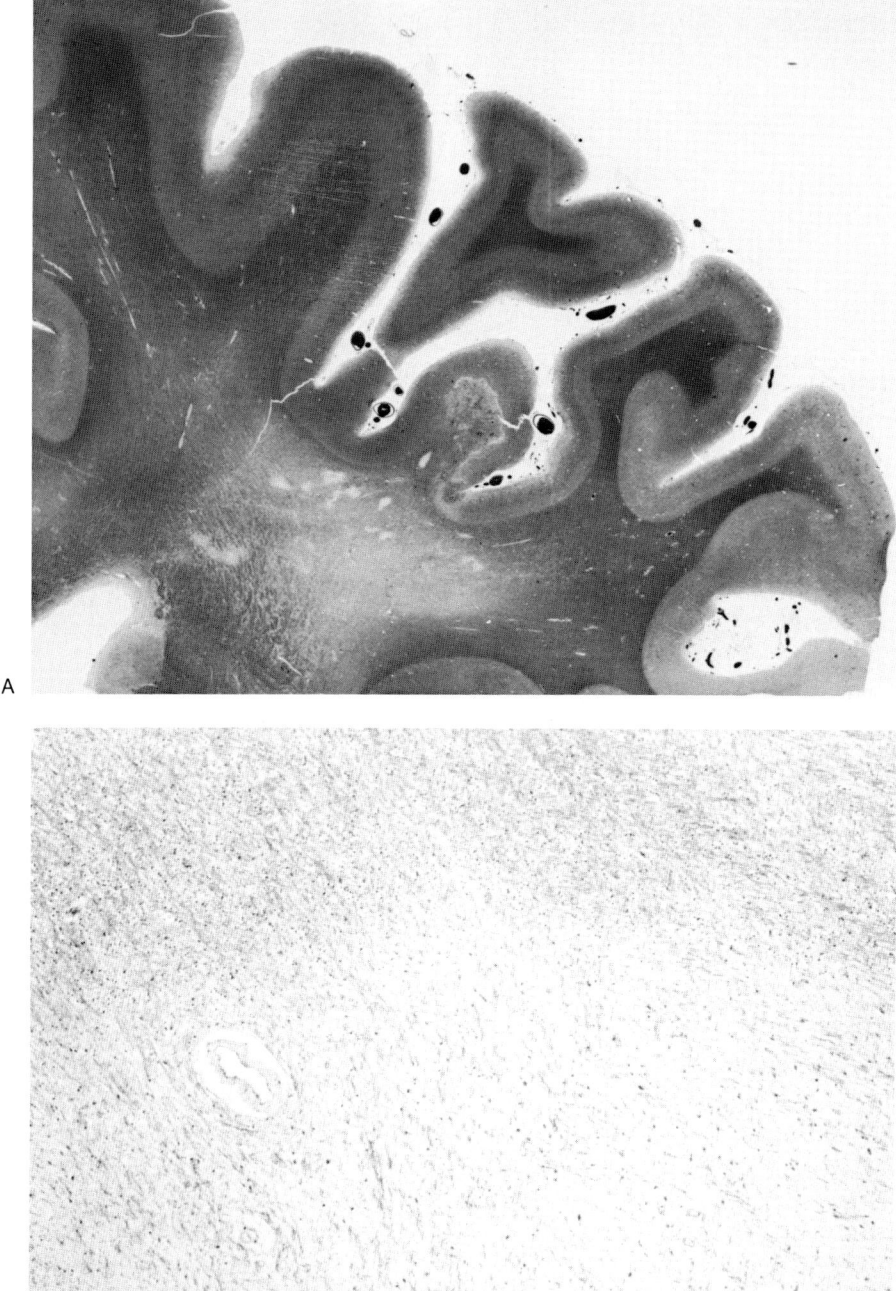

FIG. 15. Subcortical arteriosclerotic encephalopathy/Binswanger's disease. **A:** Section of hemisphere showing attenuation of deep white matter. Luxol fast blue stain for myelin. **B:** Low power photomicrograph at edge of affected periventricular area showing attenuation of white matter (*bottom right*).

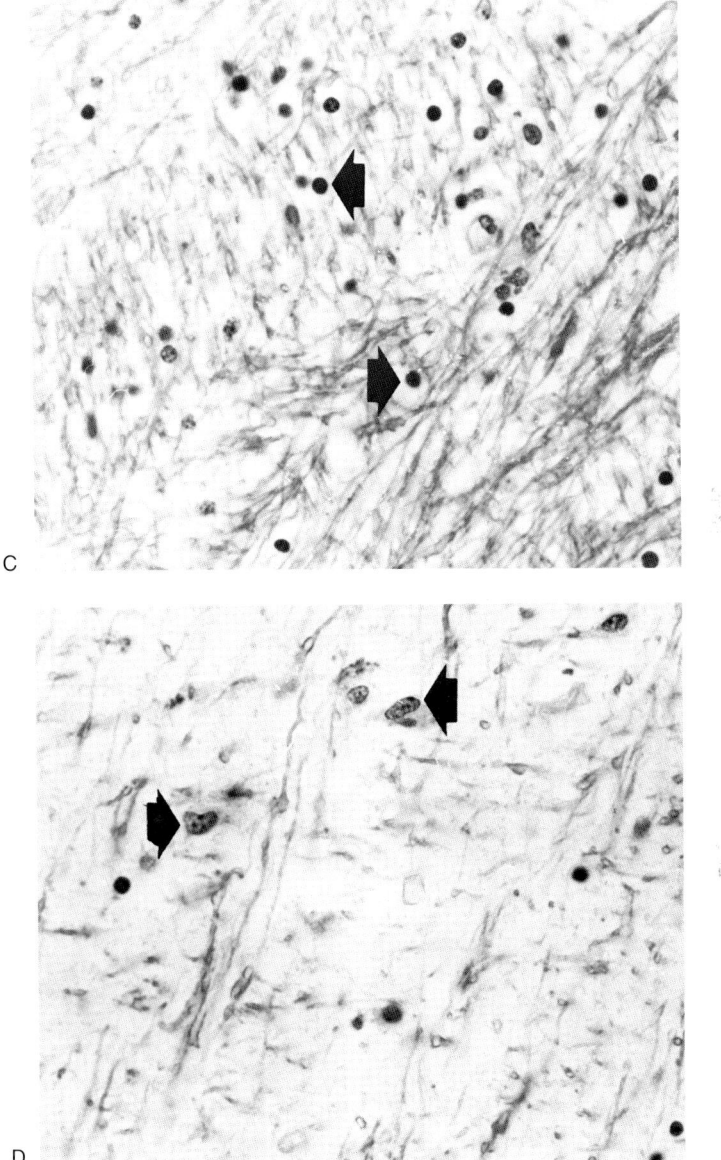

FIG. 15. *Continued.* **C:** Intact white matter showing normal density of myelin sheaths and numerous oligodendroglial cells (arrows). **D:** Affected white matter, showing reduction of myelin sheaths and oligodendroglial cells, and reactive astrocytes (arrows).

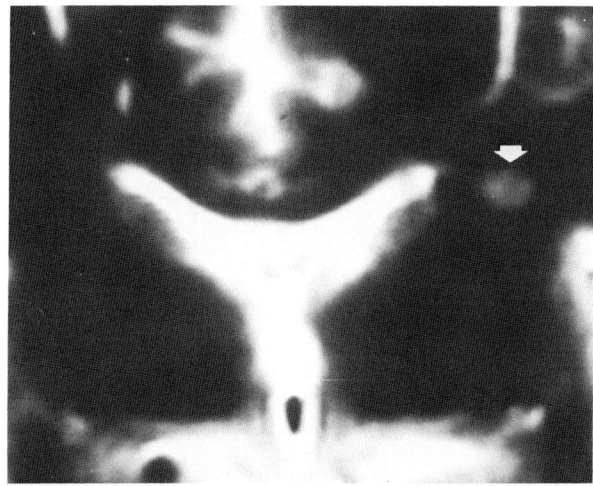
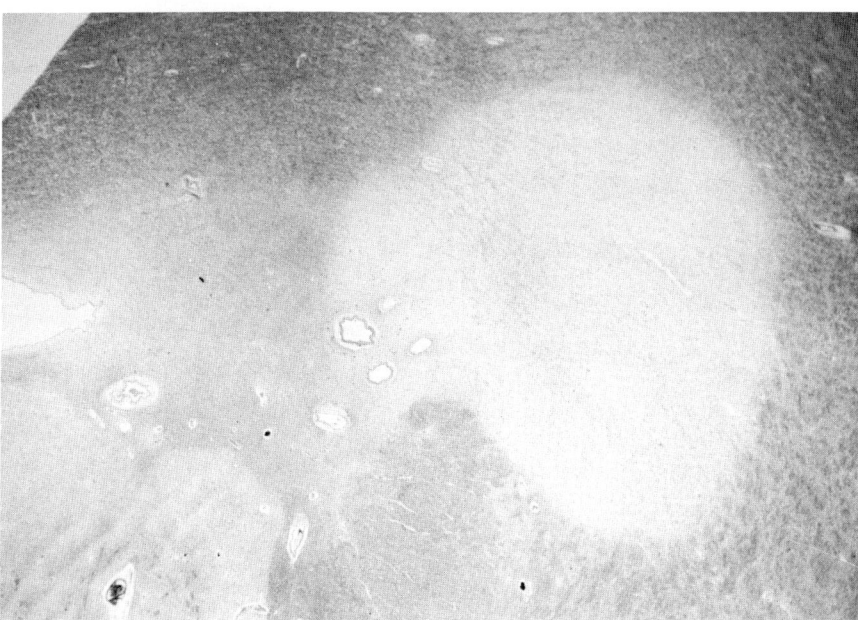

FIG. 16. "Leukoaraiosis" (**A** and **B**) vs. border zone infarct (lacune?) in white matter (**C, D,** and **E**). **A:** MR image showing focal hyperintensity in periventricular zone. **B:** Low power photomicrograph showing rarefaction of white matter similar to that in Figure 15. **C:** MR image showing lesion in white matter. **D:** Photograph of section of hemisphere showing acute infarct. **E:** Angiogram of slice showing that the infarct is in the border zone between basal perforators and pial circulation from anterior and middle cerebral arteries.

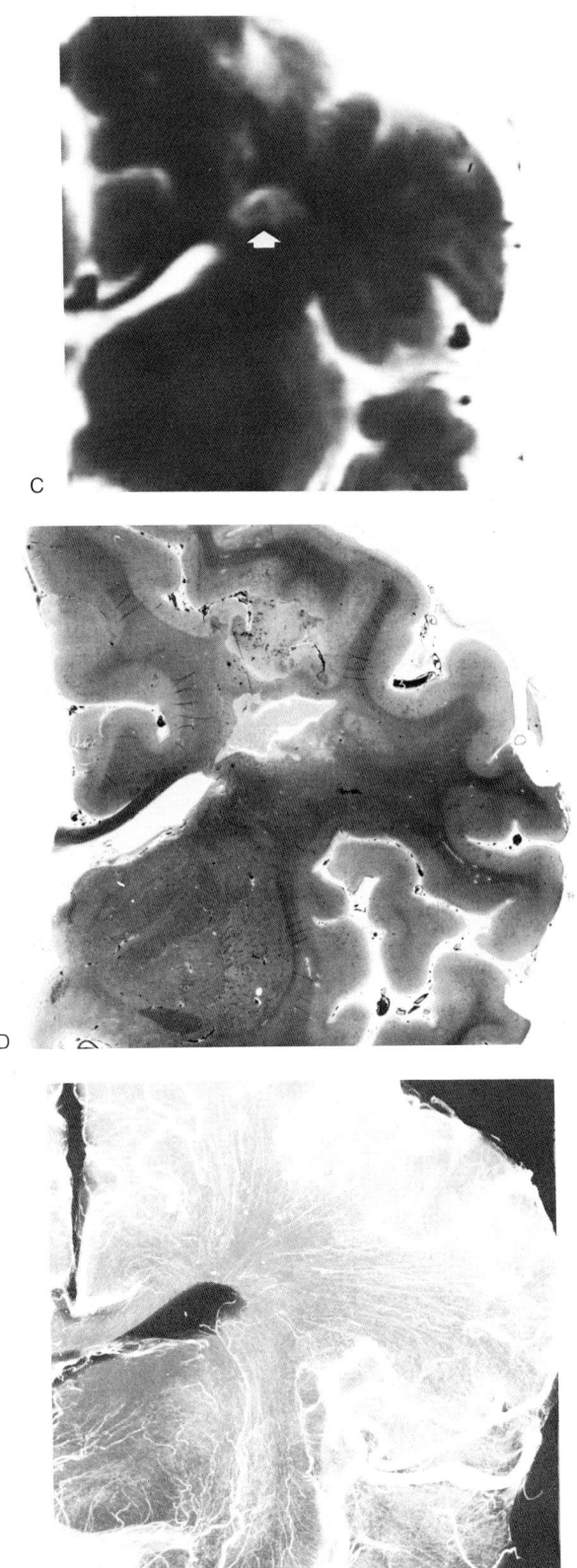

FIG. 16. Continued.

mild reactive gliosis, and arteriosclerosis in the deep white matter (medullary) penetrators (Fig. 15). The lesions are typically periventricular, but may be more diffuse in the white matter, sparing the U fibers. Injection studies illustrate that these lesions are prevalent in the distal territories of the medullary penetrators or in the border zones between those vessels and the basal penetrators. This morphologic pattern is easy to comprehend as being the result of inadequate perfusion leading to the death of the most vulnerable tissue elements, followed by a characteristic glial response. The tissue becomes somewhat rarefied, and there is an increase in interstitial space, which can be seen on tissue stains as well as imaging studies. This is not cavitation, just as the original lesion is not infarction. Brun and Englund have called these lesions "incomplete infarction" (1), an unfortunate and confusing term. (Is only part of the area infarcted? Is the infarction not finished yet?)

Patients with dementia due to Binswanger's disease usually also exhibit lacunar infarcts, especially in the frontal white matter (5, 52, 53). This distribution is similar to that reported by Dozono et al. (13) for lacunes alone. Furuta et al. found that arteriosclerosis in the medullary arteries is most pronounced in the frontal lobes in normal aging, somewhat increased in Alzheimer's disease, and significantly greater in Binswanger's disease, being well correlated with the degree of ischemic white matter changes (54). This continuum of pathologic alterations has found its counterpart in imaging studies, as numerous recent reports have identified asymptomatic (or only slightly symptomatic) white matter lesions, predominantly in the periventricular region (Fig. 16). Hachinski (2) suggested the term "leuko-araiosis" [Greek *leuko-* (white) and *araiosis* (rarefied)] to denote these symmetric patchy white matter lesions seen in the periventricular region and hemispheric white matter. Leukoaraiosis has been correlated with increased systolic blood pressure (55), cerebral atrophy (56), and cerebral hypoperfusion in both normal aging (56) and dementia (57). In the latter, leukoaraiosis seems to overlap with subcortical arteriosclerotic encephalopathy/Binswanger's disease. This is another example of terminology producing confusion rather than clarity. Since the lesions identified radiologically as leukoaraiosis may have a variety of pathological counterparts, ranging from dilated perivascular spaces (58) to demyelinated plaques to reactivate gliosis or infarcts (59), the term "leukoaraiosis" seems to have little to recommend it.

Why does hypoperfusion affect the white matter? We may speculate that the periventricular region, as a triple border zone (Fig. 8C), is highly vulnerable to mild systemic hypoperfusion or hypoxemia. Conditions which produce prolonged hypoxemia and/or hypotension, such as drug overdoses, have been reported to cause selective white matter lesions in a similar distribution (60). Experimental carbon monoxide poisoning in monkeys has produced a similar leukoencephalopathy (61). In general, it has been noted that an abrupt, moderate reduction in blood flow is likely to damage the cortex, while a milder sustained reduction will harm the white matter (62). Thus, patients with chronic mild hypertension and mild narrowing of medullary arteries may develop leukoencephalopathy, while those with more severe hypertensive changes will suffer lacunar infarcts.

CONCLUSION

The pathology of small cerebral arteries, and of the territories of the brain they supply, follows basic principles of vascular disease elsewhere in the body. Hypoxic/ischemic episodes may be mild or severe, local or widespread, and will lead to corresponding consequences. The brain's vascular distribution provides for collateral circulation in some instances, and delineates vulnerable border zones in others. Lesions are relatively easy to identify and categorize pathologically, but predictions of pathologic findings based upon clinical presentations and imaging studies are imperfect and have led to inconsistencies in nomenclature. In particular, the term "lacune" has been stretched so far that it has lost its identity. It is a useful term to denote a small deep infarct; however, many small deep lesions labelled as lacunes on imaging studies, and many clinical syndromes which are regarded as "lacunar" are not really due to infarcts. Further clinical-pathological correlation is called for to sort this out, and to provide a classification system based upon pathogenetic mechanisms. Studies which combine several imaging modalities with careful neuropathologic examination have begun to provide a useful framework of information toward that end. Until they are complete, we should all exercise thoughtful restraint in our use of terminology.

ACKNOWLEDGMENTS

We gratefully acknowledge the assistance of Gerald Verdi, who prepared the photographs, and Lyle Ostrow, who produced the schematic diagrams.

REFERENCES

1. Brun A, Englund E. A white matter disorder in dementia of the Alzheimer type: a pathoanatomical study. Ann Neurol 1986;19:253-262.
2. Hachinski VC, Potter P, Merskey H. Leukoaraiosis: an ancient name for a new problem. Arch Neurol 1987;44:21-23.
3. Janota I, Mirsen TR, Hachinski VC, Lee DH, Merskey DM. Neuropathologic correlates of leukoaraiosis. Arch Neurol 1989;46:1124-1128.
4. Revesz T, Hawkins CP, duBooulay EPGH, Barnard RO, McDonald WI. Pathological findings correlated with magnetic resonance imaging in subcortical arteriosclerotic encephalopathy (Binswanger's disease). J Neurol Neurosurg Psych 1989;52:1337-1344.
5. Fisher CM. Binswanger's encephalopathy: a review. J Neurol 1989;236:65-79.
6. Bamford J, Warlow CP. Evolution and testing of the lacunar hypothesis. Stroke 1988;19:1074-1082.
7. Boiten J, Lodder J. Lacunar infarcts: pathogenesis and validity of the clinical syndromes. Stroke 1991;22:1374-1378.
8. Fisher CM. The arterial lesions underlying lacunes. Acta Neuropathol (Berl) 1969;12:1-15.
9. Weiller C, Ringelstein EB, Reiche W, Thron A, Buell U. The large striatocapsular infarct: a clinical and pathophysiological entity. Arch Neurol 1990;1085-1091.
10. Moody DM, Bell MA, Challa VR. Features of the cerebral vascular pattern that predict vulnerability to perfusion or oxygenation deficiency: an anatomic study. AJNR 1990;11:431-439.
11. Adams JH, Brierly JB, Connor CR, Treip CS. The effects of systemic hypotension upon the human brain. Clinical and neuropathological observations in 11 cases. Brain 1966;89:235-268.
12. Cole FM, Yates PO. Comparative incidence of cerebrovascular lesions in normotensive and hypertensive patients. Neurology 1968;18:255-259.
13. Dozono K, Nobuyoshi I, Nishihara Y, Horie A. An autopsy study of the incidence of lacunes in relation to age, hypertension, and arteriosclerosis. Stroke 1991;22:993-996.
14. Tohgi H, Chiba K, Kimura M. Twenty-four hour variation of blood pressure in vascular dementia of the Binswanger type. Stroke 1991;22:603-608.
15. Fisher CM. Cerebral miliary aneurysms in hypertension. Am J Pathol 1972;66:313-330.
16. Cole FM, Yates PO. The occurrence and significance of intracerebral micro-aneurysms. J Pathol Bacteriol 1967;93:393-411.
17. Rosenblum WI. Miliary aneurysms and "fibrinoid" degeneration of cerebral blood vessels. Hum Pathol 1977;8:133-139.
18. Wakai S, Nagai M. Histological verification of microaneurysms as a cause of cerebral hemorrhage in surgical specimens. J Neurol Neurosurg Psych 1989;52:595-599.
19. Russell RWR. How does blood pressure cause stroke? Lancet 1975;ii:1283-1285.
20. Challa VR, Moody DM, Bell MA. The Charcot-Bouchard aneurysm controversy: impact of a new histologic technique. J Neuropathol Exp Neurol 1992;51:264-271.
21. Hughes W. Hypothesis: origin of lacunes. Lancet 1965;ii:19-21.
22. Fox JA, Hugh AE. Localization of atheroma: a theory based on boundary layer separation. Brit Heart J 1966;28:388-399.

23. Vracko R. A comparison of the microvascular lesions in diabetes mellitus with those of normal aging. *J AM Geriatr Soc* 1982;30:201.
24. Aronson SM. Intracranial vascular lesions in patients with diabetes mellitus. *J Neuropathol Exp Neurol* 1973;32:183–196.
25. Vinters HV, Miller BL, Pardridge WM. Brain amyloid and Alzheimer's disease. *Ann Int Med* 1988;109:41–54.
26. Kawai M, Kalaria RN, Harik SI, Perry G. The relationship of amyloid plaques to cerebral capillaries in Alzheimer's disease. *Am J Pathol* 1990;137:1435–1446.
27. Vinters HV, Gilbert JJ. Cerebral amyloid angiopathy: Incidence and complications in the aging brain. II. The distribution of amyloid vascular changes. *Stroke* 1983;14:924–928.
28. Vinters HV. Cerebral amyloid angiopathy. A critical review. *Stroke* 1987;18:311–324.
29. Loes DJ, Biller J, Yuh WTC, et.al. Leukoencephalopathy in cerebral amyloid angiopathy. MR imaging in four cases. *AJNR* 1990;11:485–488.
30. Sigal LH. The neurologic presentation of vasculitic and rheumatologic syndromes. A review. *Medicine* 1987;66:157–180.
31. Travers RL, Allison DJ, Brettle RP, Hughes GRV. Polyarteritis nodosa: a clinical and angiographic analysis of 17 cases. *Seminars in Arthritis and Rheumatism* 1979;8:184–199.
32. Vanderzant C, Bromberg M, MacGuire A, McCune J. Isolated small-vessel angiitis of the central nervous system. *Arch Neurol* 1988; 45:683–687.
33. Cupps TR, Moore PM, Fauci AS. Isolated angiitis of the central nervous system. Prospective diagnostic and therapeutic experience. *Am J Med* 1983;74:97–105.
34. Ellis SG, Verity MA. Central nervous system involvement in systemic lupus erythematosus: a review of neuropathologic findings in 57 cases, 1955–1977. *Seminars in Arthritis and Rheumatism* 1979;8:212–221.
35. Devinsky O, Petito CK, Alonso DR. Clinical and neuropathological findings in systemic lupus erythematosus: the role of vasculitis, heart emboli and thrombotic thrombocytopenic purpura. *Ann Neurol* 1988;23:380–384.
36. Bluestein HG, Zvaifler NJ. Antibodies reactive with central nervous system antigens. *Hum Pathol* 1983;14:424–428.
37. Long AA, Denburg SD, Carbotte RM, Singal DP, Denburg JA. Serum lymphocytotoxic antibodies and neurocognitive function in systemic lupus erythematosus. *Ann Rheum Dis* 1990; 49:249–253.
38. White PH. Antiphospholipid antibody syndrome. *Ann Allergy* 1990;65:425–426.
39. Sammaritano LR, Gharavi AE, Lockshin MD. Antiphospholipid antibody syndrome: immunologic and clinical aspects. *Seminars in Arthritis and Rheumatism* 1990;20:81–96.
40. Briley DP, Coull BM, Goodnight SH Jr. Neurologic disease associated with antiphospholipid antibodies. *Ann Neurol* 1989;25:221–227.
41. Citron BP, Halpern M, McCarron M, et al. Necrotizing angiitis associated with drug abuse. *N Engl J Med* 1970;283:1003–1011.
42. Fredericks RK, Lefkowitz DS, Challa VR, Troost BT. Cerebral vasculitis associated with cocaine abuse. *Stroke* 1991;22:1437–1439.
43. Fisher CM. Lacunes: Small deep cerebral infarcts. *Neurology* 1965;15:774–784.
44. Bogousslavsky J. Editorial: the plurality of subcortical infarction. *Stroke* 1992;23:629–631.
45. Fisher CM. Lacunar strokes and infarcts: a review. *Neurology* 1982;32:871–876.
46. Challa VR, Bell MA, Moody DM. A combined hematoxylin-eosin, alkaline phosphatase and high resolution microradiographic study of lacunes. *Clin Neuropathol* 1990;9:196–204.
47. Poirier J, Gray F, Gherardi R, Derouesne C. Cerebral lacunae. A new neuropathological classification. *J Neuropathol Exp Neurol* 1985;44: 312.
48. Fisher CM. Lacunar infarcts. A review. *Cerebrovasc Dis* 1991;1:311–320.
49. Landau D. Au clair de lacune: Holy, wholly holey logic. *Neurology* 1989;39:725–730.
50. Miller LL, Ostrow LW, Pullicino P, Ostrow PT. Small deep cerebral infarcts demonstrated by post mortem angiography and magnetic resonance imaging. *J Neuropathol Exp Neurol* 1992; 51:343.
51. Pullicino P, Miller LL, Munschauer FE, Ostrow PT. Linear subinsular MR hyperintensities. *Ann Neurol* 1992;32:267.
52. Fukuda H, Kobayashi S, Okada K, Tsunematsu T. Frontal white matter lesions and dementia in lacunar infarction. *Stroke* 1990;21:1143–1149.
53. Ishii N, Nishihara Y, Imamura T. Why do frontal lobe symptoms predominate in vascular dementia with lacunes? *Neurology* 1986;36:340–345.
54. Furuta A, Nobuyoshi N, Nishihara Y, Horie A. Medullary arteries in aging and dementia. *Stroke* 1991;22:442–446.
55. Inzitari D, Diaz F, Fox A, et al. Vascular risk factors and leukoaraiosis. *Arch Neurol* 1987; 44:42–47.
56. Kobari M, Meyer JS, Ichijo M. Leukoaraiosis, cerebral atrophy, and cerebral perfusion in normal aging. *Arch Neurol* 1990;47:161–165.
57. Kawamura J, Meyer JS, Terayama Y, Weathers S. Leukoaraiosis correlates with cerebral hypoperfusion in vascular dementia. *Stroke* 1991; 22:609–614.
58. Kirkpatrick JB, Hayman LA. White-matter lesions in MR imaging of clinically healthy brains of elderly subjects: possible pathologic basis. *Neuroradiology* 1987;162:509–511.
59. Braffman BH, Zimmerman RA, Trojanowski JQ, Gonatas NK, Hickey WF, Schlaepfer WW. Brain MR: pathologic correlation with gross and histopathology. 2. Hyperintense white-matter foci in the elderly. *AJR* 1988;151:559–566.
60. Ginsberg MD, Hedley-Whyte ET, Richardson

EP. Hypoxic-ischemic leukoencephalopathy in man. *Arch Neurol* 1976;33:5–14.
61. Ginsberg MD, Myers RE, McDonagh BF. Experimental carbon monoxide encephalopathy in the primate II. Clinical aspects, neuropathology, and physiologic correlation. *Arch Neurol* 1974;30:209–216.
62. Romanul F. Examination of the brain and spinal cord. In: Tedeschi CG, ed. *Neuropathology: methods and diagnosis*. Boston: Little, Brown, and Company, 1970;131–214.

6

Pathogenesis of Lacunar Infarcts and Small Deep Infarcts

Patrick M. Pullicino

Department of Neurology, State University of New York at Buffalo, Buffalo General Hospital, Buffalo, New York 14203

In this chapter the pathogenesis of lacunar infarcts and small deep ischemic lesions (as defined on p. 73) will be considered under three main headings: (a) occlusion of small arteries due to local arterial wall pathology, (b) embolic occlusion of small arteries, and (c) hypoperfusion in small arterial territories.

LACUNAR INFARCTS

Occlusive Disease of Small Arteries Due to Local Arterial Pathology

Fisher examined 18 brains using serial sections to investigate the entire course of the penetrating arteries supplying a total of 68 lacunar infarcts (Table 1) (1–6). Fifty-five (81%) of the infarcts were caused by an occlusion of the penetrating artery supplying the territory of the infarct. All of 45 arteries whose diameter was recorded to be less than 225 μm and that were associated with a lacunar infarct were found to be occluded, whereas only 9 (47%) of 19 arteries of 300 μm or greater that were associated with a lacunar infarct were completely occluded. This difference may be due to a significant collateral capillary circulation (7) making infarction less likely when small arteries are stenosed but not occluded.

The mechanism of occlusion in the arteries of less than 225 μm in diameter appeared to be a mechanical obstruction of the lumen by fibrous connective tissue or fibrinoid, which is part of lipohyalinosis. In two cases thrombosis in a lipohyalinotic microaneurysm occluded the artery (1). This has also been seen by other authors (8). In one case a small artery appeared to have been compressed by extrinsic pressure from a nearby microaneurysm (1). Hypertension was closely linked with the development of lipohyalinosis since hypertension was present in all the cases in which lipohyalinosis was found to be the cause of a lacunar infarct (1), and hypertension is very strongly related to lacunar infarcts of a size that would most likely be caused by a lipohyalinotic occlusion (9,10).

The pathological study in which Fisher found multiple lipohyalinotic occlusions (1) was performed over 20 years ago, at a time when the prevalence of hypertension was greater than it is now (11) and less effective treatment for hypertension was available. Since lipohyalinosis appears to be closely linked to hypertension, it is likely that lipohyalinosis, and the small, often asymptomatic lacunar infarcts that it causes, are less prevalent nowadays (7).

Thrombotic occlusion at the site of an atheromatous stenosis was the mechanism of occlusion in five (56%) of nine occluded arteries with diameter 300 μm or greater. Other mechanisms were occlusion of the ar-

TABLE 1. *Pathogenesis of lacunar infarcts with lesion demonstrated by serial section*

Reference	No. of brains	No. of lacunar infarcts	Case no.	Parent artery	Artery diameter (μm)	Arterial patency	Pathogenesis	Site of infarct	Clinical picture
1	4	36	1	?	40–200	Occluded	Lipohyalinosis (one atypical)	Multiple	?
		5	2–4	?	40–200	Occluded	Lipohyalinosis	Multiple	?
		2	3	?	?	Stenosed	Lipohyalinosis (one atypical)	?	?
		2	2	MCA	150	Occluded	Thrombosed microaneurysm	White matter	?
		2	3	MCA	300–500	Occluded	Thrombosed microaneurysm	Internal caps	PMH
		1	3	MCA	300–500	Stenosed	Microatheroma	Thalamus	?
		1	?	?	?	Stenosed	Pressure from microaneurysm	?	?
2	9	1	4	Basilar branch	?	Patent	Embolism	Pons	?
		3	3	MCA	750	95% stenosed	Microatheroma	Internal caps	PMH
			8		400	88% stenosed	Microatheroma	Internal caps	PMH
			9		400	65% stenosed	Microatheroma	Internal caps	PMH
		2	5	AChA	425	83% stenosed	Microatheroma	Internal caps	PMH
					400	90% stenosed	Microatheroma	Internal caps	PMH
		2	6	MCA	500	94% stenosed and thrombosed	Thrombosed microatheroma	Internal caps	PMH
			7		500	96% stenosed and thrombosed	Thrombosed microatheroma	Internal caps	PMH
		2	2	MCA	300	Patent	Embolism	Internal caps	PMH
			4	MCA	800	Patent	Embolism	Internal caps	PMH
		1	1	MCA	300	Occluded	Lipohyalinosis (atypical)	Internal caps	PMH
3	1	3	1	Basilar branch	500	Occluded	Microdissection/atheroma	Pons	Pontine syndrome
			2	Basilar branch	300	Stenosed	Junctional atheroma	Pons	Pontine syndrome
			3	Basilar branch	500	Thrombosed	Atheroma	Pons	PMH
4	1	2	1	Basilar branch	500	Occluded	Basilar A. atheroma	Pons	PMH
			2	Basilar branch	500	94% stenosed	Junctional atheroma	Pons	Pontine syndrome
5	1	1	1	Pica branch	350	Occluded	Large A. embolism	Pons	Pontine syndrome
6	2	2	1	PCA branch	200	Occluded	Lipohyalinosis	Thalamus	PSS
			2	PCA branch	225	Occluded	Lipohyalinosis	Thalamus	PSS

MCA, middle cerebral artery; AChA, anterior choroidal artery; PCA, posterior cerebral artery; PICA, posterior inferior cerebellar artery; PMH, pure motor hemiparesis; PSS, pure sensory stroke.

tery by atheroma (one case), microdissection (one case), probable embolism (one case), and atypical lipohyalinosis (one case) (Table 1). Atheroma that occludes a penetrating artery may be situated within the proximal part of the penetrating artery "microatheroma" (2), in the penetrating artery right at the junction with a larger artery—so-called junctional atheroma (3)—or it may be totally within the larger parent artery, obstructing the origin of the penetrating artery—so-called mural atheroma (4). Fisher commented that he had performed serial sections of the basilar artery in three further cases and found mural atheroma obstructing the origin of penetrating arteries (7), suggesting that this is a common cause for lacunar infarction.

Angelergues et al. (12) published the autopsy findings of a patient who developed a bilateral paramedian thalamic infarct in the convalescent phase of acute meningitis. Marked endarteritis of the basilar artery and a chronic meningitis were found, and were the probable cause of the lacunar infarct.

Embolic Occlusion of Small Arteries

Cardiogenic Embolism

In an autopsy series, Tuszynski et al. found that 6 (10.7%) of 56 patients had rheumatic heart disease or presumed nonbacterial thrombotic endocarditis as the sole apparent etiology for lacunar infarcts (13), but larger cortical infarcts were also present in these patients. Occlusion of small cerebral parenchymal vessels with fibrin has been found at autopsy in nonbacterial thrombotic endocarditis (14). At least 4 (8%) of Blackwood et al.'s 48 autopsy cases with a proven cardiac embolic source had cerebral infarcts of a size compatible with lacunar infarcts (15).

In 3 of the 68 lacunar infarcts studied by serial section by Fisher, the supplying artery was patent and intact, and embolism was postulated as the mechanism of infarction. In one case, a small branch was occluded at its origin by a clot in the posterior inferior cerebellar artery (5). Since there was only slight local atherosclerosis, embolism was thought to be likely. In a further case (case 9 in ref. 2), the degree of stenosis of the penetrating artery may not have been severe enough to account for the infarct, and embolism was a possible mechanism.

Artery-to-Artery Embolism

Laloux and Brucher described a patient with a dissecting aneurysm of the aorta who developed transient neurologic symptoms and who was found at autopsy to have lacunar infarcts in the left thalamus, putamen, and caudate nuclei, in addition to cortical and larger infarcts (16). Multiple perforating arteries, particularly adjacent to lacunar infarcts were occluded by cholesterol crystal emboli. The diameter of the embolized arteries varied from 14 to 480 μm. Vascular hyalinosis was not prominent. Extensive atheromatous changes with large amounts of cholesterol crystals were found in the dissected wall of the aortic arch (16). Amarenco et al. found that 13 of 17 patients with cerebral infarction of unknown cause who had ulcerated plaques in the aortic arch had lacunar or small deep infarcts at autopsy (17).

Hemodynamic Compromise in Small Arterial Territories

Lacunar Infarcts

Eight (53%) of 15 arteries studied by Fisher with lacunar infarcts caused by microatheroma or junctional atheroma were stenosed but not occluded. In five penetrating arteries (measuring 400 to 750 μm) the severity of atheromatous stenosis that led to infarction was 95%, 94%, 90%, 88%, and 83% (calculated from Fisher's measurements) (2,4). Hypoperfusion, secondary to severe stenosis in single penetrating artery territories, appears to have caused the infarct in these cases. De Reuck has also noted narrowing and poststenotic dilatation of larger perforating arteries on microangiography in brains with lacunar infarcts (18). It thus appears that atheromatous stenosis of a penetrating artery commonly leads to Fisher's lacunar infarction.

Eight of the 12 infarcts associated with pure motor hemiparesis that had a detailed history were associated with an atheromatous stenosis of the relevant penetrating artery (Table 1). Five (63%) of these eight infarcts had evidence of an unstable clinical course: preceding transient ischemic attack (TIA) (case 9), fluctuating onset (case 5, right), progressive onset associated with antihypertensives (case 7), recurrent stroke within a month (case 5, left)(2) and stepwise onset (infarct 2)(3).

Only one of four infarcts in patients who had pure motor hemiplegia without vascular stenosis had an unstable clinical course [case 1 (4)]. These cases suggest that an unstable clinical course may be associated with a critical state of low perfusion distal to a stenosed penetrating artery. Fisher remarked that severe narrowing appeared not to be tolerated as well in this size of artery as in larger (extracerebral) arteries (2).

In two patients with 94% and 96% microatheromatous stenosis of 500 μm diameter penetrating arteries [cases 6 and 7 (2)], clinical deficits were associated with the initiation of vigorous antihypertensive therapy. In these two cases hypoperfusion caused by overzealous treatment of hypertension might have caused ischemia distal to the stenosis (2).

In contradistinction, none of 45 arteries of 225 μm or less that supplied the territory of a lacunar infarct showed stenosis although 3 lipohyalinotic arteries of unstated caliber were stenosed (Table 1). Collaterals in the capillary circulation (19) may reduce the risk that hypoperfusion secondary to stenosis of small arteries of this size will give rise to lacunar infarcts.

White Matter Infarcts

Dozono et al. found that the degree of arteriolosclerosis of medullary arteries was related to the number of lacunar infarcts in 200 autopsy brains (20). These authors found occlusive lesions like lipohyalinosis to be uncommon, but they did not use serial sections, and unlike other studies found that the white matter was the most common site for lacunar infarcts. Since many of these infarcts were situated in the terminal zones of the medullary arteries, the authors speculated that hemodynamic factors may be involved in the causation of these white matter infarcts.

Reyes found deep cerebral white matter infarcts at autopsy in the brains of two patients who had sickle cell trait but no other stroke risk factors (21). In addition, one of these patients had a pontine infarct. Hypoperfusion or occlusion of small arteries by sludging of sickled cells was suggested as the mechanism for these infarctions.

Unproven Mechanisms of Perforating Artery Hypoperfusion

Spasm

Burger et al. showed that vasospasm may cause transient monocular blindness by documenting multifocal narrowing of retinal arteries on fundal photographs taken during an episode of visual loss. The vasospasm resolved at the same time that the patients' vision returned (22). The authors speculated that transient or fixed cerebrovascular events might be related to vasospasm. Friberg and Olsen noted apparently spontaneous regional hypoperfusion during cerebral blood flow measurements in six patients with a history of stroke (four had small deep infarcts) or TIA (23). During routine testing, cerebral blood flow fell to levels compatible with ischemia, and in four patients this was associated with a transient neurologic deficit. The authors suggested that spasm of small intracerebral arteries may be the primary cause of focal cerebral ischemia in some patients. This is in keeping with recent evidence that inappropriate constrictions of small resistance arteries in the heart may cause myocardial ischemia (24). A condition in which transient or persistent neurologic deficits are associated with segmental arterial constrictions of large arteries on angiography has been called reversible cerebral angiopathy (25) or isolated benign angiitis of the central nervous system (26). There has been no demonstration, however, of involvement of small cerebral arteries in this condition.

Hypoperfusion Secondary to Carotid Turbulent Flow

Hughes et al. put forward a hemodynamic explanation for lacunar infarctions (27). They suggested that the nonexpansile portion of the carotid artery in the bony carotid canal induces turbulent flow, and that this turbulence is likely to be greater in hypertensives, possibly extending along the carotid up to the mouths of the penetrating arteries. Since turbulence is known to reduce the head of pressure in a tube, Hughes et al. hypothesized that turbulence in hypertensives might reduce flow within the penetrating arteries resulting in ischemia. This hypothesis has not been supported by any data.

PERIVASCULAR SPACE ENLARGEMENT

Van Swieten et al. measured the area of dilated perivascular spaces in square millimeters per square centimeter of white matter in the frontal and parietal white matter of nine brains of patients over 60 years of age (28). Dilated perivascular spaces were present in six (86%) of seven brains with severe demyelination and arteriolosclerosis, but also in one brain with normal white matter and normal arterioles. Senile plaques and amyloid angiopathy were found as frequently in brains with dilated perivascular spaces as in brains without. The presence and degree of dilated perivascular spaces correlated (r = 0.63, p < 0.01) with lower relative brain weight (loss of brain weight corrected for age). Van Swieten et al. suggested that arteriolosclerosis is the initiating pathology in the formation of dilated perivascular spaces. Although these authors could not exclude that dilated perivascular spaces are caused directly by the pulsatile forces of sclerotic small arteries (see Pulsations of "Unfolded" Small Arteries below), they suggested that the spaces arise secondary to brain atrophy. They concluded that in the brains they studied, brain atrophy was due to a gradual white matter demyelination secondary to sclerosis of small arteries.

Heier et al. found univariate correlations between perivascular spaces larger than 2 mm on magnetic resonance (MR) scan and age, hypertension, dementia, and white matter focal hyperintensities (29). Only age, however, remained significant using a multivariate logistic regression analysis.

Theories of Pathogenesis of Enlarged Perivascular Spaces

Alteration of Blood-Brain Barrier

Benhaiem-Sigaux et al. (30) reported expanding cerebellar lacunes due to dilatation of the perivascular spaces. These "giant" lacunes appear to have mass effect and appear to have caused hydrocephalus by obstruction of the aqueduct in one reported case (31). Benhaiem-Sigaux et al. suggested that an abnormality of arterial wall permeability was the cause of these expanding lacunes (30).

Pulsations of "Unfolded" Small Arteries

Hughes performed cine angiography of the basilar artery in patients with the lacunar state and noted that the terminal segment of the basilar artery moved about 5 mm forward and upward with each pulsation (32). He proposed that a similar "corkscrewing" movement of unfolded (tortuous and elongated) penetrating arteries was responsible for the formation of perivascular spaces by traumatizing the surrounding brain tissue (Fig. 1).

Perivascular Lytic Agent

Moore proposed the development of a lytic factor in the perivascular space to explain the perivascular changes and spaces seen around small arteries (33). He suggested that this factor was possibly a tissue catabolite arising from faulty metabolism consequent to blood flow or oxygen consumption derangements. However, he did not put forward any evidence to support this theory.

Vaginalite Destructive or Inflammation of Arterial Sheaths

This theory, which is largely of historical interest (see Chapter 1), was originally put forward by Marie (34). According to this theory, enlarged perivascular spaces were caused by damage to the surrounding brain by an inflammation of the perivascular sheaths.

State of Degeneration

The Vogts proposed that one of the elements leading to lacunes and in particular to dilated perivascular spaces was damage to the cerebral parenchyma such as neu-

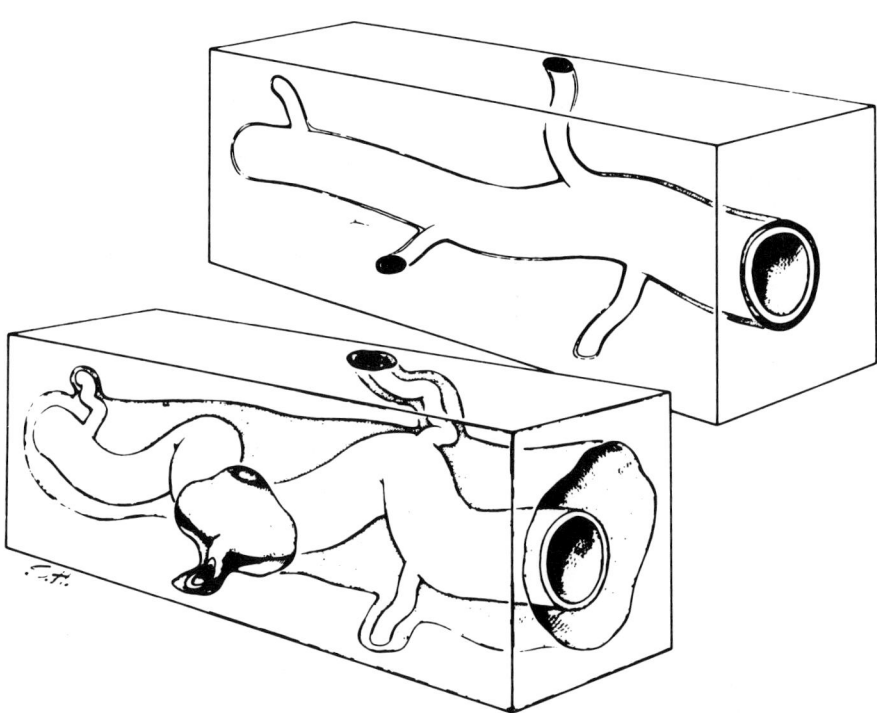

FIG. 1. Diagram illustrating how a normal artery (*above*) becomes elongated and tortuous ("unfolding"), and develops a dilated perivascular space (*below*). From ref. 128, with permission of the American Heart Association, Inc.

ronal loss and demyelination (34). Although this theory is mainly of historical interest, a correlation between cerebral atrophy, demyelination, and perivascular space area has recently been shown (28).

SMALL DEEP INFARCTS

Presumed Occlusive Etiology

Large Artery Disease

Bogousslavsky et al. found 10 (63%) of 16 patients with small deep infarcts of undetermined cause to have a relevant stenosis of the large parent artery (middle cerebral or basilar) (35). These authors suggested that occlusion of penetrating arteries by local atherosclerosis of the large parent artery may be underestimated as a cause of lacunar infarction. Fisher has also recently suggested that "mural atheroma" of the basilar artery that blocks the origin of penetrating arteries is a common cause of basilar branch infarcts (7).

Stenosis of the middle cerebral artery due to presumed granulomatous angiitis following trigeminal herpes zoster has also been associated with an ipsilateral small deep infarct (36,37). In these cases the penetrating arteries may be occluded by an angiitis that primarily affects the parent artery.

Bogousslavsky et al. (38) reported a patient with a tuberothalamic/anterior choroidal small deep infarct on computed tomography (CT) who had an internal carotid dissection extending up to the siphon. Occlusion of a combined origin of these arteries may have occurred.

Fisher reported the autopsy findings in a patient with a lacunar infarct in the cerebral peduncle caused by a saccular basilar aneurysm (39). The pathogenetic mechanisms suggested were either direct compression of the aneurysm on a penetrating artery or aneurysm-to-artery embolization. A case of pure sensory stroke secondary to a rostral basilar aneurysm shown on MR has also been reported (40). Paramedian small deep thalamic infarction on CT has been noted following surgery for posterior communicating aneurysms (41).

Coagulopathies

Levine et al. (42) found both small deep infarcts and MR hyperintensities presumed due to white matter infarcts in patients with antiphospholipid antibodies. Fibrin thrombi were found in multiple small intracerebral vessels in this and another study (43). There was no evidence of vasculitis on histopathology. The association of antiphospholipid antibody syndrome with small deep infarcts has been noted by other authors (44).

Drake reported two patients with the lupus anticoagulant who had small deep infarcts in the basal ganglia on CT (45). One of these patients had systemic lupus erythematosus. The pathogenesis of the infarcts in these patients was unknown, but lupus anticoagulant may facilitate platelet aggregation and this might have led to a small arterial occlusion. The patient of Malamut et al. with bilateral thalamic infarction probably also had a lupus anticoagulant state (46).

Devinsky et al. reported an autopsy series of patients with systemic lupus erythematosus (47). A lacunar infarct was found in one brain. Systemic lupus commonly affects arteries of very small size, giving microinfarcts that are asymptomatic and seen only on microscopy (48). Vasculitis appears to be rare, and infarction is probably due to hypercoagulability, an associated antiphospholipid antibody syndrome, or cardiogenic embolism from Libman-Sacks verrucous vegetations (49). Kitagawa et al. also implicated hypertension (50).

DiMauro et al. reported a presumed lacunar infarct in a 5-year-old with hemolytic-uremic syndrome (51). Small arterial thrombi were the postulated cause. Fibrin thrombi are also found in small cerebral arteries in disseminated intravascular coagulation (52).

Dawson et al. reported a man with a plasma cell dyscrasia who had multiple small T2 gray matter hyperintensities on MR. At autopsy numerous acute and subacute microinfarctions were found, and numerous capillaries and small arterioles adjacent to the infarcts were obstructed by fibrin-platelet thrombi (53). Fibrin thrombi have also been found in the brains of patients with metastatic carcinoma (54).

Petiot et al. reported a patient with factor V deficiency who presented with a thalamic presumed lacunar infarct (55). These authors suggested that factor V deficiency might be associated with thromboembolic complications because factor V participates in the prothrombinase complex.

Fisher described a patient with recurrent pure sensory TIAs who had thrombocythemia (56). Pearce et al. reported three patients with presumed lacunar infarcts who had polycythemia (57). Two of these patients were hypertensive, however. (Raised hematocrit is also discussed below in Hypoperfusion.)

Arteritis

Mayo et al. (58) reported a patient with periarteritis nodosa who had two small deep infarcts associated with new onset of parkinsonism. A renal biopsy showed necrotizing arteriolitis; a similar pathology presumably affected cerebral arterioles. Vasculitis has been mentioned by other authors as a cause of small deep infarcts (59).

Multiple small deep infarcts have been reported in a patient with Cogan's syndrome (60). The infarcts appeared in the setting of a high sedimentation rate, and arteritis was thought to be the cause.

Isolated angiitis of the central nervous system affects small or medium sized arteries and has been associated with subcortical infarcts on CT (61). The most frequent underlying pathology is a granulomatous angiitis (26,62). Small deep infarcts occurring days or weeks after trigeminal herpes zoster are thought to be due to granulomatous angiitis, but angiographic evidence suggests involvement of the parent large arteries rather than of the penetrating arteries (36,63).

Infectious Causes

Meningeal inflammation may extend to involve arteries lying in the subarachnoid space, and a process called endarteritis obliterans, or Heubner's arteritis, may result (64). This was originally described in association with syphilis and tuberculosis, but may be seen in several inflammatory conditions. Heubner's arteritis may lead to thrombosis of the involved artery and small deep infarcts may result, as in some of the inflammatory conditions described below.

Seven patients with neurocysticercosis were described with presumed lacunar infarcts on CT or MR (65). Cysticerci in the subarachnoid space induce a subacute or chronic meningitis, with thickening of the meninges and entrapment of blood vessels around the base of the brain, including penetrating arteries. This is thought to lead to occlusion of the penetrating arteries and lacunar infarcts (65).

Johns et al. reported two young men with meningovascular syphilis who developed pure motor hemiplegia secondary to CT-demonstrated pontine presumed lacunar infarcts (66). A syphilitic endarteritis of paramedian basilar branches was proposed as the etiology. Small deep infarcts secondary to syphilis have been reported by other authors (38,59).

May and Jabbari (67) and Kohler et al. (68) have reported patients with thalamic small deep infarcts secondary to Lyme disease. Direct spread of infection to the penetrating arteries was a suggested cause of the infarcts, but an immunologic mechanism was also possible. Other authors have mentioned Lyme disease as a cause of small deep infarcts (38).

Eda et al. reported four cases of acute hemiplegia following varicella infection in childhood (69). In three of these patients, CT showed a small deep infarct near the internal capsule. The pathogenesis may be a granulomatous angiitis similar to that seen in adults following trigeminal herpes zoster.

Engstrom et al. reported 12 patients with acquired immunodeficiency syndrome (AIDS) who had cerebral infarcts on CT (70). Twelve (68%) of 19 infarcts shown on CT were subcortical (basal ganglia, thalamus, or deep white matter). Cerebral infarcts were associated with cryptococcus (4), tuberculosis (1), zoster vasculitis (1), and cardiogenic embolism (1). Park et al. found lacunar infarcts and microinfarcts at autopsy or on CT in three of seven children with AIDS (71). An arteriopathy caused by human immunodeficiency virus infection of parenchymal or leptomeningeal blood vessels or arterial injury secondary to multiple infections were two postulated causes of infarction.

Presumed Embolic Etiology

Cardiogenic Embolism

Santamaria et al. reported eight infarcts in the basal ganglia region due to probable cardiogenic embolism (72). The infarcts were larger than the usually accepted size of lacunar infarcts and the authors suggested occlusion of multiple lenticulostriate arteries by an embolus arrested in the trunk of the middle cerebral artery as one possible pathogenetic mechanism. Twenty-two percent of Weisberg's probable cardiogenic embolic infarcts seen on CT were in the lenticulostriate territory, and at least four of these had a clinical lacunar syndrome (73). Other studies have also reported cases of presumed lacunar infarcts (74) and small deep infarcts due to probable cardiogenic embolism (59,75–78).

Embolism is the most common cause of occlusions of the top of the basilar artery, and the perforating arteries arising in this vicinity are also frequently occluded as part of the top of the basilar syndrome (79). Bogousslavsky et al. found that 30% of CT thalamic small deep infarcts had a probable embolic cause. These included a patient with a recent myocardial infarct in whom an embolus was found in a small cerebral artery at autopsy. Probable cardiogenic embolism was found in 33% of the paramedian infarcts (38). Cardiogenic embolism from prosthetic cardiac valves (38,80,81) and from a pedunculated left ventricular thrombus (41) have also been reported as causing paramedian thalamic and midbrain infarcts.

Atrial Fibrillation

Atrial fibrillation with (38,82) and without (82,83) rheumatic mitral stenosis has been associated with bilateral paramedian diencephalic small deep infarcts on CT. Twenty-one percent of asymptomatic cerebral infarcts seen in patients with nonvalvular atrial fibrillation were small deep infarcts less than 1 cm in size (84). Only 35% of these patients were hypertensive, supporting cardiogenic embolism from atrial fibrillation as the probable etiology in some of these patients. Gandolfo et al. found atrial fibrillation in normotensives to be a risk factor for presumed lacunar infarcts (85).

Artery-to-Artery Embolism

CT- or MR-proven paramedian thalamic/mesencephalic small deep infarcts have been reported in association with arch aortography (86) and coronary angioplasty (87,88), as has a capsular small deep infarct secondary to coronary angiography (89). Artery-to-artery embolism was the likely cause in these patients. Artery-to-artery embolism has been suggested as a possible cause of lacunar infarcts (77) and small deep infarcts (59,78). Possible artery-to-artery embolism was seen in 38% of ventrolateral (thalamogeniculate territory) infarcts in Bogousslavsky et al.'s series of thalamic infarcts (38). These authors also reported a paramedian thalamic infarct in a patient with a megadolicho basilar artery secondary to Marfan's syndrome (38). There may be an association between carotid stenosis and presumed lacunar infarction (90,91). Caplan et al. found a small deep infarct on CT in a patient following intravenous injection of oral preparations of pentazocine and tripelennamine (Ts and Blues) (92). This infarct was probably due to embolism of microcrystalline cellulose and talc that was injected intravenously and traversed the lungs through vascular shunts that are present in chronic drug abusers.

Hypoperfusion

There is a wide variety of ischemic lesions proven or suspected to be due to hypoperfusion injury, including:

1. Watershed infarcts between major cerebral arteries (93,94)
2. Compound granular atrophy (see Chapter 5)
3. Subcortical (93,95) or low-flow infarcts (96,97) situated in the terminal zone of the medullary arteries, particularly lateral to the lateral ventricles in the centrum semiovale, associated with severe occlusive ipsilateral carotid disease
4. White matter infarcts that are not associated with ipsilateral severe occlusive carotid disease (20,21)
5. Small deep infarcts in the head of the caudate/anterior limb of the internal capsule that are in the terminal zone of Heubner's artery, or of the lateral lenticulostriate arteries (98,99)
6. Small deep infarcts (100) or presumed lacunar infarcts (101) associated with distal middle cerebral artery occlusion
7. Internal borderzone infarcts associated with distal middle cerebral artery occlusion (102)
8. Subinsular linear infarction not associated with middle cerebral artery disease (103,104)
9. Lacunar infarcts distal to a stenosis of the relevant penetrating artery (2)
10. Periventricular white matter ischemic injury in subcortical arteriosclerotic encephalopathy (Binswanger's disease) (see Chapter 11)
11. Cortical laminar necrosis (94)

The mechanism of the hypoperfusion appears to be different in several of the above lesions. Hypotension is primarily linked with watershed infarcts between major cerebral artery territories (105,106) and with cortical laminar necrosis (see Chapter 5). Although hypotension is a suspected aggravating factor of Binswanger's disease, this has not been proven (see Chapter 11). Hypotension has been associated with lacunar infarcts distal to a penetrating artery stenosis (2). Bladin and Chambers have suggested that hypotension plays a role in watershed infarcts of the type listed in no. 3 above (107). Jacobs et al. (108) reported small bilateral infarcts of the midbrain periaqueductal gray secondary to a cardiopulmonary arrest. Sawada et al. have reported delayed onset extensive white matter injury secondary to a severe hypoxic-ischemic episode in a 44-year-old with asthma but with no vascular risk factors (94). Hemodynamically significant cardiac disease may interact with cerebrovascular stenosis to increase the risk of hypoperfusion injury (93), particularly in diabetics (109,110).

Severe stenosis or occlusion of the internal carotid are clearly linked to low-flow infarcts in the centrum semiovale (93,95–97,111) or in the caudate/anterior limb of internal capsule region (99), but also strongly associated with watershed infarcts between major arterial territories (93,112). Severe carotid stenosis or occlusion may cause diminished perfusion, a lowered hemodynamic reserve (113), and a diminished response of cerebral blood flow to hypercapnia (114). This suggests that cerebral symptoms in patients with severe carotid stenosis or occlusion are often due to hypoperfusion (114). Kobayashi et al. found a significant reduction of cerebral blood flow in patients with asymptomatic small deep infarcts compared to normal controls (115). They postulated a watershed etiology for these infarcts. Carotid artery dissection may also be a risk factor for low-flow infarcts (116), as may the reduced carotid flow in moyamoya disease (59,95).

Hypertension is the principal risk factor for Binswanger's disease (see Chapter 11), but may also be a risk factor for subinsular infarction (103).

Middle cerebral artery occlusion may produce internal borderzone infarcts or deep infarcts despite good cortical collateral flow (100). These infarcts are probably situated in the terminal zone of the white matter penetrators arising from the cortical middle cerebral branches (100).

Caplan et al. found that 5 (28%) of 18 patients with middle cerebral artery occlusive disease had subcortical infarcts (101). The course of the stroke in these patients was often fluctuating or progressive, suggesting a critical state of low perfusion in the pathogenesis of these infarcts (101). A progressive clinical course, however, can occur in the absence of middle cerebral artery stenosis or occlusion (117) and Fisher's cases summarized above suggest that the pathogenetic mechanism may be a fluctuating state of critical perfusion distal to a penetrating artery stenosis (2). Fisher and Curry found that 30% of patients with pure motor hemiplegia had TIAs prior to the onset of the stroke (118), and in 50% of patients the stroke came on gradually over the course of 12 to 72 hours. Some patients who develop pure motor hemiparesis have striking repetitive brief episodes of hemiplegia, which have been called the "capsular warning syndrome" by Donnan and Bladin (119). It is possible that many of these fluctuating clinical states relate to hypoperfusion in stenosed penetrating arteries.

LaRue et al. found the mean hematocrit to be higher in patients with presumed lacunar infarcts than in patients with thrombotic or embolic stroke (120). This was, however, only significant for patients with systolic hypertension. This study suggested that a high hematocrit may increase the risk of lacunar infarction and that there may be an interaction between hypertension and a high hematocrit on the risk of lacunar infarction. LaRue et al. speculated that a lower blood flow and a higher blood viscosity secondary to a high hematocrit might reduce the oxygen uptake of tissue supplied by penetrating arteries to a greater extent than that of tissue supplied by larger arteries, where collateral circulation is possible. A high hematocrit has also been linked to Binswanger's disease (see Chapter 11), as well as to watershed infarcts between the major cortical arterial territories (93).

Unknown Mechanisms

Lacunar Transient Ischemic Attacks

About 30% of lacunar infarcts have a preceding TIA (118) and the Dutch TIA study group found that small vessel disease is probably the most common cause of TIA (121). Although artery-to-artery embolism from a carotid source is accepted as the usual cause of cortical TIAs, both spasm (23) and hypoperfusion distal to a penetrating artery stenosis (2) are potential causes of lacunar TIAs. There may be an association between arterial spasm and atherosclerotic stenosis. In the coronary circulation, abnormal paradoxical constriction of larger coronary arteries in response to stress occurs at sites of atheromatous stenosis (122) and Faraci et al. have shown that atherosclerosis potentiates constrictor responses of primate cerebral arteries (123).

Migraine

Ferbert et al. found a higher frequency of T2 white matter hyperintensities on MR in patients with migraine as compared to matched controls (124). These lesions were thought to be of probable ischemic origin. Five percent of Ghika et al.'s patients with small deep infarcts in the territory of the deep carotid perforators had migraine (78) and 10% of Bogousslavsky et al.'s cases of thalamic infarcts occurred during a migraine attack and were probably due to migraine (38).

Oral Contraceptives

Mills and Swanson reported a patient on oral contraceptives who developed bilateral paramedian thalamic infarction (125). Other authors have mentioned the association of oral contraceptives with thalamic infarcts (38,81,126).

Cocaine Abuse

Rowley et al. reported that two of three patients with stroke after cocaine abuse had bilateral paramedian infarction of the thalamus (127). One of these patients had focal narrowing of the P1 segments of the posterior cerebral arteries bilaterally. The authors thought that vessel wall injury secondary to defective autoregulation during cocaine-induced hypertension was the possible cause of the infarcts. Adrenergic-mediated vasospasm was thought an unlikely cause because of the sparse perivascular sympathetic supply of the P1 segment.

CONCLUSION

This chapter has discussed many possible causes for lacunar infarcts and small deep infarcts, some well established by careful autopsy study, others based on the association of a clinical or laboratory-supported diagnosis with the finding of a small deep infarct on imaging. Small deep infarcts that have the same imaging appearance as autopsy-proven lacunar infarcts have been associated with many different conditions, including cardiogenic and artery-to-artery embolism. It is therefore important to look for a potential embolic source or an underlying general medical condition in patients with small deep infarcts who are normotensive or who have any other atypical features. Epidemiological studies (see Chapter 12) indicate, however, that the majority of lacunar infarcts are probably due to microatheroma or lipohyalinosis.

A review of Fisher's work shows that lacunar infarcts were frequently associated with a microatheromatous stenosis of the relevant penetrating artery, suggesting that hypoperfusion secondary to penetrating artery stenosis may be a common cause of lacunar infarction. The cause of lacunar TIA is still unknown, but evidence reviewed here suggests that hypoperfusion in the territory of a stenosed penetrating artery, possibly associated with local spasm, may be a cause.

REFERENCES

1. Fisher CM. The arterial lesions underlying lacunes. *Acta Neuropathol* 1969;12:1–15.
2. Fisher CM. Capsular infarcts. The underlying vascular lesions. *Arch Neurol* 1979;36:65–73.
3. Fisher CM. Bilateral occlusion of basilar artery branches. *J Neurol Neurosurg Psychiatry* 1977;40:1182–1189.
4. Fisher CM, Caplan LR. Basilar artery branch occlusion: a cause of pontine infarction. *Neurology* 1971;21:900–905.
5. Fisher CM, Tapia J. Lateral medullary infarction extending to the lower pons. *J Neurol Neurosurg Psychiatry* 1987;50:620–624.
6. Fisher CM. Thalamic pure sensory stroke: a pathologic study. *Neurology* 1978;28:1141–1144.
7. Fisher CM. Lacunar infarcts—a review. *Cerebrovasc Dis* 1991;1:311–320.
8. Benhaiem-Sigaux N, Gherardi R, Salama J,

Gray F, Amouroux J, Poirier J. Thrombosis of a saccular microaneurysm causing cerebral (pontine) lacunae. *Acta Neuropathol* 1986; 69:332–336.
9. Gautier JC. Cerebral ischaemia in hypertension. In: Russell RWR, ed. *Cerebral arterial disease.* London: Churchill Livingstone; 1976: 181–209.
10. Orgogozo JM, Bogousslavsky J. Lacunar syndromes. In: Toole JF, ed. *Handbook of clinical neurology, Vol 10 (54): vascular diseases part II.* Amsterdam: Elsevier Scientific; 1989:235–269.
11. Garraway WM, Whisnant JP. The changing pattern of hypertension and the declining incidence of stroke. *JAMA* 1987;258:214–217.
12. Angelergues R, De Ajuriaguerra J, Hécaen H. Paralysie de la verticalité du regard d'origine vasculaire. *Rev Neurol (Paris)* 1957;4:301–319.
13. Tuszynski MH, Petito CK, Levy DE. Risk factors and clinical manifestations of pathologically verified lacunar infarctions. *Stroke* 1989; 20:990–999.
14. Rogers LR, Cho ES, Kempin S, Posner JB. Cerebral infarction from non-bacterial thrombotic endocarditis. *Am J Med* 1987;83:746–756.
15. Blackwood W, Hallpike JF, Kocen RS, Mair WGP. Atheromatous disease of the carotid arterial system and embolism from the heart in cerebral infarction: a morbid anatomical study. *Brain* 1969;92:897–910.
16. Laloux P, Brucher JM. Lacunar infarctions due to cholesterol emboli. *Stroke* 1991;22:1440–1444.
17. Amarenco P, Duyckaerts C, Tzourio C, Hénin D, Bousser M-G, Hauw J-J. The prevalence of ulcerated plaques in the aortic arch in patients with stroke. *N Engl J Med* 1992;326:221–225.
18. De Reuck J. Neuropathology of cerebral ischemia: topographic and angioarchitectural features. *Cerebrovasc Dis* 1991;1[Suppl 1]: 69–72.
19. Moody DM, Bell MA, Challa VR. Features of the cerebral vascular pattern that predict vulnerability to perfusion or oxygenation deficiency: an anatomic study. *AJNR* 1990;11:431–439.
20. Dozono K, Ishii N, Nishihara Y, Horie A. An autopsy study of the incidence of lacunes in relation to age, hypertension and atherosclerosis. *Stroke* 1991;22:993–996.
21. Reyes MG. Subcortical cerebral infarctions in sickle cell trait. *J Neurol Neurosurg Psychiatry* 1989;52:516–518.
22. Burger SK, Saul RF, Selhorst JB, Thurston SE. Transient monocular blindness caused by vasospasm. *N Engl J Med* 1991;325:870–873.
23. Friberg L, Olsen TS. Cerebrovascular instability in a subset of patients with stroke and transient ischemic attack. *Arch Neurol* 1991; 48:1026–1031.
24. Maseri A. Coronary vasoconstriction: visible and invisible. *N Engl J Med* 1991;325:1579–1580.
25. Bogousslavsky J, Pierre P. Ischemic stroke in patients under 45. *Neurol Clin* 1992;10:113–124.
26. Hankey GJ. Isolated angiitis/angiopathy of the central nervous system. *Cerebrovasc Dis* 1991;1:2–15.
27. Hughes W, Dodgson MCH, MacLennan DC. Chronic cerebral hypertensive disease. *Lancet* 1954;2:770–774.
28. Van Swieten JC, Van den Hout JHW, Van Ketel BA, Hijdra A, Wokke JHJ, Van Gijn J. Periventricular lesions in the white matter on magnetic resonance imaging in the elderly. A morphometric correlation with arteriolosclerosis and dilated perivascular spaces. *Brain* 1991;114: 761–774.
29. Heier LA, Bauer CJ, Schwartz L, Zimmerman RD, Morgello S, Deck MDF. Large Virchow-Robin spaces: MR-clinical correlation. *AJNR* 1989;10:929–936.
30. Benhaiem-Sigaux N, Gray F, Gherardi R, Roucayrol AM, Poirier J. Expanding cerebellar lacunes due to dilatation of the perivascular space associated with Binswanger's subcortical arteriosclerotic encephalopathy. *Stroke* 1987; 18:1087–1092.
31. Poirier J, Barbizet J, Gaston A, Meyrignac C. Démence thalamique. Lacunes expansives du territoire thalamo-mésencéphalique paramédian. Hydrocéphalie par stenose de l'aqueduc de Sylvius. *Rev Neurol* 1983;139:349–358.
32. Hughes W. Origin of lacunes. *Lancet* 1965;2: 19–21.
33. Moore MT. Perivascular encephalolysis. *Arch Neurol Psychiatry* 1954;71:344–357.
34. Poirier J, Derouesné C. Le concept de lacune cérébral de 1838 à nos jours. *Rev Neurol (Paris)* 1985;141:3–17.
35. Bogousslavsky J, Regli F, Maeder P. Intracranial large-artery disease and "lacunar" infarction. *Cerebrovasc Dis* 1991;1:154–159.
36. Kuroiwa Y, Furukawa T. Hemispheric infarction after herpes zoster ophthalmicus: computed tomography and angiography. *Neurology* 1981;31:1030–1032.
37. Pullicino P, Fava S. Recurrent cerebral infarction and central retinal artery occlusion following mandibular zoster. *Can J Neurol Sci* 1991; 18:105.
38. Bogousslavsky J, Regli F, Uske A. Thalamic infarcts: clinical syndromes, etiology, and prognosis. *Neurology* 1988;38:837–848.
39. Fisher M, Smith TW, Jacobs R. Pure motor hemiplegia secondary to a saccular basilar artery aneurysm. *Stroke* 1988;19:104–107.
40. Nicolai A, Lazzarino LG. Transient pure sensory strokes in patient with aneurysm of rostral basilar artery. *J Neurol Neurosurg Psychiatry* 1992;55:72–73.
41. Meissner I, Sapir S, Kokmen E, Stein SD. The paramedian diencephalic syndrome: a dynamic phenomenon. *Stroke* 1987;18:380–385.
42. Levine SR, Deegan MJ, Futrell N, Welch KMA. Cerebrovascular and neurologic disease associated with antiphospholipid antibodies: 48 cases. *Neurology* 1990;40:1181–1189.

43. Woodard C, Brey R, Hart R, Kagen-Hallett K. Neuropathological findings in stroke associated with antiphospholipid antibodies (aPL). *Neurology* 1991;41:296(abst)
44. Biller J, Merchut M, Emanuele M. Nonhemorrhagic infarction of the thalamus. *Neurology* 1984;34:1269–1270.
45. Drake ME. Lupus anticoagulant and lacunar infarctions. *Eur Neurol* 1988;28:174–176.
46. Malamut BL, Graff-Radford NR, Chawluk J, Grossman RI, Gur RC. Memory in a case of bilateral thalamic infarction. *Neurology* 1992; 42:163–169.
47. Devinsky O, Petito CK, Alonso DR. Clinical and neuropathological findings in systemic lupus erythematosus: the role of vasculitis, heart emboli, and thrombotic thrombocytopenic purpura. *Ann Neurol* 1988;23:380–384.
48. Johnson RT, Richardson EP. The neurological manifestations of systemic lupus erythematosus. A clinical-pathological study of 24 cases and review of the literature. *Medicine (Baltimore)* 1968;47:337–369.
49. Futrell N, Millikan C. Frequency, etiology, and prevention of stroke in patients with systemic lupus erythematosus. *Stroke* 1989;20:583–591.
50. Kitagawa Y, Gotoh F, Koto A, Okayasu H. Stroke in systemic lupus erythematosus. *Stroke* 1990;21:1533–1539.
51. DiMario FJ Jr, Bronte-Stewart H, Sherbotie J, Turner ME. Lacunar infarction of the basal ganglia as a complication of hemolytic-uremic syndrome. *Clin Pediatr* 1987;26:586–590.
52. Schwartzman RJ, Hill JB. Neurological complications of disseminated intravascular coagulation. *Neurology* 1982;32:791–797.
53. Dawson TM, Lavi E, Raps EC, Goldberg HI. Thrombotic microangiopathy isolated to the central nervous system. *Ann Neurol* 1991; 30:843–846.
54. Lohrmann HP, Adam W, Heymer B, Kubanek B. Microangiopathic hemolytic anemia in metastatic carcinoma: report of eight cases. *Ann Intern Med* 1973;79:368–375.
55. Petiot P, Croisile B, Confavreux C, et al. Thalamic stroke and congenital factor V deficiency. *Stroke* 1991;22:1606.
56. Fisher CM. Pure sensory stroke and allied conditions. *Stroke* 1982;13:434–447.
57. Pearce MS, Chandrasekera CP, Ladusans EJ. Lacunar infarcts in polychthaemia with raised packed cell volumes. *Br Med J* 1983;287:935–936.
58. Mayo J, Arias M, Leno C, Berciano J. Vascular parkinsonism and periarteritis nodosa. *Neurology* 1986;36:874–875.
59. Pullicino P, Nelson RF, Kendall BE, Marshall J. Small deep infarcts diagnosed on computed tomography. *Neurology* 1980;30:1090–1096.
60. Karni A, Sadeh M, Blatt I, Goldhammer Y. Cogan's syndrome complicated by lacunar brain infarcts. *J Neurol Neurosurg Psychiatry* 1991; 54:169–171.
61. Moore PM. Diagnosis and management of isolated angiitis of the central nervous system. *Neurology* 1989;39:167–173.
62. Koo EH, Massey EW. Granulomatous angiitis of the central nervous system: protean manifestations and response to treatment. *J Neurol Neurosurg Psychiatry* 1988;51:1126–1133.
63. Gjerstad L, Nyberg-Hansen R, Bjorland O, Nakstad P, Russell D, Rootwelt K. Herpes zoster ophthalmicus with cerebral angiitis and reduced cerebral blood flow. *Acta Neurol Scand* 1986;74:460–466.
64. Harriman DGF. Bacterial infections of the central nervous system. In: Blackwood W, Corsellis JAN, eds. *Greenfield's neuropathology*. 3rd ed. London: Edward Arnold; 1976:238–268.
65. Barinagarrementeria F, Del Brutto OH. Lacunar syndrome due to nerocysticercosis. *Arch Neurol* 1989;46:415–417.
66. Johns DR, Tierney M, Parker SW. Pure motor hemiplegia due to meningovascular syphilis. *Arch Neurol* 1987;44:1062–1065.
67. May EF, Jabbari B. Stroke in neuroborreliosis. *Stroke* 1990;21:1232–1235.
68. Kohler J, Kern U, Kasper J, Rhese-Kupper B, Thoden U. Chronic central nervous system involvement in Lyme borreliosis. *Neurology* 1988;38:863–867.
69. Eda I, Takashima S, Takeshita K. Acute hemiplegia with lacunar infarction after varicella infection in childhood. *Brain Dev* 1983;5:494–499.
70. Engstrom JW, Lowenstein DH, Bredesen DE. Cerebral infarctions and transient neurologic deficits associated with acquired immunodeficiency syndrome. *Am J Med* 1989;86:528–532.
71. Park YD, Belman AL, Kim TS, et al. Stroke in pediatric acquired immunodeficiency syndrome. *Ann Neurol* 1990;28:303–311.
72. Santamaria J, Graus F, Rubio F, Arbizu T, Peres J. Cerebral infarction of the basal ganglia due to embolism from the heart. *Stroke* 1983;14:911–914.
73. Weisberg LA. Nonseptic cardiogenic cerebral embolic stroke: clinical-CT correlations. *Neurology* 1985;35:896–899.
74. Landi G, Cella E, Baccardi E, Musicco M. Lacunar versus non-lacunar infarcts: pathogenetic and prognostic differences. *J Neurol Neurosurg Psychiatry* 1992;55:441–445.
75. Rascol A, Clanet M, Manelfe C, Guiraud B, Bonafe A. Pure motor hemiplegia: CT study of 30 cases. *Stroke* 1982;13:11–17.
76. Gorsselink EL, Peeters HPM, Lodder J. Causes of small deep infarcts detected by CT. *Clin Neurol Neurosurg* 1984;86:271–273.
77. Horowitz DH, Tuhrim S, Weinberger JM, Rudolph SH. Mechanisms in lacunar infarction. *Stroke* 1992;23:325–327.
78. Ghika J, Bogoussalvsky J, Regli F. Infarcts in the territory of the deep perforators from the carotid system. *Neurology* 1989;39:507–512.
79. Caplan LR. "Top of the basilar" syndrome. *Neurology* 1980;30:72–79.
80. Wall M, Salmovits TL, Weisberg LA, Trufant SA. Vertical gaze ophthalmoplegia from infarction in the area of the posterior thalamo-subthalamic paramedian artery. *Stroke* 1986;17:546–555.

81. Masdeu JC, Rosenberg M. Midbrain-diencephalic horizontal gaze paresis. *J Clin Neuro Ophthalmol* 1987;7:227–234.
82. Biller J, Sand JJ, Corbett JJ, Adams HP Jr, Dunn V. Syndrome of the paramedian thalamic arteries: clinical and neuroimaging correlation. *J Clin Neuro Ophthalmol* 1985;5:217–223.
83. McKee AC, Levine DN, Kowall NW, Richardson EP Jr. Peduncular hallucinosis associated with isolated infarction of the substantia nigra pars reticularis. *Ann Neurol* 1990;27:500–504.
84. Feinberg WM, Seeger JF, Carmody RF, Anderson DC, Hart RG, Pearce LA. Epidemiologic features of asymptomatic cerebral infarction in patients with nonvalvular atrial fibrillation. *Arch Intern Med* 1990;150:2340–2344.
85. Gandolfo C, Caponetto C, Del Sette M, Santoloci D, Loeb C. Risk factors in lacunar syndromes: a case-control study. *Acta Neurol Scand* 1988;77:22–26.
86. Kompf D, Opperman J, Konig F, Talmon-Gros S, Babaian E. Vertikale Blickparese und thalamische Demenz. *Nervenarzt* 1984;55:625–636.
87. Liu GT, Carrazana EJ, Charness ME. Unilateral oculomotor palsy and bilateral ptosis from paramedian midbrain infarction. *Arch Neurol* 1991;48:983–986.
88. Biller J, Shapiro R, Evans LS, Haag JR, Fine M. Oculomotor nuclear complex infarction. Clinical and radiological correlation. *Arch Neurol* 1984;41:985–987(abst).
89. Cacciatore A, Russo LS Jr. Lacunar infarction as an embolic complication of cardiac and arch angiography. *Stroke* 1991;22:1603–1605.
90. Norris JW, Zhu CZ. Silent stroke and carotid stenosis. *Stroke* 1992;23:483–485.
91. Tegeler CH, Shi F, Morgan T. Carotid stenosis in lacunar stroke. *Stroke* 1991;22:1124–1128.
92. Caplan LR, Thomas C, Banks G. Central nervous system complications of addiction to "T's and Blues." *Neurology* 1982;32:623–628.
93. Bogousslavsky J, Regli F. Unilateral watershed cerebral infarcts. *Neurology* 1986;36:373–377.
94. Sawada H, Udaka F, Seriu N, Shindou K, Kameyama M, Tsujimura M. MRI demonstration of cortical laminar necrosis and delayed white matter injury in anoxic encephalopathy. *Neuroradiology* 1990;32:319–321.
95. Bruno A, Yuh WTC, Biller J, Adams HP Jr, Cornell SH. Magnetic resonance imaging in young adults with cerebral infarction due to Moyamoya. *Arch Neurol* 1988;45:303–306.
96. Yamauchi H, Fukuyama H, Yamaguchi S, Miyoshi T, Kimura J, Konishi J. High-intensity area in deep white matter indicating hemodynamic compromise in internal carotid artery occlusive disorders. *Arch Neurol* 1991;48:1067–1071.
97. Weiller C, Ringelstein EB, Reiche W, Buell U. Clinical and hemodynamic aspects of low-flow infarcts. *Stroke* 1991;22:1117–1123.
98. Zülch K-J. *The cerebral infarct. Pathology, pathogenesis and computed tomography.* Berlin: Springer-Verlag; 1985.
99. Waterston JA, Brown MM, Butler P, Swash M. Small deep cerebral infarcts associated with occlusive internal carotid artery disease. *Arch Neurol* 1990;47:953–957.
100. Bozzao L, Fantozzi LM, Bastianello S, Bozzao A, Fieschi C. Early collateral blood supply and late parenchymal brain damage in patients with middle cerebral artery occlusion. *Stroke* 1989;20:735–740.
101. Caplan L, Babikian V, Helgason C, et al. Occlusive disease of the middle cerebral artery. *Neurology* 1985;35:975–982.
102. Angeloni U, Bozzao L, Fantozzi L, Bastianello S, Kushner M, Fieschi C. Internal borderzone infarction following acute middle cerebral artery occlusion. *Neurology* 1990;40:1196–1198.
103. Cobb SR, Mehringer CM, Itabashi HH, Pribram H. CT of subinsular infarction and ischemia. *AJNR* 1987;8:221–227.
104. Pullicino P, Miller LL, Munschauer FE, Ostrow PT. Linear subinsular MR hyperintensities. *Ann Neurol* 1992;32:267–268(abst).
105. Torvik A. The pathogenesis of watershed infarcts in the brain. *Stroke* 1984;15:221–223.
106. Howard R, Trend P, Russell RWR. Clinical features of ischemia in cerebral arterial borderzones after periods of reduced cerebral blood flow. *Arch Neurol* 1987;44:934–940.
107. Bladin CF, Chambers BR. Partial internal watershed infarction. *J Neurol* 1990;147:149 (abst).
108. Jacobs L, Heffner RR Jr, Newman RP. Selective paralysis of downward gaze caused by bilateral lesions of the mesencephalic periaqueductal gray matter. *Neurology* 1985;35:516–521.
109. Dobkin BH. Orthostatic hypotension as a risk factor for symptomatic occlusive cerebrovascular disease. *Neurology* 1989;39:30–34.
110. Pullicino PM, Xuereb M, Aquilina J, Piedmonte MR. Stroke following acute myocardial infarction in diabetics. *J Intern Med* 1992;231:287–293.
111. Wodarz R. Watershed infarctions and computed tomography. A topographical study in cases with stenosis or occlusion of the carotid artery. *Neuroradiology* 1980;19:245–248.
112. Ringelstein EB, Zeumer H, Angelou D. The pathogenesis of strokes from internal carotid artery occlusion. Diagnostic and therapeutical implications. *Stroke* 1983;14:867–875.
113. Leblanc R, Yamamoto YL, Tyler JL, Diksic M, Hakim A. Borderzone ischemia. *Ann Neurol* 1987;22:707–713.
114. Brown MM, Wade JPH, Bishop CCR, Russell RWR. Reactivity of the cerebral circulation in patients with carotid occlusion. *J Neurol Neurosurg Psychiatry* 1986;49:899–904.
115. Kobayashi S, Okada K, Yamashita K. Incidence of silent lacunar lesion in normal adults and its relation to cerebral blood flow and risk factors. *Stroke* 1991;22:1379–1383.
116. Weiller C, Mullges W, Ringelstein EB, Buell U, Reiche W. Patterns of brain infarctions in internal carotid artery dissections. *Neurosurg Rev* 1991;14:111–113.
117. Halsey JH. Progressive lacunar infarction with

demonstrated patency of the middle cerebral artery. *Stroke* 1986;1028:1030.
118. Fisher CM, Curry HB. Pure motor hemiplegia of vascular origin. *Arch Neurol* 1965;13:30–44.
119. Donnan GA, Bladin PF. Capsular warning syndrome: repetitive hemiplegia preceding capsular stroke. *Stroke* 1987;18:296(abst).
120. LaRue L, Alter M, Lai SM, et al. Acute stroke, hematocrit, and blood pressure. *Stroke* 1987; 18:565–569.
121. Kappelle LJ, Van Latum JC, Koudstaal PJ, Van Gijn J. Transient ischaemic attacks and small-vessel disease. *Lancet* 1991;337:339–341.
122. Yeung AC, Vekshtein VI, Krantz DS, et al. The efffect of atherosclerosis on the vasomotor response of coronary arteries to mental stress. *N Engl J Med* 1991;325:1551–1556.
123. Faraci FM, Williams JK, Breese KR, Armstrong ML, Heistad DD. Atherosclerosis potentiates constrictor responses of cerebral and ocular blood vessels to thromboxane in monkeys. *Stroke* 1989;20:242–247.
124. Ferbert A, Busse D, Thron A. Microinfarction in classic migraine? A study with magnetic resonance imaging findings. *Stroke* 1991;22:1010–1014.
125. Mills RP, Swanson PD. Vertical oculomotor apraxia and memory loss. *Ann Neurol* 1978; 4:149–153.
126. Petit H, Rousseaux M, Clarisse J, Delafosse A. Troubles oculo-céphalomoteurs et infarctus thalamo-sous-thalamique bilatéral. *Rev Neurol* 1981;137:709–722.
127. Rowley HA, Lowenstein DH, Rowbotham MC, Simon RP. Thalamomesencephalic strokes after cocaine abuse. *Neurology* 1989;39:428–430.

7

Lacunar Syndromes

Gérard Besson and Marc Hommel

Department of Clinical and Biological Neurosciences, Stroke Unit, Centre Hospitalier Universitaire Regional de Grenoble, 38043 Grenoble, France

When lacunes were first described, they were considered to be fortuitous autopsy findings. Raymond stated that they were too small and too common to produce any clinical signs or symptoms (1). Although lacunar infarcts are now known to cause clinical syndromes, the great majority of lacunar infarcts probably remain asymptomatic (2–4). Eighty-eight (77%) of the 114 patients in Fisher's study had no history of neurological deficit and a clinicopathological correlation could be made in only eight patients (7%) (2). Fang confirmed this lack of clinicopathological correlation in a study of 51 brains that had lacunar infarcts (3).

The concept of lacunar syndromes was established in the 1960s with the works of C.M. Fisher and his colleagues. By correlating clinical features with the anatomical sites of lacunes at autopsy, Fisher and colleagues were able to ascribe five clinical syndromes to lacunar infarcts. Since these clinical lacunar syndromes were first reported, the number of clinical syndromes has grown to at least 70 (5). In this chapter we have divided the lacunar syndromes into two groups: a classic group (pure motor hemiplegia, pure sensory stroke, ataxic hemiparesis, dysarthria–clumsy hand syndrome, sensorimotor stroke) and a miscellaneous group including all other lacunar syndromes. We have focused on the clinical syndromes associated with lacunar infarcts confirmed at autopsy whatever the etiology of the underlying arterial occlusion.

THE CLASSIC LACUNAR SYNDROMES

Pure Motor Hemiplegia and Pure Motor Hemiparesis

In 1965, Fisher and Curry (6) coined the term pure motor hemiplegia to define the first and most frequent lacunar syndrome. This syndrome was not new, since Dechambre had reported two cases (his cases 4 and 6) of motor hemiparesis without other clinical findings, each due to an infarct located in the centrum ovale (7). Fisher and Curry defined pure motor hemiplegia as a paralysis involving the face, arm, and leg on one side not accompanied by sensory signs, visual field defect, or neuropsychological disturbance. In the case of brain stem lesions, the hemiplegia must be free of vertigo, deafness, tinnitus, diplopia, cerebellar ataxia, and nystagmus.

The age-adjusted annual incidence of pure motor stroke has recently been evaluated at 26.6 per 100,000 inhabitants in a population-based study in Sweden (8). The percentage of strokes presenting as pure motor hemiparesis has been estimated at 3% of stroke patients admitted to Harlem Hospital (9), at 9.1% in Oxford (10), at 12.6% in Sweden (8), and at 14.2% in the Stroke Data Bank and in the Lausanne stroke registry (11,12). The mean age of onset was 61 years for Richter et al. (9), 63.1 years for Melo et al. (12), 63.5 years for Soisson et al. (13), and 72 years for Norrving and Staaf (8). Although this syndrome is frequent in the elderly, it has also been reported in childhood (14–16).

Prodromal transient ischemic attacks (TIAs) were recorded in 16.1% (8) to 57% of patients (17). TIAs occurred within 24 hours (57% for Norrving and Staaf), within 48 hours (87% for Fisher and Curry), or within 1 week (17, 18) of the onset of the motor deficit. They infrequently occurred more than 1 week (24%) before the stroke (8). Recurrent transient pure motor hemiparesis supports the hypothesis of reduced flow in a penetrating artery, and may indicate impending small artery occlusion (19). The terms capsular claudication (20) and capsular warning syndrome (21) were coined to describe this phenomenon.

For Rascol et al. the onset of pure motor hemiparesis was sudden in 47% and progressed gradually in 6% (17). The progression occurred within the first 24 hours in 38.4% of patients with progressing pure motor stroke (8). The motor weakness progressed from one limb to the other during several hours (22–24).

The motor weakness may be incomplete (pure motor hemiparesis), affecting particularly the proximal parts of the limbs (6). The severity of the motor deficit has been studied by Richter et al. (9). These authors reported that the motor deficit was equal in the upper and lower limbs in 61%, mostly affected the upper limb in 35%, and mostly affected the lower limb in 4%.

The diagnosis of pure motor stroke is theoretically dependent on the exclusion of even minor involvement of sensory pathways, which may be difficult in practice. Using somatosensory evoked responses, Chokroverty and Rubino (25) reported evidence of involvement of the lemniscal pathway in 7 of 15 patients with clinical pure motor hemiplegia. These results were supported by two clinical studies in which abnormalities of somatosensory evoked response were recorded in patients with pure motor stroke (26,27). These patients with apparent clinical pure motor hemiplegia with abnormal somatosensory responses may be considered as having sensorimotor stroke. Although the motor deficit in pure motor stroke must be isolated, transient hypesthesia or paresthesias have been reported and are compatible with the diagnosis of pure motor hemiparesis (6,21). Dysarthria, which was noted by Fisher and Curry, was considered as very common by Schott and Laurent (28).

The clinical outcome of pure motor stroke is probably better than that of hemiplegia due to a cortical infarct. Norrving and Staaf reported that at 3 weeks after a pure motor hemiparesis, 61.3% of their patients had recovered completely or had minor motor deficits, 26.3% had moderate motor deficits, and 11.3% had major motor deficit (8). Only one elderly patient died within 1 month. The motor outcome is better when the initial motor deficit is incomplete (29).

Clinicopathological correlations are rare in lacunar stroke because of the very low case fatality. Six of the nine autopsy cases of Fisher and Curry were lacunar infarcts involving the posterior limb of the internal capsule, and three were lacunar infarcts involving the basis pontis (6). The production of pure motor hemiparesis by lacunar infarcts in either capsular (30,31) or pontine (30,32) locations (33) has been known since the early 20th century. Although some of these earlier reports are incomplete (34,35), there are several well-documented case reports in old French theses. In 1874, Veyssière reported a case of pure motor hemiplegia due to capsulolenticular infarct (case 20) (36). In 1875, Lépine reported a 44-year-old woman with the sudden onset of a left pure motor hemiplegia preceded by transient homolateral paresthesias (37). At autopsy 26 months later, a cortical infarct was found that involved the first and the second frontal convolutions and destroyed the corona radiata but spared the parietal lobe. This is, to our knowledge, the only autopsy case report of pure motor hemiplegia due to a cortical infarct. Raymond (case 18), in 1875, and Pitres (cases 4 and 5), in 1884, reported cases of pure motor hemiparesis due to capsular infarcts with or without lenticular involvement (38,39). In 1877, Landouzy reported one case of pure motor hemiplegia due to a hemorrhagic lacune located in the centrum semiovale (40). Since the report of Fisher and Curry, lacunes associated with pure motor stroke have been reported in the internal capsule (8,21,23,41), the cerebral peduncle (42,43), the basis pontis (22,44,45) (Fig. 1), and the medulla oblongata (24). Chokroverty and Rubino reported a pure motor stroke due to a cortical infarct (46), but a thalamocapsular lacune that might also have explained the clinical findings was present.

Partial Pure Motor Stroke

Partial pure motor stroke is a common variant of pure motor hemiparesis, making up 33.3% of Norrving and Staaf's 180 cases of pure motor stroke (8). Partial can be used to refer to less severe degrees of weakness (hemiparesis) or to sparing of face, arm, or leg. The occurrence of partial pure motor strokes may be explained by the anteroposterior face-arm-leg somatotopic organization of the pyramidal tract (19).

Brachiocrural weakness is the most common type of partial pure motor stroke (47) associated with a presumed lacunar infarct on computed tomography (CT) (82%) (8). Brachiocrural weakness with early development of spasticity has been associated with a medullary infarct at autopsy (6,25,48,49). The first reported clinical-anatomical correlation of a brachiocrural motor deficit was, however, in 1877 by Charcot and Pitres (case 12) (50), who found a small cortical infarct at autopsy. A few years later, Pitres reported a case of brachiocrural motor deficit due to a lacunar infarct in the anterior limb of the internal capsule (51).

Norrving and Staaf found a brachiocrural motor deficit to be the second most common form of partial pure motor stroke that was associated with a presumed lacunar infarct on CT (25%) (8). Melo et al., however, found it to be the most common (58%) (12). Only two cases have been reported with pathologic confirmation (52,53). Case 31 of

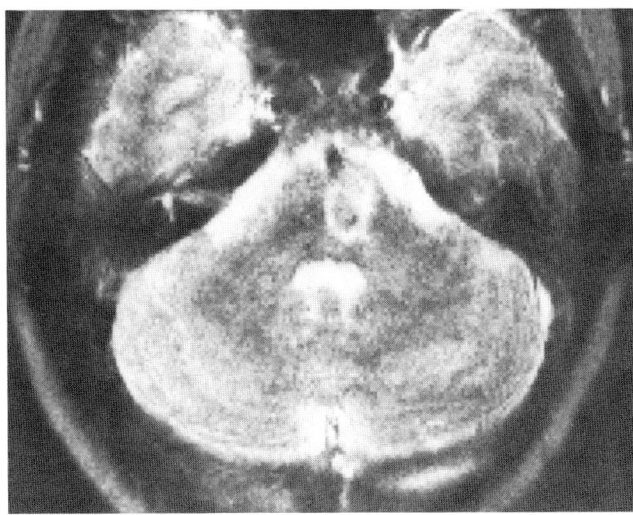

FIG. 1. Axial T2-weighted MR image of a 55-year-old hypertensive and diabetic woman presenting with a right pure motor hemiplegia. MR shows a lacunar infarct in the left pons.

Pitres's thesis was due to a lacunar infarct in the centrum semiovale (52) and the case of Gauche was due to a small cortical infarct (53).

Isolated lower facial palsies have occasionally been reported. Cruveilhier (book 20, vol. 1) reported the only case with autopsy correlation (54). In 1834, Professor Dupuytren developed a left lower facial palsy during a lecture. He continued the lecture, supporting his weakened lip with a finger (54). No sensory examination was noted. He died a few months later after having had two transient ischemic attacks. At autopsy, a small yellow scar was found in the right corona radiata near the lateral ventricle. This was compatible with an old infarct and was in a location that could have produced the lower facial palsy. A lower facial palsy can be associated with dysarthria (55) and dysphagia (55). Although there is an autopsy report of a hemorrhage in the genu of the internal capsule giving this syndrome, there is no autopsy report of an infarct giving rise to it (56). Presumed lacunar infarcts causing a lower facial palsy have been shown on imaging studies to have a capsular (17,21,55) or pontine (57,58) location.

Isolated brachial monoplegia is a rare manifestation of a supratentorial infarct (3%) (59). At least three cases due to a capsular lacunar infarct (60,61) and one due to a small cortical infarct (62) have been reported at autopsy. A case of isolated brachial monoparesis due to a pontine infarct has been reported on CT (63). Isolated crural monoparesis has only been reported on CT studies (17,21).

Unilateral vocal cord palsy is a very unusual partial pure motor stroke described by Garel and Dor in 1890 (64). An isolated palsy of the left vocal cord was found in a 35-year-old man with endocarditis. He died 8 days later from cardiac failure, and at autopsy the authors found a small deep infarct 8 mm in diameter in the anterior limb of the right internal capsule.

Bilateral Pure Motor Stroke

Bilateral pure motor hemiplegia (i.e., pure motor quadriplegia) is due to bilateral pyramidal tract lesions. It must be differentiated from the "locked-in syndrome," in which a bilateral horizontal gaze palsy is present in addition to quadriplegia. The locked-in syndrome is usually due to a basilar occlusion, although Fisher has reported a case due to occlusion of two small basilar branch arteries (65). Two cases of bilateral pure motor hemiplegia with autopsy confirmation have been reported. The motor deficit was partial in both, and was due to bilateral capsular infarcts in one (65a) and to bilateral medullary infarcts in the other (66). A bilateral faciobrachial paresis has recently been related to bilateral capsular infarcts shown on CT (67). Three patients with bilateral infarction of the medullary pyramids have been reported with almost pure motor quadriplegia. Transient involvement of deeper medullary structures was, however, present in all cases. Additional neurologic signs included abnormalities of eye movement (68), paralysis of the tongue and palate (69), and nausea and confusion (70).

Ataxic Hemiparesis and Dysarthria–Clumsy Hand Syndrome

Ataxic Hemiparesis

Ataxic hemiparesis is a syndrome in which pyramidal and cerebellar signs occur on the same side. This association is explained by interruption of the cerebello-thalamo-cortico-ponto-cerebellar loop. Cerebellar ataxia is defined as a disturbance in amplitude of movement (hypermetria), in combining movements (asynergia), in the speed of alternating movements (adiadokokinesia), in the speed of initiation and arrest of movement (dyschronometria), and in the continuity of contraction (tremor)

(71). It may be difficult to demonstrate cerebellar ataxia in patients with severe weakness, and for this reason ataxic hemiparesis is sometimes recognized only after partial recovery of a pure motor hemiplegia (13,72). Fisher and Cole first described the syndrome of homolateral ataxia and crural paresis in 1965 (73). This syndrome is a combination of lower limb weakness with a striking dysmetria of the arm and leg on the same side. Thirteen years later, Fisher coined the term ataxic hemiparesis to describe the combination of pure motor hemiparesis with cerebellar incoordination on the same side (74). Fisher wondered whether the incoordination was due to weakness or to cerebellar ataxia.

The percentage of strokes presenting as ataxic hemiparesis was 1.9% of strokes in Oxford (10) and 2.6% of strokes in the Stroke Data Bank (11). The mean age of onset is 69.1 years according to Magrotti et al. (75).

The most common cerebellar sign in ataxic hemiparesis is dysmetria, which may be slight (20%), moderate (15%), or severe (65%) (76). Adiadokokinesia occurs in about 40% of patients. Hypotonia has only been described in a few cases (73,77–80) as has tremor (73,79,81–83). Motor weakness is usually proportional in the face, arm, and leg (55%); however, it may be more severe in the leg (42%) or in the arm (3%) (76).

Fisher and Cole noted that mild hypesthesia may be found in association with ataxic hemiparesis (73). Since their report, hypesthesia has often been reported as an associated sign, and Sanguineti et al. found that 36% of patients with ataxic hemiparesis had hypethesia (76). The sensory loss in these cases is always slight, and usually only involves lemniscal sensation, with loss of pinprick sensation (80,84,85), but there may also be loss of vibratory and joint position sensation in the foot. Using somatosensory evoked responses, involvement of the lemniscal pathway has been demonstrated in four patients with ataxic hemiparesis (26). Anisocoria (73), tongue deviation (74,86), and nystagmus have also been recorded in patients with ataxic hemiparesis (73,74,81,86). Huang and Lui suggested that nystagmus, dysarthria, and normal sensory testing suggest a brainstem lesion (84).

There are only a few reports of patients with ataxic hemiparesis with autopsy correlation of the infarct site. The first was by Foix and Hillemand in 1926 (32), who reported a patient with hemiparesis and mild cerebellar signs due to a pontine infarct. In 1930, Nicolesco, Cretu, and Demetresco suggested that crural monoplegia with cerebellar incoordination could be due to a lacune located in the upper part of the anterior limb of the internal capsule (87). Unfortunately, in this very short paper it is impossible to know whether the conclusion these authors reached was based on a clinicopathological correlation or if it was a hypothesis. In 1955, Garcin reported the first well-documented observation (88) of a thalamic lacune (possibly a hemorrhagic scar) that spared the internal capsule but gave rise to ataxic hemiparesis. In 1969, he published a further similar autopsy case report with Lapresle (89). In their first autopsy-proven case, Fisher and Cole suggested that a lacunar infarct in the posterior limb of the internal capsule was responsible for the syndrome of homolateral ataxia and crural paresis (73). Unfortunately, 11 lesions were found in the brain in this case, so the authors could not be sure which of these was the relevant one. Fisher subsequently reported three patients with ataxic hemiparesis in each of whom a lacunar infarct was found at the junction of the upper third and lower two thirds of the basis pontis at autopsy (74). The only proven anatomic allocations for ataxic hemiparesis are therefore the internal capsule, the thalamus, and the upper pons. Imaging studies using CT scan and magnetic resonance imaging (MRI) have confirmed these locations (Fig. 2) and have also suggested that ataxic

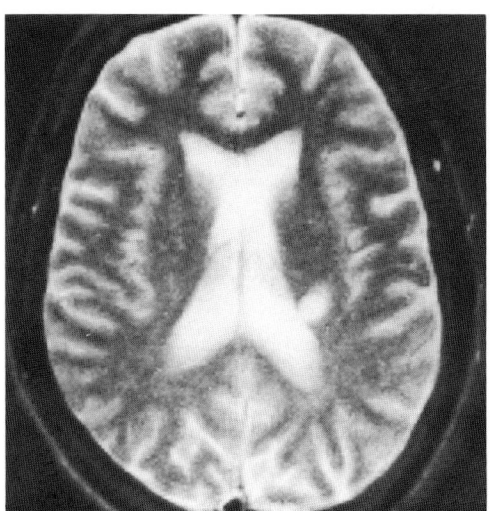

FIG. 2. Axial T2-weighted MR image of a 39-year-old hypertensive man presenting with right ataxic hemiparesis. MR shows a lacunar infarct in the upper part of the left internal capsule.

hemiparesis may be caused by cortical infarcts (90), or by a presumed lacunar infarct in the corona radiata (77), the anterior limb of the internal capsule extending to the head of the caudate nucleus (91), the posterior limb of the internal capsule extending to the thalamus (72), the median part of the pons (92), or the lower pons (93).

Variants of Ataxic Hemiparesis

Slight hypesthesia is acceptable as part of the ataxic hemiparesis syndrome. The term hypesthetic ataxic hemiparesis is used when prominent sensory symptoms are present (94). This syndrome has been reported in thalamocapsular infarcts, in which case the hypesthesia is caused by involvement of the ventral posteromedial nucleus of the thalamus by the infarct. A diagnosis of "painful ataxic hemiparesis" was made in a patient with ataxic hemiparesis, with ipsilateral pain and normal sensory and neuropsychological examination. CT showed an infarct in the contralateral thalamus (95).

A case of ataxic hemiparesis with contralateral trigeminal distribution weakness involvement (moderate weakness of the masseter and temporalis muscles, with normal sensation and corneal reflexes) has been related to a small infarct in the basis pontis (96).

When ataxic hemiparesis occurs bilaterally it is called an ataxic tetraparesis. In the single case report in the literature, the two sides were affected sequentially. CT demonstrated an infarct in the basis pontis (97).

The Dysarthria–Clumsy Hand Syndrome

In 1967, Fisher described a syndrome characterized by dysarthria and clumsiness of one hand (98). The clumsiness, which was particularly marked in writing, was thought to be due to cerebellar incoordination (99). This explanation is, however, controversial (100) because the finger-to-nose test may be normal (98) or may show dysmetria (98,99,101,102). Several additional signs may be present, such as lower facial paralysis (98,99,101–103), ipsilateral brisk tendon reflexes and a Babinski sign (98,102,104), dysphagia (98,103), or deviation of the protruded tongue (98,102).

The percentage of strokes due to the dysarthria–clumsy hand syndrome has been estimated at 1.4% of the strokes in the Stroke Data Bank (11). The single case in the literature with autopsy confirmation showed a lacunar infarct in the upper 5 mm of the basis pontis (98). Imaging studies using CT or MRI have confirmed this location and have also suggested that the dysarthria–clumsy hand syndrome can be due to a lacunar infarct in the corona radiata (21) or in the genu of the internal capsule (103,104). This syndrome can be considered a variant of ataxic hemiparesis because there is often an association of ipsilateral pyramidal (lower facial paralysis, Babinski sign, brisk tendon reflexes) and cerebellar signs (dysmetria).

Pure Sensory Stroke

In 1965, Fisher characterized pure sensory stroke as a persistent or transient subjective numbness with slight sensory loss involving face, arm, and leg, unaccompanied by motor weakness, dysarthria, vertigo, diplopia, nystagmus, visual field deficit, or neuropsychological disturbance (105).

The percentage of strokes due to pure sensory stroke was estimated to be 1.2% of strokes in Oxford (10) and 1.8% of strokes in the Stroke Data Bank (11). Prodromal TIAs were recorded in 17% of patients with pure sensory stroke (106). In patients without TIA, the onset was sudden in 38% and the deficit progressed in a stepwise fashion in 33% (106). The symptoms were discovered on awakening in 29% of cases (106).

Sensory loss in pure sensory stroke may involve protopathic sensibility, epicritic sensibility, or, more commonly, both. Isolated proprioception loss (107,108), or isolated pin and light touch abnormalities are rare (109). Paresthesias are frequent and the affected areas may be described as "numb, asleep, hot, frozen, tingling, gripping, pricking, stiff, tight, pressing, bandaged, cold, hard, itching, or dead" (105). Unpleasant numbness may be reminiscent of the thalamic syndrome of Déjérine and Roussy (110). Fisher used the term pure paresthetic stroke when there was no objective sensory loss (105).

Although involvement of face, arm, and leg is the most common type of pure sensory stroke (83%), sensory loss can affect face and arm (7%), arm and leg (8%), or face, trunk, and leg (1%) (106). A cheirooral sensory loss has recently been reported in relation to small infarcts in the thalamus and in the pons (111). Fisher has proposed the following clinicotopographic correlations (106):

Isolated paresthesias of the face, arm, and leg indicate a thalamic lesion.
Sensory loss in the hand involving only some of the fingers indicates a cortical lesion.
Involvement of the abdomen indicates a thalamic lesion.
None of these patterns occur in brainstem lesions.

Involvement of the abdomen, however, has been reported in a patient with a pontine infarct (107).

The prognosis of pure sensory stroke is good. Paresthesias and dysesthesias may disappear within 2 or 3 days, or persist for weeks and months (106). There is no disability due to the stroke, a chronic pain problem being rare (2 out of 39 patients) according to Fisher (106). The first autopsy correlation of pure sensory stroke was by Bourneville in 1873. He found numerous lacunes involving the thalamocortical pathways but sparing the thalamus (112). In his thesis, De Ajuriaguerra quoted an observation of Lhermitte and himself in which isolated limb pain was due to a thalamic infarct (113). Hemialgic (pain syndrome on one side of the body) syndrome without sensory loss in another patient was related to a thalamic infarct shown at autopsy (114). Fisher reported six cases of pure sensory stroke due to lacunar infarcts in the posteroventral thalamus (105, 106,115). Imaging studies have confirmed these locations (Fig. 3) and suggest that pure sensory stroke can also be due to cortical infarcts (116) and to pontine lacunar infarcts (107).

Sensorimotor Stroke

In 1977, Mohr et al. described a patient with an isolated sensorimotor deficit caused by a thalamocapsular lacunar infarct (117). Two different studies found the mean age of onset in sensorimotor stroke to vary from 63.8 (118) to 66 years (119). Previous TIA occurred in 8.8% of cases (118). In view of the fact that sensory loss and motor weakness may be affected to differ-

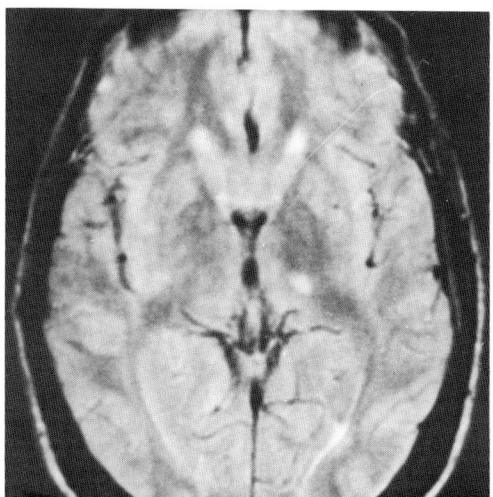

FIG. 3. Axial T2-weighted MR image of a 65-year-old hypertensive and hypercholesterolemic man presenting with a right pure sensory stroke. MR shows a lacunar infarct in the left thalamus.

ent extents, Huang et al. classified sensorimotor stroke into four types according to the extent and nature of the sensory loss (119):

Type 1: all sensory modalities are affected.
Type 2: only nociceptive deficits are present.
Type 3: only proprioceptive deficits are present.
Type 4: only one limb is involved.

Each type was classified into two groups according to whether the motor or sensory deficit was complete or not: group A, submaximal motor and sensory impairment; group B, total paralysis or total sensory loss in at least one limb.

The percentages in each subgroup in these series was as follows: 1A (29%), 1B (16%), 2A (13%), 2B (4%), 3A (20%), 3B (13%), 4 (4%). Sensorimotor stroke has a favorable short-term prognosis for further major vascular events (118), and there is good recovery in nearly 80% of patients (10,118).

Dechambre was the first to describe the association of a sensorimotor stroke and a thalamocapsular lacune (7). Türck described the autopsy findings in two well-documented cases of sensorimotor stroke in 1859 (120). His case 4 correlated with a 20 x 10 mm infarct in the thalamo-capsular region, and his case 1 was associated with a 25 x 10 mm infarct in the same region. Only two other patients with sensorimotor stroke in whom the sensory deficits were of similar severity have had autopsy correlation. In one, a paramedian medullary infarct was found (69), and in the other a pontomedullary infarct was found (121). Garcin and Lapresle, however, reported two cases of cheiro-oral sensory loss, one associated with a hemiparesis (122) and the other with weakness of the first three fingers (123). At autopsy, the authors found a thalamic lacunar infarct (123), involving the internal capsule in both cases (122). Imaging studies show that sensorimotor stroke can be due to small deep infarcts in the corona radiata (124,125), the anterior limb of the internal capsule (119) extending to the caudate nucleus (125), the posterior limb of the internal capsule (125) extending to the lenticular nucleus (125), the pons (126), and the medulla (127).

MISCELLANEOUS LACUNAR SYNDROMES

Many syndromes, resulting either from brainstem or hemispheric strokes, have been related to small deep infarcts. Although some of these may be due to genuine lacunar infarcts, many have not been studied pathologically and could either be due to occlusion of more than one perforating artery or could be of embolic origin. We have, therefore, included them in a group of miscellaneous or atypical lacunar syndromes. The number of these has recently been increasing rapidly (5,128).

Lacunar Syndromes with Oculomotor Palsies

Pure Hemiplegia Plus Contralateral Oculomotor Nerve Palsy (Weber's Syndrome)

The underlying lesion at autopsy in Weber's classic description of this midbrain syndrome was a hematoma (129). Most of the older cases were due to hematomas, tumors, or tuberculomas. Mayor was first to describe an infarct as the cause of this syndrome (130). The size of the pontine and midbrain infarct in the case of Marrotte was too large to be called a lacune (131). Other cases have been reported with autopsy (132,133) or CT (134) correlation. Sieben et al. found occlusions of the mesencephalic artery in patients with midbrain infarcts whose clinical findings included Weber's syndrome (135).

Pure Hemiplegia Plus Abducens Nerve Palsy

The first case of this syndrome was due to a pontine infarct (136). This syndrome is rare in its classic form. A lacune located in the ventral part of the pons may interrupt the sixth nerve fasciculus and the pyramidal tract (128,137). This syndrome is very similar to Landry's syndrome, in which hypesthesia is associated with a hemiplegia and abducens palsy.

Pure Motor Hemiplegia Plus Horizontal Gaze Palsy

The association of pure motor hemiplegia and horizontal gaze palsy was reported by Fisher (128). An isolated horizontal gaze palsy due to a lesion selectively affecting the paramedian pontine reticular formation (PPRF) (Foville's syndrome) is diagnosed by the absence of saccades toward the side of the lesion, associated with the preservation of oculocephalic movements. A horizontal gaze palsy is, however, often associated with hemiplegia and hemianesthesia, and can be related to small pontine infarcts (138). An infarct that involves the abducens nucleus or the PPRF, as well as the pyramidal tract, is usually larger than a lacune, and is usually caused by an occlusion of either the basilar artery or of the ostia of several paramedian arteries.

Pure Motor Hemiplegia Plus Horizontal One-and-a-Half Syndrome

This syndrome was first described by Fisher et al. (44), who described four patients with a unilateral dorsal pontine tegmentum infarct at autopsy who had an ipsilateral lateral gaze palsy, an internuclear ophthalmoplegia, and a contralateral hemiplegia. The oculomotor deficit was attributable to damage to the ipsilateral medial longitudinal fasciculus, the ipsilateral PPRF, and/or the abducens nucleus. The ipsilateral eye is fixed in mid position and the contralateral eye can only abduct. This syndrome is usually caused by unilateral pontine infarcts or lacunar infarcts, and correlations with imaging have been reported (139). Ataxic hemiparesis plus internuclear ophthalmoplegia is due to a lacunar infarct affecting the pyramidal tract, the cerebellar connections, and the medial longitudinal fasciculus (140).

Isolated Eye Movement Disorders

Isolated Oculomotor Nerve Palsy

Intra-axial lesions of the third nerve are supposedly rare. The signs are identical to those found in peripheral third nerve palsies. Two cases have been reported in which a lacunar infarct was found in the midbrain (141,142); dysarthria was, however, associated. A pupil-sparing third nerve palsy has been reported (142), as have cases with imaging correlation (134).

Nuclear Syndrome of the Third Nerve

In the nuclear syndrome of the third nerve, a contralateral superior rectus palsy is associated with an ipsilateral oculomotor palsy. Pierrot-Deseilligny et al. (143) and Bogousslavsky et al. (134) reported cases studied with CT.

Nuclear Oculomotor Syndrome Plus Contralateral Cerebellar Ataxia

In Claude's syndrome, contralateral limb ataxia is due to a lesion of the cerebellar loop at the level of the red nucleus. The early descriptions of this rare syndrome were based on autopsy findings of small midbrain infarcts (144–146). More recently, cases due to infarcts have been described with CT (134,143,147) and MRI (148–150) correlation (Fig. 4).

Nuclear Oculomotor Syndrome Plus Involuntary Movements [Benedikt's Syndrome (151)]

This syndrome associates a third nerve palsy with abnormal contralateral movements. The nature of the involuntary movement is difficult to classify, as it may be a combination of tremor and chorea as in the autopsy case of Souques et al. (152).

Internuclear Ophthalmoplegia

A small infarct of the medial longitudinal fasciculus is a common cause of unilateral internuclear ophtalmoplegia. Cases due to small infarcts have been found at autopsy with both unilateral (153) and bilateral (154) internuclear ophtalmoplegia.

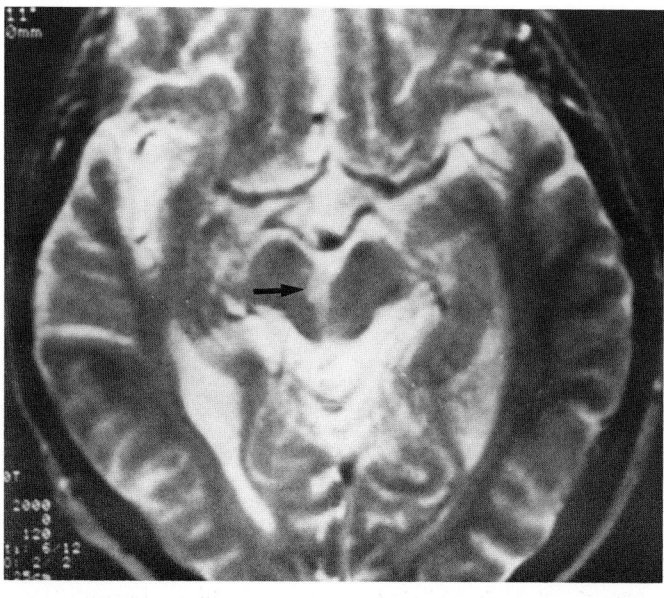

FIG. 4. Axial T2-weighted MR image of a 61-year-old hypertensive hypercholesterolemic man presenting with a right Claude syndrome. MR shows a lacunar infarct in the right mesencephalon (arrow).

Vertical Gaze Palsy

Upgaze palsy and combined up- and downgaze palsy are often related to bilateral midbrain infarcts in the territory of the paramedian mesencephalic arteries. Although downgaze palsy is always caused by bilateral lesions, small unilateral infarcts may give rise to upgaze palsy (155–157). Dissociated vertical gaze palsy, the vertical one-and-a-half syndrome, and monocular elevation palsies may be caused by small unilateral infarcts (157,158). Vertical gaze palsies may be isolated or associated with ataxia (159,160), an altered level of consciousness, and neuropsychological dysfunction, including confusion, altered level of consciousness, memory and language disturbances, and abulia (160).

Miscellaneous Oculomotor Disorders

Other oculomotor disorders caused by small infarcts include ptosis (161), skew deviation, Horner's syndrome (162), horizontal one-and-a-half syndrome plus peripheral ipsilateral facial palsy (163), ocular overshoot associated with dysarthria, staggering gait, ipsilateral ataxia, facial weakness and contralateral sensory loss to pain and temperature (164), and isolated sixth nerve palsy (165).

Movement Disorders

Chorea

Chorea is an involuntary arrhythmic movement of a forcible, rapid, jerky type, associated with hypotonia. Early publications, however, do not distinguish clearly between chorea, athetosis, and ballism. For example, Bidon, in his extensive review of posthemiplegic chorea before 1886, called chorea "all incoordinated and involuntary movements, that may be exacerbated during voluntary movements" (166,167). In patients with chorea and unilateral or bilateral lacunar infarcts in the deep striatum at autopsy, chorea may be unilateral and affect both (168–172) or one limb (173,174), or may be bilateral (175,176). Other cases studied with imaging have been reported (177–182). Combarros et al. (183) reported a case of oral dyskinesia associated with dysarthria and ataxia due to bilateral thalamocapsular infarction.

Ballism

In ballism, the movements are more forceful than in chorea, have a larger amplitude, and begin proximally in the limbs. They also have a strong rotational component. Before the advent of neuroleptic therapy, the prognosis was poor, and for this reason the number of old autopsy cases is large. Ballism due to stroke is usually unilateral (hemiballism) and has been studied at autopsy (184,185) by CT (184,186) and by MRI (187). Infarction is an extremely rare cause of bilateral ballism (188,189).

Dystonia

Dystonia is characterized by inappropriately prolonged muscle contractions that forcefully distort the body into characteristic postures. Focal lesions may give rise to dystonia (190). Marsden et al. (191) in their review noted 48 cases of dystonia due to focal lesions, either found at autopsy or by CT. Clinically the dystonia is often secondary to cerebral palsy, and when the thalamus is affected, there is often hypesthesia. Both lacunar infarcts (191–196) and larger infarcts may cause contralateral dystonia (192,197–201). The dystonia may be focal, affecting one limb or may cause blepharospasm (192) or hemifacial spasm (193), and may have a rhythmic character (194).

Asterixis

Asterixis is a flapping tremor classically affecting both upper extremities and associated with metabolic disturbances. Asterixis may, however, be caused by an infarct and may be unilateral. Degos showed that parietal or midbrain infarcts may cause asterixis, but there was no autopsy or imaging demonstration of a lacunar infarct in this study (202). Shuttleworth reported one case of transient asterixis of both feet associated with bilateral lacunar infarcts in the basal ganglia (203). Lacunar infarcts in the rostral midbrain (204), thalamus (205,206), internal capsule (205,207), and basal ganglia (207) have been reported to cause asterixis.

Parkinsonism

Critchley introduced the concept of vascular parkinsonism and stated that rigidity and akinesia were the prominent features, that tremor was usually absent, and that pseudobulbar palsy, focal signs, dementia, and spasticity were frequent (208). Vascular or "arteriosclerotic" parkinsonism remains controversial because of its rarity and the paucity of clinicopathologic correlations. The main problem is the difficulty of excluding coincidental Parkinson's disease as the cause of parkinsonism in a patient with lacunar infarcts. Criteria have been proposed for the diagnosis of vascular parkinsonism: an acute onset, spontaneous improvement, no other cause for a parkinsonian syndrome, and a pathological examination showing neither neuronal loss in the substantia nigra nor Lewy bodies (209). Lhermitte and Cornil reported a case of a progressive parkinsonian syndrome with tremor due to multiple lacunar infarcts affecting both the putamen and pallidum (210). Hughes et al. (211) described a case of acute parkinsonism following a stroke. Bilateral caudate infarcts were found at autopsy. Friedman et al. also described a patient who developed acute parkinsonism following a stroke. Bilateral putaminal small deep infarcts were found on CT, and there was a relatively high homovanillic acid level in the cerebrospinal fluid (209). Mayo et al. (212) reported a progressive parkinsonian syndrome in a patient with periarteritis nodosa. A patient with a small deep infarct in the head of the caudate nucleus on CT presented with parkinsonism of subacute onset. The parkinsonism improved and there was no subsequent deterioration (213). Bornstein et al. reported five patients studied with CT, with unilateral infarcts and predominantly contralateral parkinsonism (214). Tolosa et al. reported three patients who had parkinsonism with spontaneous partial recovery, and whose CT showed basal ganglia infarcts (215). Quinn et al. reported a patient with progressive parkinsonism, who had a modest response to levodopa. Autopsy revealed lacunar infarcts of the putamen that were related to amyloid angiopathy (216). Murrow et al. reported a patient with parkinsonism who responded to levodopa. At autopsy, several lacunar infarcts were found in the basal ganglia in the absence of the usual pathology of idiopathic Parkinson's disease (217). Fitzgerald et al. (218) reported a series of patients with lower body parkinsonism characterized by predominant and disproportionate gait difficulty, in which risk factors and imaging suggested a vascular etiology. In summary, several autopsy and imaging reports support the concept of vascular parkinsonism. (See Chapters 9 and 11 for other syndromes due to multiple small deep infarcts.)

Curative Effects of Small Deep Infarcts

Brain infarcts almost always cause loss of function. However, in some rare cases, benefit may result from deep infarcts affecting functionally strategic areas. Essential tremor has resolved secondary to a small deep infarct adjacent to the thalamus (219) and following a cerebellar infarct

(220). Signs of parkinsonism have disappeared following a thalamopeduncular (221) or a lenticular infarct (222).

Lacunar Syndromes with Neuropsychological Disturbances

Aphasia

The left thalamus has a well-established role in language function. A lacunar infarct affecting the anteropolar thalamus and the anterior part of the posterior limb of the internal capsule can produce disturbances of vocal volume and of language characterized by defective comprehension, with perseveration, paraphasias and decreased spontaneous speech, but with normal repetition (223). Acalculia or apraxia may also be present (224). Similar features can be observed with small infarcts in the territory of the anterior choroidal artery (225–227). Perseveration, apathy, and disorientation are seen in the unilateral tuberothalamic artery syndrome, and moderate contralateral weakness may also be present. Transcortical aphasia, verbal and visual memory abnormalities, and acalculia may be found in left-sided thalamic infarcts. Hemispatial neglect, visual memory impairments, and disturbed visuospatial processing may be seen in right-sided thalamic infarcts (228, 229).

Hallucinosis and "Top of the Basilar" Syndrome

Lhermitte (230) and Van Bogaert (231) described peduncular hallucinosis as vivid, nonstereotyped, colorful images that are nonthreatening to the patient. Rostral midbrain infarcts have been found at autopsy (232) or on imaging (233,234) in these cases. In the "top of the basilar" syndrome, hallucinosis may be associated with amnesia, somnolence, confusion, and eye movement disturbances. Infarcts in the territories of the rostral part of the basilar artery are mostly due to an embolic mechanism (235).

Isolated Dysarthria

Isolated transient or progressive dysarthria has been related to presumed lacunar infarcts on CT (236–238). Some patients had associated slight accompanying signs, including facial weakness, asymmetrical finger-tapping, or increased unilateral muscle stretch reflexes. This lacunar syndrome may be a variant of the dysarthria–clumsy hand syndrome.

CONCLUSION

The lacunar syndromes cover a wide range of neurological signs and symptoms. A lacunar syndrome may be suggested by clinical examination, and this usually correlates with a specific anatomical lesion site. The clinical findings are, however, neither specific for the nature of the lesion, nor for the mechanism of the arterial occlusion in the case of infarction. Some lacunar syndromes have been clearly shown at autopsy to be caused by genuine lacunar infarcts; others have only imaging evidence of presumed lacunar infarcts. Fisher's criteria for a lacune (small deep infarct due to the occlusion of a single perforating artery) can never be strictly applied in clinical settings, even with the use of the most sophisticated imaging techniques. Although autopsy is considered the gold standard for the diagnosis of lacunar infarcts, most reported autopsy cases have not included a meticulous search for the site and cause of the vascular occlusion. Autopsy rates are now declining, and the low fatality rate in lacunar syndromes also makes autopsy confirmation more difficult. As a result, imaging has become increasingly important, and imaging and ultrasonography studies are now almost mandatory in patients with clinical syndromes compatible with lacunar infarcts. Commonly used diagnostic criteria for lacunes are moving from the necessity for autopsy proof toward the probabilities provided by imaging. A less strict but more pragmatic view is that a lacunar infarct should be diagnosed when the clinical findings suggest a lacunar syndrome, the imaging studies show an appropriate small deep infarct (<1.5 mm) that appears to be related to a single perforating artery occlusion, and the noninvasive cardiac and ultrasound tests (or magnetic resonance angiography) do not show a comparable large artery occlusion or embolic process (239).

REFERENCES

1. Raymond F. Sur la pathogénie de certains accidents paralytiques observé chez des vieillards. Leurs rapports probables avec l'urémie. *Rev Med* 1885;5:705–738.
2. Fisher CM. Lacunes: small, deep cerebral infarct. *Neurology* 1965;15:774–784.
3. Fang H. Lacunar infarction: a clinico-pathologic correlation study. *J Neuropathol Exp Neurol* 1972;31:212.
4. Weisberg LA, Stazio A. Neurologically asymptomatic patients with a single cerebral lacuna. *South Med J* 1989;82:981–984.
5. Fisher CM. Lacunar infarcts—a review. *Cerebrovasc Dis* 1991;1:311–320.
6. Fisher CM, Curry B. Pure motor hemiplegia of vascular origin. *Arch Neurol* 1965;13:30–44.
7. Dechambre A. Mémoire sur la curabilité du ramollissement cérébral. *Gaz Med Paris* 1838;6:305–314.
8. Norrving B, Staaf G. Pure motor stroke from presumed lacunar infarct. Incidence, risk factors and initial course. *Cerebrovasc Dis* 1991;1:203–209.
9. Richter RW, Brust JCM, Bruun B, Shafer SQ. Frequency and course of pure motor hemiparesis: a clinical study. *Stroke* 1977;8:58–60.
10. Bamford JM, Sandercock P, Jones L, Warlow C. The natural history of lacunar infarction: the Oxfordshire community stroke project. *Stroke* 1987;18:547–551.
11. Chamorro A, Sacco RL, Mohr JP, et al. Clinical-computed tomographic correlations of lacunar infarction in the Stroke Data Bank. *Stroke* 1991;22:175–181.
12. Melo TP, Bogousslavsky J, Van Melle G, Regli F. Pure motor stroke: a reappraisal. *Neurology* 1992;42:789–798.
13. Soisson T, Cabanis EA, Iba-Zizen MT, Bousser MG, Laplane D, Castaigne P. Pure motor hemiplegia and computed tomography. *J Neuroradiology* 1982;9:304–322.
14. Scholten DJ, Alberzts C, Snijders CJ, Balks AG. Renovascular hypertension as a cause of cerebrovascular accident in childhood: a case report. *Neuropadiatria* 1977;8:311–318.
15. Young RSK, Coulter DI Allen RJ. Capsular stroke as a cause of hemiplegia in infancy. *Neurology* 1983;33:1044–1046.
16. Kappelle LJ, Willemse J, Ramos LMP, Van Gijn J. Ischaemic stroke in the basal ganglia and internal capsule in childhood. *Brain Dev* 1989;11:283–292.
17. Rascol A, Clanet M, Manelfe C, Guiraud B, Bonafe A. Pure motor hemiplegia: CT study of 30 cases. *Stroke* 1982;13:11–17.
18. Mohr JP, Caplan LR, Melski JW, et al. The Harvard cooperative stroke registry: a prospective registry. *Neurology* 1978;28:754–762.
19. Orgogozo JM, Bogousslavsky J. Lacunar syndromes. In: Vinken PJ, Bruyn GW, Klawans HL, eds. *Handbook of clinical neurology. Vascular diseases,* part II, vol. 54. Amsterdam: Elsevier Science; 1989:235–269.
20. Chambers BR, Donnan GA, Bladin PF. Patterns of stroke. An analysis of the first 700 consecutive admissions to the Austin hospital stroke unit. *Aust NZ Med* 1983;13:57–64.
21. Donnan GA, Tress BM, Bladin PF. A prospective study of lacunar infarction using computerized tomography. *Neurology* 1982;32:49–56.
22. Rafalowska J, Rowinska-Marcinska K. On pure motor hemiplegia (Fisher's syndrome). *Pol Med Sci History Bull* 1975;15:3–8.
23. Hanaway J, Young RR. Localization of the pyramidal tract in the internal capsule of man. *J Neurol Sci* 1977;34:63–70.
24. Ho KL, Meyer KR. The medial medullary syndrome. *Arch Neurol* 1981;38:385–387.
25. Chokroverty S, Rubino FA. "Pure" motor hemiplegia. *J Neurol Neurosurg Psychiatry* 1975;38:896–899.
26. Kelly MA, Perlik SJ, Fisher MA. Somatosensory evoked potentials in lacunar syndromes of pure motor and ataxic hemiparesis. *Stroke* 1987;18:1093–1097.
27. Abbruzzese G, Bino G, Dall'Agata D, Morena M, Primavera A, Favale E. Somatosensory evoked potentials in lacunar syndromes. *J Neurol* 1988;235:300–303.
28. Schott B, Laurent B. Les lacunes cérébrales. *Rev Prat* 1984;34:1125–1131.
29. Mohr JP, Kase CS, Wolf PA, Price TA, Heyman A, Dambrosia JH, Kunitz S. Lacunes in the NINCDS pilot stroke data bank. *Ann Neurol* 1982:12:84.
30. Ferrand J. *Essai sur l'hémiplégie des vieillards. Les lacunes de desintégration cérébrale* [Thesis]. Paris, 1902.
31. Foix C, Lévy M. Les ramollissements sylviens. Syndromes des lésions en foyer du territoire de l'artère sylvienne et de ses branches. *Rev Neurol* 1927;2:1–51.
32. Foix C, Hillemand P. Contribution l'étude des ramollissements protubérantiels. *Rev Med* 1926;43:287–305.
33. Marie P, Guillain G. Existe-t-il en clinique des localisations dans la capsule interne? *Semaine Med* 1902;22:209–213.
34. Picot. Le on sur un cas d'hémiplégie. Lésions corticales du cerveau (zone motrice et zone la-

tente). *Gaz Hebd Sc Med Bordeaux* 1881; 2:403–406.
35. Rendu J. Observation de lésion des couches corticales; ramollissement limité et chute de la paupière supérieure. *Lyon Med* 1877;24:446–451.
36. Veyssière R. *Recherches cliniques et expérimentales sur l'hémianesthésie de cause cérébrale* [Thesis]. Paris, 1874.
37. Lépine R. *De la localisation dans les maladies cérébrales* [Thesis]. Paris, 1875.
38. Raymond F. *Etude anatomique, physiologique et clinique sur l'hémianesthésie, l'hémichorée et les tremblements symptomatiques* [Thesis]. Paris, 1876.
39. Pitres A. *Recherche sur les lésions du centre ovale des hémisphères cérébraux étudiées du point de vue des localisations cérébrales* [Thesis]. Paris, 1877.
40. Landouzy P. Hémiplégie droite. Contracture tardive et atrophie musculaire des membres droits. *Prog Med* 1877;5:992–994.
41. Fisher CM. Capsular infarcts. The underlying vascular lesions. *Arch Neurol* 1979;36:65–73.
42. Ho KL. Pure motor hemiplegia due to infarction of the cerebral peduncle. *Arch Neurol* 1982;39:524–526.
43. Fisher M, Smith TW, Jacobs R. Pure motor hemiplegia secondary to a saccular basilar artery aneurysm. *Stroke* 1988;19:104–107.
44. Fisher CM, Caplan LR. Basilar artery branch occlusion: a cause of pontine infarction. *Neurology* 1971;21:900–905.
45. Besson G, Hommel M, Clavier I, Perret J. Failure of magnetic resonance imaging in the detection of pontine lacune. *Stroke* 1992;23:1535–1536.
46. Chokroverty S, Rubino F, Haller C. Pure motor hemiplegia due to cerebral cortical infarction. *Arch Neurol* 1977;34:93–95.
47. Arboix A, Marti-Vilalta JL, Garcia JH. Clinical study of 227 patients with lacunar infarcts. *Stroke* 1990;21:842–847.
48. Leestma JE, Noronha A. Pure motor hemiplegia, medullary pyramid lesion, and olivary hypertrophy. *J Neurol Neurosurg Psychiatry* 1979;36:877–884.
49. Ropper AH, Fisher CM, Kleinmann GM. Pyramidal infarction in the medulla: a cause of pure motor hemiplegia sparing the face. *Neurology* 1979;29:91–95.
50. Charcot JM, Pitres A. Contribution l'étude des localisations dans l'écorce des hémisphères du cerveau. Observations relatives aux paralysies et aux convulsions d'origine corticale. *Rev Mensuelle Med Chir* 1877;1:180–195.
51. Pitres A. A propos d'un cas de monoplégie persistante du membre inférieur gauche causée par une lésion trés limitée de la capsule interne droite. *Arch Clin Bordeaux* 1893:1–14.
52. Pitres A. *Recherche sur les lésions du centre ovale des hémisphéres cérébraux étudiées du point de vue des localisations cérébrales* [Thesis]. Paris, 1877.
53. Gauché JB. Note sur un cas de monoplégie brachiale avec hémiplégie faciale incomplete; foyer de ramollissement rouge au milieu de la circonvolution frontale ascendante du côté oppose. *Gaz Med Paris* 1879:309.
54. Cruveilhier J. *Atlas d'anatomie pathologique du corps humain.* Paris: JB Bailliere; 1829–1842.
55. Huang C, Broe G. Isolated facial palsy: a new lacunar syndrome. *J Neurol Neurosurg Psychiatry* 1984;47:84–86.
56. Daland J. A case of dysphagia and dysphasia resulting from a lesion in the internal capsule. *J Nerv Ment Dis* 1897:614–619.
57. Huang CY, Woo E, Yu YL, Chan FL. Lacunar syndromes due to brainstem infarct and haemorrhage. *J Neurol Neurosurg Psychiatry* 1988;51:509–515.
58. Hopf HC, Tettenborn B, Kramer G. Pontine supranuclear facial palsy. *Stroke* 1990;21:1754–1757.
59. Boiten J, Lodder J. Isolated monoparesis is usually caused by superficial infarction. *Cerebrovasc Dis* 1991;1:337–340.
60. Benett AH, Campbell CM. Case of brachial monoplegia, due to lesion of the internal capsule. *Brain* 1885;8:78–84.
61. Prince M. A case of incipient locomotor ataxia and monoplegia from focal lesion of the internal capsule in the same patient. *J Nerv Ment Dis* 1895:685.
62. Poulin A. Oblitération par embolie d'une branche de l'artè re sylvienne se rendant aux circonvolutions frontale et pariétale ascendante. Monoplégie brachiale transitoire. Rétablissement de la fonction au bout de deux jours. *Bull Soc Anat Paris* 1878:577–579.
63. Iwasaki Y, Kinoshita M, Ikeda K, Takamiya K, Shiojima T. A case of pure motor monoparesis due to pontine infarction. *Intern J Neurosci* 1990;55:157–159.
64. Garel J, Dor L. Du centre cortical moteur laryng et du trajet intra-cérébral des fibres qui en émanent. *Ann Maladies Oreille Larynx* 1890;16:209–235.
65. Fisher CM. Bilateral occlusion of basilar artery branches. *J Neurol Neurosurg Psychiatry* 1977;40:1182–1189.
65a. Fisher CM. Bilateral capsular infarcts—the mechanism of recovery from hemiplegia. *J Neuropathol Exp Neurol* 1978;37:613.
66. Jagiella WM, Sung JH. Bilateral infarction of the medullary pyramids in humans. *Neurology* 1989;39:21–24.
67. Michielsen B, Van den Bergh R. Bilateral faciobrachial paresis as a consequence of symmetrical capsular infarcts. *Acta Neurol Belg* 1991;91:280–287.
68. Meyer JS, Herndon RM. Bilateral infarction of the pyramidal tracts in man. *Neurology* 1962;12:637–642.
69. Trelles JO, Trelles L, Urquiaca C. Le ramollissement médian du bulbe. A propos de 2 cas anatomo-cliniques. *Rev Neurol* 1973;129:91–104.
70. Paulson GW, Yates AJ, Paltan-Ortiz JD. Does

infarction of the medullary pyramid lead to spasticity? *Arch Neurol* 1986;43:93–95.
71. Garcin R. The ataxias. In: Vinken PJ, Bruyn GW, eds. *Handbook of clinical neurology*, vol. 1. Amsterdam: North-Holland Publishing Company 1975:309–355.
72. De Renzi E, Nichelli P, Crisi G. Hemiataxia and crural hemiparesis following capsular infarct. *J Neurol Neurosurg Psychiatry* 1983; 46:561–563.
73. Fisher CM, Cole M. Homolateral ataxia and crural paresis: a vascular syndrome. *J Neurol Neurosurg Psychiatry* 1965;28:48–55.
74. Fisher CM. Ataxic hemiparesis a pathologic study. *Arch Neurol* 1978;35:126–128.
75. Magrotti E, Borutti G, Mariani G, Donati E, Faggi L. Ataxic hemiparesis syndrome. Clinical and CT study of 20 new cases. *Funct Neurol* 1990;5:65–71.
76. Sanguineti I, Tredici G, Beghi E, et al. Ataxic hemiparesis syndrome: clinical and CT study of 20 new cases and review of the literature. *Ital J Neurol Sci* 1986;7:51–59.
77. Biller J, Scardigli K. Ataxic hemiparesis from lesions of the corona radiata. *Arch Neurol* 1984;41:136.
78. Iragui VJ, MacCutchen CB. Capsular ataxic hemiparesis. *Arch Neurol* 1982;39:528–529.
79. Mori E, Yamadori A, Kudo Y, Tabuchi M. Ataxic hemiparesis from small capsular hemorrhage. Computed tomography and somatosensory evoked potentials. *Arch Neurol* 1984;41:1050–1053.
80. Perman GP, Racy A. Homolateral ataxia and crural paresis: case report. *Neurology* 1980; 30:1013–1015.
81. Delgado G, Gallego J, Zubieta JL. High resolution CT-scan in pontine ataxic hemiparesis. *J Neurol Neurosurg Psychiatry* 1985;48:1069.
82. Murthy JMK. Ataxic hemiparesis—ventrolateral nucleus of the thalamus: yet another site of lesion. *Stroke* 1988;19:122.
83. Boiten J, Lodder J. Ataxic hemiparesis following thalamic infarction. *Stroke* 1990;21:339–340.
84. Huang CY, Lui FS. Ataxic hemiparesis, localisation and clinical features. *Stroke* 1984;15: 363–366.
85. Hommel M, Gaïo JM, Pollak P, Borgel F, Perret J. Hémiparésie ataxique par lacune thalamique. *Rev Neurol* 1987;143:602–604.
86. Nabatame H, Fukuyama H, Akigushi I, Kameyama M, Nishimura K, Torizuka K. Pontine ataxic hemiparesis studied by high resolution magnetic resonance imaging system. *Ann Neurol* 1987;21:204–207.
87. Nicolesco I, Cretu V, Demetresco L. Syndrome de l'artère cérébrale antérieure. Monoplégie crurale droite avec symptologie cérébelleuse prépondérante. *Bull Soc Med Hop Bucarest* 1930:276.
88. Garcin R. Syndrome cérébello-thalamique par lésion localisée du thalamus avec une digression sur le "signe de la main creuse" et son intéret seméiologique. *Rev Neurol* 1955;93:143–149.
89. Garcin R, Lapresle J. Incoordination cérébelleuse du membre inférieur par lésion localisée dans la région interne du thalamus contro-latéral. *Rev Neurol* 1969;120:5–13.
90. Yagnik PM, Dhaduk V, Huen L. Parietal ataxic hemiparesis. *Eur Neurol* 1988;28:164–166.
91. Rosa A, Mizon JP, Betermiez P. Hémiparésie crurale avec ataxie homolatérale propos d'un cas avec étude tomodensitomé trique. *Rev Otoneuroophtalmol* 1983;55:283–288.
92. Biller J, Adams HP, Dunn V, Simmons Z, Jacoby CG. Dichotomy between clinical findings and MR abnormalities in pontine infarction. *J Comput Assist Tomogr* 1986;10:379–385.
93. Perret J, Hommel M, Pollak P, Gaio JM, Lebas JF, Crouzet G. Clinical and radiological correlations in ishemic brainstem infarcts: a magnetic resonance imaging study. In: Gouaze A, Salamon G, eds. *Brain anatomy and magnetic resonance imaging*. Springer-Verlag, Berlin 1988:169–177.
94. Lee N, Roh JK, Myung H. Hypesthetic ataxic hemiparesis in a thalamic lacune. *Stroke* 1989; 20:819–821.
95. Bogousslavsky J, Regli F, Ghika J, Feldmeyer JJ. Painful ataxic hemiparesis. *Arch Neurol* 1984;41:892–893.
96. Sakai T, Murakami S, Ito K. Ataxic hemiparesis with trigeminal weakness. *Neurology* 1981; 31:635–636.
97. Van Gijn J, Vermeulen M. Ataxic tetraparesis from lacunar infarction in the pons. *J Neurol Neurosurg Psychiatry* 1983;46:669–670.
98. Fisher CM. A lacunar stroke. The dysarthria–clumsy hand syndrome. *Neurology* 1967;17: 614–617.
99. Tuhrim S, Yang WC, Rubinowitz H, Weinberger J. Primary pontine hemorrhage and the dysarthria–clumsy hand syndrome. *Neurology* 1982;32:1027–1028.
100. Decamps A, Dordain G. Les syndromes lacunaires. *Rev Med* 1982;19:1021–1025.
101. Koppel BS, Weinberger G. Pontine infarction producing dysarthria–clumsy hand syndrome and ataxic hemiparesis. *Eur Neurol* 1987;26:211–215.
102. Glass JD, Levey AI, Rothstein JD. The dysarthria–clumsy hand syndrome: a distinct clinical entity related to pontine infarction. *Ann Neurol* 1990;27:487–494.
103. Spertell RB, Ransom BR. Dysarthria–clumsy hand syndrome produced by capsular infarct. *Ann Neurol* 1979;6:263–265.
104. De Vries L, Sno HN. Atactische hemiparese en "dysarthria–clumsy hand," twee vervante syndromen veroorzaakt door een lacunair herseninfarct. *Ned Tijdschr Geneeskd* 1985;129:1628–1631.
105. Fisher CM. Pure sensory stroke involving face, arm and leg. *Neurology* 1965;15:76–80.
106. Fisher CM. Pure sensory stroke and allied conditions. *Stroke* 1982;13:434–447.
107. Hommel M, Besson G, Pollak P, Borgel F, Le Bas JF, Perret J. Pure sensory stroke due to a pontine lacune. *Stroke* 1989;20:406–408.
108. Sacco RL, Bello JA, Traub R, Brust J. Selec-

tive proprioceptive loss from a thalamic lacunar stroke. *Stroke* 1987;18:1160–1163.
109. Rosenberg NL, Koller R. Computerized tomography and pure sensory stroke. *Neurology* 1981;31:217–220.
110. Kim JS. A lenticulocapsular lacune producing pure sensory stroke. *Cerebrovasc Dis* 1991;1:302–304.
111. Kawakami Y, Chikama M, Tanimoto T, Shimamura Y. Radiological studies of the cheirooral syndrome. *J Neurol* 1989;236:177–181.
112. Bourneville A. De l'hémianesthésie liée une lésion d'un hémisphère du cerveau. *Prog Med* 1873;1:244–246.
113. De Ajuriaguerra J. *La douleur centrale* [Thesis]. Paris, 1937:66–67.
114. Lhermitte J, Fumet. Syndrome hémialgique pur d'origine thalamique chez un lacunaire. *Rev Neurol* 1921;37:468–473.
115. Fisher CM. Thalamic pure sensory stroke. *Neurology* 1978;28:1141–1144.
116. Derouesné C, Mas JL, Bolgert F, Castaigne P. Pure sensory stroke caused by a small cortical infarct in the middle cerebral artery territory. *Stroke* 1984;15:660–662.
117. Mohr JP, Kase CS, Meckler RJ, Fisher CM. Sensorimotor stroke due to thalamocapsular ischemia. *Arch Neurol* 1977;34:739–741.
118. Landi G, Anzalone N, Cella E, Boccardi E, Mussico M. Are sensorimotor strokes lacunar strokes? A case-control study of lacunar and non-lacunar infarcts. *J Neurol Neurosurg Psychiatry* 1991;54:1063–1068.
119. Huang CY, Woo E, Chan FL. When is sensorimotor stroke a lacunar syndrome? *J Neurol Neurosurg Psychiatry* 1987;50:720–726.
120. Türck L. Über die Beziehung gewisser Krankheitsherde des grossen Gehirnes zur Anästhesie. Sitzungsberichte der Mathematisch Naturunissenschaftlichen. *Classe Kaiserlichen Akademie Wissenschaften* 1859;36:191–199.
121. Brown WJ, Fang HCH. Spastic hemiplegia in man associated with unilateral infarct of the cortico spinal tract at the pontomedullary juncture. *Trans Am Neurol Assoc* 1956:22–26.
122. Garcin R, Lapresle J. Syndrome sensitif de type thalamique et topographie cheiro-orale par lésion localisée du thalamus. *Rev Neurol* 1954;90:124–129.
123. Garcin R, Lapresle J. Deuxième observation personnelle de syndrome sensitif de type thalamique et topographie cheiro-orale par lésion localisée du thalamus. *Rev Neurol* 1960;103:474–481.
124. Miyashita K, Naritomi H, Sawada T, et al. Identification of recent lacunar lesions in cases of multiple small infarctions by magnetic resonance imaging. *Stroke* 1988;19:834–839.
125. Boiten J, Lodder J. Discrete lesions in the sensorimotor control system. A clinico-topographical study of lacunar infarcts. *J Neurol Sci* 1991;105:154.
126. Rothrock JF, Lyden PD, Hesselink JR, Brown JJ, Healy ME. Brain magnetic resonance imaging in the evaluation of lacunar stroke. *Stroke* 1987;18:781–786.
127. Milandre L, Arnaud O, Khalil R. Infarction of the medullary pyramid identified on MRI. *Cerebrovasc Dis* 1992;2:183–184.
128. Fisher CM. Lacunar strokes and infarcts: a review. *Neurology* 1982;32:871–876.
129. Weber H. A contribution to the pathology of the crura cerebri. *Med Chir Trans* 1863;46:121–139.
130. Mayor. Paralysie alterne portant sur le moteur oculaire commun. *Bull Soc Anat* 1877;16:239–240.
131. Marrotte. Observation de ramollissement du pédoncule cérébral gauche, avec lésion du nerf moteur oculaire commun. *Union Med* 1853:407–408.
132. Devic A, Paufique, Girard P, Guinet P. Observations anatomocliniques d'un syndrome de parinaud (paralysie volontaire et réflexe). Considérations sur le rôle de la région commissurale. *Rev Neurol* 1945;77:37–39.
133. Kobayashi S, Mukuno K, Tazaki Y, Ishikawa S, Okada K. Oculomotor nerve complex syndrome. A case with clinico-pathological correlation. *Neuro Ophthalmol* 1986;6:55–59.
134. Bogousslavsky J, Regli F. Atteint intra-axiale du nerf moteur oculaire commun dans les infarctus mésencéphaliques. *Rev Neurol* 1984;140:263–270.
135. Sieben G, De Reuk J, Vander Eecken H. Thrombosis of the mesencephalic artery. A clinico-pathological study of two cases and its correlation to the arterial vascularisation. *Acta Neurol Belg* 1977;77:151–162.
136. Landry M. *Bull Soc Anat Paris* 1858;33:406–410.
137. Hommel M, Besson G, Tarel V, et al. L'imagerie par résonance magnétique dans les paralysies de l'oculomotricité horizontale par infarctus. *Rev Neurol* 1988;144:18–24.
138. Pierrot-Deseilligny C, Chain F, Gray F, Escourolle R, Castaigne P. Paralysies supranucléaires de la latéralité d'origine protubérantielle. *Rev Neurol* 1979;135:741–762.
139. De Witt LD, Wray S, Kistler JP, Davis KR, Brady TJ, Buonanno F. Nuclear magnetic resonance in neuro-ophthalmologic syndromes. *Neurology* 1984;34:96–97.
140. Hommel M, Besson G, Le Bas JF, et al. Prospective study of lacunar infarcts using magnetic resonance imaging. *Stroke* 1990;21:546–554.
141. Achard C, Levi L. Paralysie totale et isolée du moteur oculaire commun par foyer de ramollissement pédonculaire. *Rev Neurol* 1901;12:646–648.
142. Breen LA, Hopf HC, Farris BK, Gutman L. Pupil-sparing oculomotor nerve palsy due to midbrain infarction. *Arch Neurol* 1990;48:105–106.
143. Pierrot-Deseilligny C, Schaison M, Bousser MG, Brunet P. Syndrome nucléaire du nerf moteur oculaire commun: à propos de deux observations cliniques. *Rev Neurol* 1981;137:217–222.
144. Claude H. Syndrome pédonculaire de la région du noyau rouge. *Rev Neurol* 1912;4:311–313.

145. Claude H, Loyez. Ramollissement du noyau rouge. *Rev Neurol* 1912;13:49–51.
146. Van Bogaert L. Syndrome inférieur du noyau rouge, troubles psycho-sensoriels d'origine mésocéphalique. *Rev Neurol* 1924:417–423.
147. Gaymard B, Saudeau D, de Toffol B, Larmande P, Autret A. Two mesencephalic lacunar infarcts presenting as Claude's syndrome and pure motor hemiparesis. *Eur Neurol* 1991; 31:152–155.
148. Kistler JP, Buonanno FS, De Witt LD, Davis KR, Brady TJ, Fisher CM. Vertebral basilar posterior cerebral territory stroke delineation by proton nuclear magnetic resonance. *Stroke* 1984;15:417–426.
149. Iwatsubo T, Iwata M, Inoue K, Mannen T. Imagerie par résonance magnétique dans un cas d'infarctus mésencéphalique paramédian. *Rev Neurol* 1987;143:605–607.
150. Sanguineti I, Tagliabue M, Boglium G, Cavaletti G, Crespi V, Delodovici ML. Correspondance. *Rev Neurol* 1988;144:840–841.
151. Benedikt M. Tremblement avec paralysie croisée du moteur oculaire commun. *Bull Med* 1889;3:547–548.
152. Souques, Crouzon, Bertrand I. Révision du syndrome de Benedikt à propos de l'autopsie d'un cas de ce syndrome trémoro-choréo-athétoide et hypertonique du syndrome du noyau rouge. Mémoire original. *Rev Neurol* 1930; 11:378–417.
153. Cogan DG, Kubik CS, Smith WL. Unilateral internuclear ophthalmoplegia. *Arch Ophthalmol* 1950;44:783–796.
154. Jenkyn LR, Margolis G, Reeves AG. Reflex vertical gaze and the medial longitudial fasciculus. *J Neurol Neurosurg Psychiatry* 1978; 41:1084–1091.
155. Büttner-Ennever JA, Büttner U, Cohen B, Baumgartner G. Vertical gaze paralysis and the rostral interstitial nucleus of the longitudinal fasciculus. *Brain* 1982;1105:125–149.
156. Ranalli PJ, Sharpe JA, Fletcher WA. Palsy of upward and downward saccadic, pursuit, and vestibular movements with a midbrain lesion: pathologic correlations. *Neurology* 1988;38:114–122.
157. Hommel M, Bogousslavsky J. The spectrum of vertical gaze palsy following unilateral brainstem stroke. *Neurology* 1991;41:1229–1234.
158. Bogousslavsky J, Regli F. Upgaze palsy and monocular paresis of downgaze from ipsilateral thalamo-mesencephalic infarction: a vertical one-and-a-half syndrome. *J Neurol* 1984;231: 43–45.
159. Chiray M, Foix C, Nicolesco J. Hémitremblement du type de la sclérose en plaques par lésion rubro-thalamo-sous thalamique. Syndrome de la région supéro-externe du noyau rouge avec atteinte silencieuse ou non du thalamus. *Ann Med* 1923;14:173–191.
160. Castaigne P, Lhermitte F, Buge A, Escourolle R, Hauw JJ, Lyon-Caen O. Paramedian thalamic and midbrain infarcts: clinical and neuropathological study. *Ann Neurol* 1981;10:127–148.
161. Growdon JH, Winkler GF, Wray SH. Midbrain ptosis. A case with clinicopathologic correlation. *Arch Neurol* 1974;30:179–181.
162. Austin CP, Lessel S. Horner's syndrome from hypothalamic infarction. *Arch Neurol* 1991;48: 332–334.
163. Dumas G, Charachon R, Hommel M, Perret J, Le Bas JF. Apport de l'oculographie et de l'IRM aux corrélations clinico-topographiques dans les accidents vasculaires ischémiques du tronc cérébral. *Ann Otolaryngol* 1988;105:47–57.
164. Fisher CM. Lacunar infarct of the tegmentum of the lower lateral pons. *Arch Neurol* 1989; 46:566–567.
165. Donaldson D, Rosenberg NL. Infarction of abducens nerve fascicle as a cause of isolated sixth nerve palsy related to hypertension. *Neurology* 1988;38:1654.
166. Bidon H. Essai sur l'hémichorée symptomatique des maladies de l'encéphale. *Rev Med* 1886:667–698.
167. Bidon H. Essai sur l'hémichorée symptomatique des maladies de l'encéphale. *Rev Med* 1886:838–854.
168. Austregesilo A, Borges-Forte A. Sur un cas d'hémichorée avec lésion du noyau caudé. (Contribution anatomo-clinique aux localisations du striatum.) *Rev Neurol* 1937;67:477–488.
169. Austregesilo A, Gallotti O. Sur un cas d'hémiparésie et d'hémichorée avec lésion du noyau caudé. *Rev Neurol* 1924:41–43.
170. Martin JP. Hemichorea (hemiballismus) without lesions in the corpus luysii. *Brain* 1957;80:2–10.
171. Goldblatt D, Markesbery W, Reeves AG. Recurrent hemichorea following striatal lesions. *Arch Neurol* 1974;31:51–54.
172. Dooling EC, Adams RD. The pathological anatomy of posthemiplegic athetosis. *Brain* 1975;98:29–48.
173. Davison C, Goodhart SP. Monochorea and somatotopic localization. *Arch Neurol Psychiatry* 1940;43:792–803.
174. Ikeda M, Tsukagoshi H. Monochorea caused by a striatal lesion. *Eur Neurol* 1991;31:257–258.
175. Folstein S, Abbott M, Moser R, Parhad I, Clark A, Folstein M. A phenocopy of Huntington's disease: lacunar infarcts of the corpus striatum. *Johns Hopkins Med J* 1981;148:104–108.
176. Goldblatt J, White NW, Wright MGE. Bilateral chorea associated with caudate nuclei lacunar infarcts. *S Afr Med J* 1989;75:443–445.
177. Kase CS, Maulsby GO, deJuan E, Mohr JP. Hemichorea-hemiballism and lacunar infarction in the basal ganglia. *Neurology* 1981; 31:452–455.
178. Saris S. Chorea caused by caudate infarction. *Arch Neurol* 1983;40:590–591.
179. Tabaton M, Mancardi G, Loeb C. Generalized

chorea due to bilateral small, deep cerebral infarcts. *Neurology* 1985;35:588–589.
180. Kawamura M, Takahashi N, Hirayama K. Hemichorea and its denial in a case of caudate infarction diagnosed by magnetic resonance imaging. *J Neurol Neurosurg Psychiatry* 1988;51:590–591.
181. Drake ME. Lupus anticoagulant and lacunar infarctions. *Eur Neurol* 1988;28:174–176.
182. Bruno A, Rosenberg GA. The spectrum of lacunar infarction in the elderly. *Clin Geriatr Med* 1991;7:443–453.
183. Combarros O, Gutierrez A, Pascual J, Berciano J. Oral dyskinesias associated with bilateral thalamo-capsular infarction. *J Neurol Neurosurg Psychiatry* 1990;53:168–169.
184. Salama J, Gray F, Kanaan HY, Delaporte P. Le syndrome du corps de Luys. In: *Encycl Med Chir Paris Neurologie* 17037 G10, 6–1988, pp. 1–8.
185. Segal R, Sroka H, Sandbank U, Kott E. Hemiballismus with lesion of the subthalamic nucleus and neuroaxonal degeneration of the homolateral substantia nigra. *Ann Neurol* 1977;2:169–172.
186. Mas JL, Launay M, Derouesné C. Hemiballism and CT-documented lacunar infarct in the lenticular nucleus. *J Neurol Neurosurg Psychiatry* 1987;50:104–105.
187. Biller J, Graff-Radford NR, Smoker WKR, Adams HP, Johnston P. MR imaging in "lacunar" hemiballismus. *J Comput Assist Tomogr* 1986;10:793–797.
188. Château R, Tommasi M, Groslambert R, Pasqier B, Perret J. Une observation de diballisme. Etude clinique et anatomo-pathologique. *Rev Neurol* 1973;129:257–274.
189. Lodder J, Baard WC. Paraballism caused by bilateral hemorrhagic infarction in the basal ganglia. *Neurology* 1981;31:484–486.
190. Zeman W, Whitlock CC. Symptomatic dystonia. In: Vinken PJ, Bruyn GW, eds. *Handbook of clinical neurology*, vol. 6. Amsterdam: North-Holland; 19xx:517–543.
191. Marsden CD, Obeso JA, Zarranz JJ, Lang AE. The anatomical basis of symptomatic hemidystonia. *Brain* 1985;108:463–483.
192. Jankovic J, Patel SC. Blepharospasm associated with brainstem lesions. *Neurology* 1983;33:1237–1240.
193. Vermersch P, Petit H, Marion MH, Montagne B. Hemifacial spasm due to pontine infarction. *J Neurol Neurosurg Psychiatry* 1991;54:1018.
194. Sunohara N, Mukoyama M, Mano Y, Satoyoshi E. Action-induced rhythmic dystonia: an autopsy case. *Neurology* 1984;34:321–327.
195. Grimes JD, Hassan MN, Quarrington AM, D'Alton. Delayed-onset posthemiplegic dystonia: CT demonstration of basal ganglia pathology. *Neurology* 1982;32:1033–1035.
196. Russo LS. Focal dystonia and lacunar infarction of the basal ganglia. *Arch Neurol* 1983;40:61.
197. Burton K, Farrel K, Li D, Calne DB. Lesions of the putamen and dystonia: CT and magnetic resonance imaging. *Neurology* 1984;34:962–965.
198. Demierre B, Rondot P. Dystonia caused by putamino-capsulo-caudate vascular lesions. *J Neurol Neurosurg Psychiatry* 1983;46:404–406.
199. Giroud M, Dumas R. Dystonie secondaire à un infarctus putamino-capsulo-caudé chez l'enfant. *Rev Neurol* 1988;144:375–377.
200. Obeso JA, Martinez-Vila E, Delgado G, Vaamonda J, Maravi E, Martinez-Lage JM. Delayed onset dystonia following hemiplegic migraine. *Headache* 1984;24:266–268.
201. Boylan KB, Chin JH, DeArmond SJ. Progressive dystonia following resuscitation from cardiac arrest. *Neurology* 1990;40:1458–1461.
202. Degos JD, Verroust J, Bouchareine A, Serdaru M, Barbizet J. Asterixis in focal brain lesions. *Arch Neurol* 1979;36:705–707.
203. Shuttleworth EC, Drake ME. Asterixis after lacunar infarctions. *Eur Neurol* 1987;27:62–63.
204. Bril V, Sharpe JA, Ashby P. Midbrain asterixis. *Ann Neurol* 1979;6:362–364.
205. Massey EW, Goodman JC, Stewart C, Brannon WL. Unilateral asterixis: motor integrative dysfunction in focal vascular disease. *Neurology* 1979;29:1188–1190.
206. Feldmeyer JJ, Bogousslavsky J, Regli F. Asterixis uni- ou bilatéral en cas de lésion thalamique ou pariétale: un trouble moteur afférentiel? *Schweiz Med Wochenschr* 1984;114:167–171.
207. Yagnik P, Dhopesh V. Unilateral asterixis. *Arch Neurol* 1981;38:601–602.
208. Critchley M. Arteriosclerotic parkinsonism. *Brain* 1929;52:23–83.
209. Friedman A, Kang UJ, Tatemichi TK, Burke R. A case of parkinsonism following striatal lacunar infarction. *J Neurol Neurosurg Psychiatry* 1986;49:1087–1088.
210. Lhermitte J, Cornil L. Un cas de syndrome parkinsonien: lacunes symétriques dans le globus pallidus. *Rev Neurol* 1921;37:189–191.
211. Hughes W, Dodgson MCH, MacLennan DC. Chronic cerebral hypertensive disease. *Lancet* 1954;2:770–774.
212. Mayo J, Arias M, Leno C, Berciano J. Vascular parkinsonism and periarteritis nodosa. *Neurology* 1986;36:874–875.
213. Lazzarino LG, Nicolai A, Toppani D. Subacute parkinsonim from a single lacunar infarct in the basal ganglia. *Acta Neurol (Napoli)* 1990;12:292–295.
214. Bornstein NM, Reider-Grosswasser I, Korczyn AD. Clinical correlates of lacunar infarcts in the basal ganglia. *Stroke* 1989;20:136 (abst).
215. Tolosa ES, Santamaria J. Parkinsonism and basal ganglia infarcts. *Neurology* 1984;34:1516–1518.
216. Quinn N, Parkes D, Janota I, Marsden CD. Preservation of the substantia nigra and locus coeruleus in a patient receiving levodopa (2kg) plus decarboxylase inhibitor over a four-year period. *Movement Disorders* 1986;1:45–49.
217. Murrow RW, Schweiger GD, Kepes JJ, Koller WC. Parkinsonism due to a basal ganglia lacu-

nar state: clinicopathologic correlation. *Neurology* 1990;40:897–900.
218. Fitzgerald PM, Jankovic J. Lower body parkinsonism: evidence for vascular etiology. *Movement Disorders* 1989;4:249–260.
219. Duncan R, Bone I, Melville ID. Essential tremor cured by infarction adjacent to the thalamus. *J Neurol Neurosurg Psychiatry* 1988;51: 591–592.
220. Dupuis MJM, Delwaide PJ, Boucquey D, Gonsette RE. Homolateral disappearancee of essential tremor after cerebellar stroke. *Movements Disorders* 1989;4:183–187.
221. Dubois B, Pillon F, De Saxe H, Lhermitte F, Agid Y. Disappearance of parkinsonian signs after spontaneous "thalamotomy." *Arch Neurol* 1986;43:815–817.
222. Scoditti U, Rustichelli P, Calzetti S. Spontaneous hemiballism and disappearance of parkinsonism following contralateral lenticular lacunar infarct. *Ital J Neurol Sci* 1989;10:757–577.
223. Gorelick PB, Hier DB, Benevento L, Levitt S, Tan W. Aphasia after left thalamic infarction. *Arch Neurol* 1984;41:1296–1298.
224. Cambier J, Graveleau P. Clinical neuropsychology. Thalamic syndromes. Vol. 1 (45). In: Fredericks JMA, ed. *Clinical Neurology* Amsterdam: Elsevier; 1985:87–98.
225. Van Gijn J, Kraaijeveld CL. Blood pressure does not predict lacunar infarction. *J Neurol Neurosurg Psychiatry* 1982;45:147–150.
226. Pullicino P, Nelson RF, Kendall BE, Marshall J. Small deep infarcts diagnosed on computed tomography. *Neurology* 1980;30:1090–1096.
227. Puel M, Demonet JF, Cardebat D, et al. Aphasies sous-corticales. Etude neurolinguistique avec scanner X de 25 cas. *Rev Neurol* 1984; 140:695–710.
228. Graff-Radford NR, Eslinger PJ, Damasio AR, Yamada T. Non-hemorrhagic infarction of the thalamus: behavioral, anatomic, and physiologic correlates. *Neurology* 1984;34:14–23.
229. Bogousslavsky J, Regli F, Assal G. The syndrome of unilateral tuberothalamic artery territory infarction. *Stroke* 1986;17:434–441.
230. Lhermitte J. Syndrome de la calotte du pédoncule cérébral. Les troubles psycho-sensoriels dans les lésions du mésocéphale. *Rev Neurol* 1922;38:1359–1365.
231. Van Bogaert L. Syndrome inférieur du noyau rouge, troubles psycho-sensoriels d'origine mésocéphalique. *Rev Neurol* 1924;40:417–423.
232. McKee AC, Levine DN, Kowall NW, Richardson EP. Peduncular hallucinosis associated with isolated infarction of the substantia nigra pars reticulata. *Ann Neurol* 1990;27:500–504.
233. Geller TJ, Bellur SN. Peduncular hallucinosis: magnetic resonance imaging confirmation of mésencéphalic infarction during life. *Ann Neurol* 1987;21:602–604.
234. Feinberg WM, Rapcsak SZ. "Peduncular hallucinosis" following paramedian thalamic infarction. *Neurology* 1989;39:1535–1536.
235. Caplan LR. "Top of the basilar" syndrome. *Neurology* 1980;30:72–79.
236. Ozaki I, Baba M, Narita S, Matsunaga M, Takebe K. Pure dysarthria due to anterior internal capsule and/or corona radiata infarction: a report of five cases. *J Neurol Neurosurg Psychiatry* 1986;49:1435–1437.
237. Arboix A, Marti-Vilalta JL. Lacunar infarctions and dysarthria. *Arch Neurol* 1990;47:127.
238. Ichikawa K, Kageyama Y. Clinical anatomic study of pure dysarthria. *Stroke* 1991;22:809–812.
239. Bogousslavsky J. The plurality of subcortical infarction. *Stroke* 1992;23:629–631.

8

Clinical Features of Lacunar and Small Deep Infarcts at Specific Anatomical Sites

Marc Hommel and Gérard Besson

Department of Clinical and Biological Neurosciences, Stroke Unit, Centre Hospitalier Universitaire Régional de Grenoble, 38043 Grenoble, France

In contradistinction to Chapter 7, this chapter approaches lacunar syndromes from an anatomical point of view. Here we relate infarcts at specific anatomical sites and infarcts caused by occlusion of specific small arteries to different clinical syndromes. We discuss the different syndromes that may be caused by lacunar infarcts or small deep infarcts in the following specific cerebral locations: (a) corona radiata, (b) internal capsule, (c) caudate nucleus, (d) lenticular nucleus, (e) thalamus, and (f) brainstem (midbrain, pons, and medulla). We have included syndromes due to lacunar infarcts secondary to perforating artery occlusion as well as secondary to branch occlusion (1,2). We have included cases studied at autopsy or imaging that are attributed to occlusive vascular disease, and have excluded infarcts attributed to hemodynamic causes. For each site we first present the classic lacunar syndromes and then describe other syndromes that have been related to infarction at that site.

Due to the wide use of computed tomography (CT) and magnetic resonance (MR) there has been a rapid increase in the number of reports of syndromes due to lacunar infarcts. However, it may be difficult to draw clinico-topographical correlations in patients presenting with either classical or miscellaneous lacunar syndromes (see Chapter 7). Not only may imaging fail to detect the responsible infarct, but because edema, necrosis, gliosis, or demyelination may have similar imaging appearances to infarcts, it is often difficult to be sure of the precise anatomical limits of an infarct. Moreover, patients may have either multiple strokes or an infarct affecting contiguous structures, making it difficult to attribute the clinical syndrome to any single structure. This is the case, for example, in striatal and striatocapsular infarcts, which in some cases can be associated with cortical infarcts.

CORONA RADIATA

Classic Syndromes

The corona radiata is a broad band of white matter projection fibers conveying impulses to and from the entire cortex (3). At its lower end, the corona radiata is continuous with the internal capsule. Since many pathways pass through the corona radiata, small infarcts located there can produce multiple syndromes. The blood supply of the lower part of the corona radiata and arteries of the corona radiata/internal capsule junctional region is mainly provided by arteries of the lateral deep middle cerebral artery territory (see Chapter 3).

Pure Motor Stroke

Proportional (equal in face, arm, and leg) pure motor hemiparesis may be due to presumed lacunar infarctions located in the corona radiata (4–8) with or without coexistent involvement of the internal capsule (9) or the putamen (8,10). The motor weakness may occasionally be partial, affecting the face and arm as in case 31 of Pitres's thesis (11), the face alone as in the case of Professor Dupuytren recorded by Cruveilhier (book 20, vol 1) (12), or may even be restricted to one limb (13).

Ataxic Hemiparesis and the Dysarthria–Clumsy Hand Syndrome

Lacunar infarcts located in the corona radiata can produce both ataxic hemiparesis (8) and the dysarthria–clumsy hand syndrome (6). In ataxic hemiparesis, the motor weakness can affect the face, arm, and leg equally (14–20) or can be limited to the face and arm (17). When the lacunar infarct is located in the anterior part of the corona radiata, the cerebellar signs are explained by interruption of the frontopontine tract of Arnold. When the lacunar infarct is more posterior, the cerebellar signs are explained by the interruption of the parieto-and occipitopontine tracts forming Türck's bundle (17).

Pure Sensory Stroke

Infarction of the thalamocortical pathway in the corona radiata, producing pure sensory stroke, has only been reported once on CT (21).

Sensorimotor Stroke

When the presumed lacunar infarct located in the corona radiata involves the thalamocortical pathway and the pyramidal tract simultaneously, it produces a sensorimotor stroke (8,22,23).

Other Lacunar Syndromes

Dysarthria

Rare cases of pure dysarthria have been related to small deep infarcts located in the corona radiata on imaging studies (24,25). The question whether this dysarthria was due to motor weakness or related to a cerebellar pathway dysfunction has still not been answered.

INTERNAL CAPSULE

Classic Syndromes

Since the beginning of the 20th century, there have been frequent clinicopathological correlations of small deep infarcts in the internal capsule. Abadie summarized those cases reported before 1900 (26). The internal capsule is divided into three parts: the anterior limb, the genu, and the posterior limb. It is made up of all the afferent and efferent fibers that go to or come from the cortex (3). Thus, all classic and many miscellaneous lacunar syndromes can be produced by small deep infarcts affecting the internal capsule. Capsular infarcts have been classified into six topographic types (27). The anterior type involves the anterior limb of the internal capsule and is usually supplied by Heubner's artery (see Chapter 3). The lateral type involves the lenticular nucleus and the highest part of the internal capsule at its junction with the corona radiata. This area is supplied by the lateral deep middle cerebral artery branches. The posterior type involves the posterior limb of the internal capsule, which is mainly supplied by the anterior choroidal artery. The superior type involves the body of the caudate nucleus and the superior part of the internal capsule. This area is supplied by the lateral deep middle cerebral artery branches. In the inferior type, the infarct is located around the hypothalamus close to the third ventricle. This area is supplied by several different arteries (see Chapter 3). The multiple type consists of multiple small deep infarcts.

Pure Motor Stroke

Although the pyramidal tract is situated in the posterior limb of the internal capsule, it does not maintain a fixed position in the internal capsule throughout its rostrocaudal course (28). Ross showed that the pyramidal tract shifts from the anterior to the posterior part of the internal capsule during its rostrocaudal course (28). There is, however, an anteroposterior face-arm-leg somatotopic organization in the internal capsule, and this could explain how small infarcts produce partial pure motor deficits (29).

Proportional pure motor stroke occurs in the lateral, posterior, and superior types of Kashihara and Matsumoto (see above) (27). Rascol et al. have classified small deep infarcts involving the internal capsule that are responsible for pure motor stroke into three types (30). The first type are capsulo-putamino-caudate infarcts. These infarcts extend from the anterior limb of the internal capsule through the putamen to the posterior limb of the internal capsule and also to the adjacent striatum. These "giant lacunes" may be due to embolism or other mechanisms that are unusual causes of small deep infarcts (31). They are situated predominantly in the territory of the lateral lenticulostriate arteries. The second type are capsulopallidal infarcts. These involve the posterior limb of the internal capsule and, in many cases, the internal portion of the globus pallidus. They are situated in the territory of the anterior choroidal artery. The third type are anterior capsulocaudate infarcts. These involve the anterior limb of the internal capsule and the head of the caudate nucleus and are mainly situated in the lateral lenticulostriate territory. Although these three types of infarct also involve adjacent structures, CT studies have shown that pure motor stroke can be due to infarcts restricted to the internal capsule (6–9, 29, 30, 32–35). While the posterior limb of the internal capsule is most commonly associated with pure motor stroke, a presumed lacunar stroke in the anterior limb (30) or in the genu (5) may also give rise to a pure motor stroke.

Partial pure motor strokes have rarely been reported to be caused by a lacunar infarct affecting the internal capsule. A brachiofacial motor deficit, however, has been related to a presumed lacunar infarct located in the genu or in the posterior limb of the internal capsule (29).

Pitres reported a patient with a brachiocrural motor deficit that was related at autopsy to a lacunar infarct in the anterior limb of the internal capsule (36). Imaging studies have confirmed that a brachiocrural motor deficit may be caused by a presumed lacunar infarct involving the posterior limb of the internal capsule (6, 29, 30).

Isolated facial palsy has been related to a presumed lacunar infarct in the internal capsule (6, 37). Isolated brachial monoplegia is a rare lacunar syndrome that has also been reported to be caused by a capsular lacunar infarct at autopsy (38, 39) and by a presumed lacunar infarct located in the posterior limb of the internal capsule on CT (29). Isolated crural monoplegia has been reported secondary to a presumed lacunar infarct of the posterior limb of the internal capsule (6). Unilateral vocal cord palsy is a type of pure motor deficit described by Garel and Dor in 1890 that they attributed to a lacunar infarct in the anterior limb of the right internal capsule (40).

Fisher reported a patient with bilateral pure motor hemiparesis (i.e., pure motor quadriparesis) due to bilateral internal capsule lesions found at autopsy (41). A bilateral faciobrachial paresis has recently been related to bilateral infarcts in the genu and the posterior limb of the internal capsule on CT (42).

Ataxic Hemiparesis and the Dysarthria–Clumsy Hand Syndrome

The superior cerebellar peduncle constitutes one of the major cerebellar efferent systems. Cerebellar efferent fibers arise from the dentate, emboliform, and globose nuclei. These fibers decussate at the level of the inferior colliculus, enter and surround the red nucleus, and project to the ventral lateral nucleus of the thalamus (3). The corticopontine fibers, on the other hand, are one of the cerebellar afferent systems, and they arise from all the cerebral lobes and travel in the internal capsule (3). Thus, the cerebellar signs in a capsular ataxic hemiparesis syndrome may be due either to a thalamic lesion (cerebellar efferent fibers) and/or to a capsular lesion (cerebellar afferent fibers).

A presumed lacunar infarct located in the anterior limb of the internal capsule has been found to be responsible for ataxic hemiparesis (43). In this case, the infarct also involved the head of the caudate nucleus and probably interrupted the frontopontine tract of Arnold.

Presumed lacunar infarcts of the posterior limb of the internal capsule have been reported on CT (6,8,15,18,19,44–51) and on magnetic resonance imaging (MRI) (52). The infarct may extend to the thalamus (8,53,54) and to the lenticular nucleus (8).

Hypesthetic ataxic hemiparesis can be due to a presumed lacunar infarct located in the posterior limb of the internal capsule with or without thalamic involvement (55).

The dysarthria–clumsy hand syndrome has been reported from a presumed lacunar infarct in the internal capsule (56), especially the genu (44,57).

Pure Sensory Stroke

The afferent lemniscal pathway relays in the ventroposterolateral thalamic nucleus and joins the thalamocortical pathway, which ascends through the posterior limb of the internal capsule (3). A pure sensory stroke related to a presumed lacunar infarct in the posterior limb of the internal capsule has only been reported once on CT (58).

Sensorimotor Stroke

Mohr et al. described the lacunar syndrome of isolated sensorimotor deficit, due to a thalamic lacunar infarct extending into the posterior limb of the internal capsule, in 1977 (59). Thalamocapsular lacunes had been reported to cause sensorimotor syndromes prior to that time, however (60–62). Imaging studies have suggested that sensorimotor stroke can be due to a presumed lacunar infarct in the anterior limb of the internal capsule (22) extending to the caudate nucleus (8), the posterior limb of the internal capsule (8,22,27,63), the thalamus (22,63,64), and to the lenticular nucleus (8,22,51).

Other Lacunar Syndromes

Infarction in the anterior limb of the internal capsule can cause pure dysarthria (24), and if the infarction extends to the genu of the internal capsule the combination of dysarthria, facial weakness, and abulia can be observed (65). Alteration of motor activity can be produced by a lesion of the anterior limb of the internal capsule extending into the putamen or pallidum, namely appearance of hemiballism or disappearance of parkinsonism (66).

Bogousslavsky et al. (67) reported four patients with small deep infarcts in the genu of the internal capsule giving contralateral facial weakness, lingual paresis, unilateral mastication-palatal-pharyngeal weakness, slight hand weakness, and dysarthria. This was called the capsular genu syndrome. Asterixis has been associated with small deep infarcts either limited to the genu of the internal capsule (68) or which extended into the thalamus and pallidum (69).

Deep infarcts affecting the posterior limb of the internal capsule are related to occlusions in the territory of the anterior choroidal artery and its branches (70) (see Chapter 3). Hemiparesis, hemisensory loss, and hemianopia are the common manifestations of anterior choroidal artery infarcts (71). Sometimes the presence of a homonymous sectoranopia suggests an infarct in this arterial territory (72); however, it is not a very reliable sign (72,73). Cognitive defects sometimes mimicking cortical dysfunction can be associated with the sensorimotor deficit. In left-sided infarctions, aphasia with preserved repetition, perseverations, paraphasia, and impairment in comprehension, as well as decrease of vocal volume, dysarthria, apraxia, and an impairment of verbal memory, have been reported (73–76). In right-sided lesions, unilateral neglect, anosognosia, constructional apraxia, and drowsiness can be observed (25,74, 77,78). Stuttering (79) and cure of essential tremor (80) are very unusual manifestations of infarcts in the posterior limb of the internal capsule.

CAUDATE NUCLEUS

Classic Syndromes

Isolated infarcts limited to the caudate nucleus are not responsible for classic lacunar syndromes.

Other Syndromes

The caudate nucleus has a role in behavior, cognition, and affective reactions. Mendez et al. reported 11 cases of unilateral and one case of bilateral caudate infarcts (81). Although infarcts involving the adjacent anterior limb of the internal capsule were not excluded, some presumed lacunar infarcts were limited to the caudate nucleus. The clinical picture was characterized by acute and often transient minor deficits. Confusion and behavioral changes were prominent and often led to primary psychiatric diagnoses. These authors divided the behavioral changes into three groups:

Group 1 was characterized by apathy with decreased spontaneous verbal and motor activity, reduced initiative, and cessation of activities performed prior to the stroke.

Group 2 was characterized by disinhibition, inappropriate and impulsive behavior, and agitation.

Group 3 was characterized by affective symptoms: anxiety, depression, panic, insomnia, and psychotic features with hallucinations.

The neuropsychological changes that are most frequently observed include an impairment of problem-solving ability, an attention deficit, and an impairment of immediate and delayed recall. Recognition memory is, however, intact. Fromm et al. (25) reported a small deep infarct in the caudate that presented with dysarthria, anomia, and confusion. In the two cases of Habib et al. (82) of bilateral caudate presumed lacunar infarcts, there were prominent behavioral abnormalities with apathy, a lack of curiosity, and a flattened affect. The patients did not have a cognitive deficit and had features similar to those seen in some psychotics. Trillet et al. (83) reported two similar cases related to bilateral small deep infarcts in the head of the caudate nuclei extending to the anterior limb of the internal capsule. Caplan et al. (84) reported 18 small deep infarcts, nine of which extended to the anterior limb of the internal capsule. Slight hemiparesis, dysarthria, and dysphonia were frequent. The behavioral changes were similar to those reported by other authors. The patients with right caudate infarcts also often had a minor neglect syndrome (78,84).

Various abnormal movements have been described with caudate nucleus lesions: chorea (85–95), parkinsonism (96), dystonia (97, 98), and hemiballism (99).

LENTICULAR NUCLEUS (PUTAMEN AND GLOBUS PALLIDUS)

The blood supply of the lenticular nucleus derives from the lateral and medial lenticulostriate arteries, the recurrent artery of Heubner, and the anterior choroidal artery (see Chapter 3). This vascular supply explains why in some patients the infarct is not limited to the lenticular nucleus itself and why it is difficult to attribute specific symptoms to infarction of the lenticular nucleus. For this reason, certain clinical features caused by infarcts in this region may have been erroneously attributed to the head of the caudate nucleus, the anterior limb of the internal capsule, or the lenticular nucleus in some case reports.

Classic Syndromes

Isolated infarcts limited to the lenticular nucleus do not cause classic lacunar syndromes.

Other Lacunar Syndromes

Lacunar infarcts in the lenticular nucleus often appear to be asymptomatic (100). However, some infarcts affecting the lenticular nucleus may have neuropsychological and behavioral consequences, although these infarcts are usually larger than lacunes. The infarcts that involve the lenticular nucleus most frequently are striatocapsular infarcts. These have a subcortical comma shape and extend from the head of the caudate nucleus and the anterior limb of the internal capsule to the striatum. These infarcts are caused by occlusion of several perforating arteries due to either embolism to the trunk of the middle cerebral artery or to intrinsic pathology of this artery. Due to good collateral blood supply to the cortex, the infarct usually only affects the subcortical areas (34,101). Clinically there is often the sudden onset of hemiplegia mainly affecting the face and upper limb.

Neuropsychological testing in patients with striatocapsular infarction reveals cognitive abnormalities, including dysphasia, neglect, apraxia, and sometimes perseveration and frontal lobe type abnormalities (101,102). Naeser et al. (103) described eight patients with aphasia in whom left-sided subcortical infarcts were shown on CT. They divided the aphasia pattern into three categories: those with anterior superior extension had good comprehension, slow dysarthric speech, and hemiplegia; those with posterior extension had poor comprehension and fluent Wernicke-type aphasia and hemiplegia; those with both anterior and posterior extensions had global aphasia and hemiplegia. The internal capsule and overlying cortex was, however, often involved by these infarcts. Alexander et al. (104) reported 12 deep infarcts seen on CT and suggested that small lesions of the striatum and/or lateral anterior limb of the internal capsule caused at most slight word-finding difficulty or hesitancy. Word-finding difficulties were not seen when the infarct extended to the head of the caudate nucleus. The aphasia associated with infarcts extending beyond the striatum depended more on the white matter pathways affected than on striatal structures. However, it has been suggested that associated cortical infarcts that can be detected by MR, but could not previously be seen with CT, are the cause of frontal lobe abnormalities in striatocapsular infarcts (105). The syndrome of pure psychic akinesia related to bilateral lenticular nuclear necrosis to our knowledge has not been reported as a consequence of small artery occlusions

(106). Recently a patient with a striatocapsular infarct was reported to have complex visual hallucinations (107).

Small deep infarcts and lacunar infarcts of the lenticular nucleus may present with abnormal movements, either in the acute stage or later on in the clinical course. A large variety of abnormal movements has been reported: asterixis (69,108), parkinsonism (109–114), dystonia (115–120), ballism (66, 121–123), chorea (123–127) or abnormalities of posture responsible for falls (128).

THALAMUS

The thalamic blood supply arises from several sources. The thalamotuberal artery supplies the anterior thalamus, the paramedian thalamic and mesencephalic arteries supply the medial thalamus, the thalamogeniculate artery supplies the lateral thalamus, and the posteromedial and posterolateral choroidal arteries supply the posterior thalamus (see Chapter 3). Lacunar syndromes due wholly or partly to involvement of the thalamus may be caused by lacunar infarcts either in the posterior limb of the internal capsule and extending into the thalamus (sensorimotor stroke) or to infarcts within the thalamus (pure sensory stroke).

Classic Syndromes

Pure Sensory Stroke

Pure sensory stroke is produced by a lacunar infarct in the ventroposterolateral thalamic nucleus (129–133). Although thalamic lacunes causing pure sensory stroke may be seen on CT (63,134–140), they are often not detected by CT because of their small size. MRI is likely to be better at detecting these small presumed lacunar infarcts (138,141).

Fisher proposed that isolated paresthesias of the face, arm, and leg or involvement of the abdomen indicate a thalamic lesion (130), but a pontine infarct has also given rise to abdominal involvement (142).

Sensorimotor Stroke and Ataxic Hemiparesis

Mohr et al. reported the autopsy finding of a thalamic lacunar infarct with an adjacent zone of pallor extending into the posterior limb of the internal capsule that was responsible for a sensorimotor stroke (59). Garcin and Lapresle on the other hand reported a case of cheiro-oral sensory loss associated with weakness in the first three fingers due to an isolated thalamic lacunar infarct (143).

Ataxic hemiparesis has also been reported secondary to a lacunar infarct (144) or to a presumed lacunar infarct of the thalamus (8, 145–147). The painful ataxic hemiparesis and the hypesthetic ataxic hemiparesis syndromes have also been described secondary to presumed lacunar infarcts of the thalamus (148,149). The cause of the motor deficit in lacunar infarcts that are apparently restricted to the thalamus is unclear. However, since the corticospinal tract does not pass through the thalamus, it must be assumed that there must be transient ischemia or edema of the internal capsule or compression of the internal capsule by edema.

Other Lacunar Syndromes

Thalamic lesions have been reported to cause neuropsychological signs and symptoms. These features depend upon the site of the infarction.

Small presumed lacunar infarcts in the anterior thalamus in the territory of the thalamotuberal artery (thalamic polar artery) give rise to contralateral facial weakness or "emotional" facial paralysis, limb clumsiness, and slight sensory changes. Neuropsychological features predominate and are characterized by apathy, a fluctuating level of attention, perseveration, disorientation, personality change, euphoria, and lack of insight. In left-sided infarcts, transcortical aphasia is reported with reduction of spontaneous speech, paraphasias, anomia, and reduced fluency with preservation of repetition and moderate impairment of comprehension. In addition there is a reduction of vocal volume, visual memory impairments, and acalculia. In some cases the neuropsychological abnormalities are more widespread. In right-sided infarcts, hemispatial neglect, visual memory impairment, and disturbed visuospatial function are common, and are often associated with constructional apraxia (136,150–152). Austin et al. reported an association of Horner's syndrome, contralateral faciobrachial weakness, and dysarthria caused by a small deep infarct extending from the anterior thalamus to the genu of the internal capsule (153).

Castaigne et al. reported 28 autopsy-proven cases of paramedian thalamic infarcts (occlusion of the paramedian thalamic and mesencephalic arteries). Four had a unilateral small deep infarct. The most prominent features in these patients were mood and behavioral changes. Agitation and aggression alternated with apathy and immobility, and the patients were disoriented (154). Five patients had bilateral small deep infarcts, and these presented with disturbances of consciousness, deep coma, hypersomnia, disturbances of behavior, apathy, akinetic mutism, or mood or memory disturbances. These features were often associated with a vertical gaze palsy (154). The three patients with small deep infarcts reported by Graff-Radford et al. (136) had similar clinical features. Friedman's patient presented with a diffuse encephalopathy (155). Watson reported a right-sided small deep infarct presenting with neglect, associated with flattened affect and difficulty in recognizing the emotional content of facial expression, and affectively intoned speech (156). Davous et al. reported a lacunar infarct seen at autopsy in a patient presenting with aphasia, reduced fluency and paraphasias, but normal repetition and comprehension (157). Louarn et al. reported an autopsy-proven thalamic infarct giving rise to hemiplegia, hemianesthesia, and hemianopia associated with visual neglect, constructional apraxia, and kinesthetic illusions (158).

Graff-Radford et al. (136) reported eight cases of lateral thalamic infarcts extending into the posterior internal capsule. Hemiparesis and hypoesthesia were associated with construction apraxia and impairments of verbal and visual memory, visual perception, and spatial discrimination. Fromm et al.'s two patients had dysarthria and a disturbance of affect (i.e., joviality) (158a). Laplane et al.'s (159) two patients with thalamic infarcts had motor hemineglect.

In summary, right thalamic lesions may lead to a neglect syndrome, left-sided lesions to aphasia (160), and uni- or bilateral lesions to a dementia syndrome characterized by perseveration and loss of initiative, and by severe deficits of attention and memory (161, 162).

Movement disorders are a rare consequence of thalamic infarcts. Rare cases of asterixis (69,163,164), tremor (93), chorea (127), dystonia (117,165,166), oral dyskinesia (167) have been reported. The spontaneous disappearance of parkinsonian signs (168) also has been reported.

BRAINSTEM

Involvement of the penetrating arteries in the brainstem gives rise to many miscellaneous lacunar syndromes. In the brainstem, the classic syndromes are usually due to pontine lacunes.

Midbrain

Classic Syndromes

A midbrain lacune can produce a pure motor stroke (169,170). Gaymard et al. recently reported a presumed lacunar infarct seen on MR that was responsible for a pure motor stroke (171).

Other Lacunar Syndromes

The paramedian mesencephalic/thalamic arteries supply the upper medial midbrain and the medial thalamus. A distal occlusion of these arteries leads to a medial thalamic infarct. If the occlusion is more proximal, there may be a combination of midbrain and thalamic infarcts, which are often bilateral. In these mesencephalothalamic infarcts, patients often present with an association of upper midbrain and thalamic clinical features. Castaigne et al. (154) reported 19 patients with autopsy confirmation of the infarct site. The onset of the clinical features was sudden, with initial coma and subsequent hypersomnia, akinetic mutism, disorientation in time and place, and memory difficulties. Unilateral or bilateral third nerve palsy and delayed athetoid or clonic movements were also seen. Bogousslavsky et al. (172) reported a patient who presented with motor hemineglect, faciobrachial hypesthesia, motor transcortical aphasia, anterograde amnesia, and vertical gaze palsy who had a mesencephalothalamic infarct at autopsy. Guberman et al. reported two patients with both thalamic and midbrain clinical features who had an infarct in this arterial territory on CT (173).

Infarcts restricted to the upper midbrain may rarely give rise to peduncular hallucinosis (174–179). Subthalamic small deep infarcts may be associated with abnormal movements and asterixis (164,180,181). Infarction of the midbrain territory of the superior cerebellar artery has been associated with blepharospasm (182). Midbrain infarcts seen at autopsy (179,183) or on imaging (184,185) have been associated with unilateral or bilateral ballistic movements (186).

Oculomotor disturbances are frequent manifestations of midbrain infarcts. The clinical features depend on the site of the lesion and may be divided into supranuclear, nuclear, and fascicular. The supranuclear gaze palsies are due to infarction in the medial upper midbrain, usually in the territory of the paramedian mesencephalic arteries:

Combined Up and Down Vertical Gaze Palsy

This syndrome has been related to bilateral midbrain infarcts both at autopsy (154, 187–195) and with imaging (196–199). It has also been shown to be due to unilateral infarcts at autopsy (200–205) or with imaging (206).

Upward Gaze Palsy

This has also been shown to be caused by bilateral infarcts both at autopsy (191,207, 208) and with imaging (193), as well as by unilateral infarcts at autopsy (172,191,209–212) or with imaging (193,213,214).

Down Gaze Palsy

In down gaze palsy the lesion at autopsy (187,193,212,215–222) and imaging (223–225) is always bilateral.

Other Vertical Gaze Palsies

The dysconjugate vertical gaze palsies, monocular elevation palsy (206,226,227), and vertical "one-and-a-half" syndrome (206,228–231) are usually related to a unilateral infarct ipsilateral or contralateral to the clinical signs.

Third Nerve Palsy

Isolated third nerve nuclear syndromes are rare and have been related to small deep midbrain infarcts on CT (232,233). Infarction of the fascicles of the third nerve in the midbrain has been shown at autopsy (233,234) or on imaging (235). These patients may have preserved pupillary function (236,237).

An oculomotor palsy can be associated with contralateral cerebellar signs secondary to a lesion of the red nucleus. This combination is known as Claude's syndrome and has been reported at autopsy (238–240) and on imaging (171,232,235,241–243). The combination of a third nerve palsy with contralateral abnormal movements is known as Benedikt's syndrome (244,245). The third nerve is not always affected by infarcts affecting the red nucleus and Chiray et al. have reported an isolated lateral and rostral red nucleus infarct presenting with a cerebellar tremor (246).

The association of an oculomotor palsy with a contralateral hemiplegia is known as Weber's syndrome, and this syndrome has been related to a midbrain infarct at autopsy (247–251) and on imaging (177,235).

There are other uncommon neuroophthalmological features that can suggest a midbrain lesion. Halmagyi et al. described three patients studied with imaging who had tonic contraversive ocular tilt reactions secondary to midbrain infarcts on imaging (252). Selhorst et al. reported a patient with intermittent corectopia (eccentric pupil) who had a midbrain infarct at autopsy (253).

Ptosis suggests a medial tegmental midbrain infarction. It has been reported in associated with internuclear ophthalmoplegia and convergence retractory nystagmus (254), oculomotor and trochlear nuclear involvement (255), and with a dissociated vertical gaze palsy and asterixis (181).

Bilateral isolated lateral midbrain small deep infarcts involving the corticospinal tract have been responsible for tetraplegia and mutism, allowing the conscious patient to communicate only with eye movements (mesencephalic locked-in syndrome) (256).

Pons

Classic Syndromes

Pure Motor Stroke

Pure motor stroke involving the face, arm, and leg was related to a lacunar infarct in the ventral part of the basis pontis by Fisher and Curry (257). Although this location has been confirmed as a site for pure motor stroke by only a few autopsy correlations (3,258,259), it has been confirmed by CT (30,260–263) and MRI (137,241, 261,264).

Isolated supranuclear facial palsy due to a presumed lacunar infarct of the pons has been reported on CT (260) and recently on MRI (265).

Ataxic Hemiparesis and Dysarthria– Clumsy Hand Syndrome

On the basis of three autopsy cases showing lacunar infarcts in the upper basis pontis, CM Fisher coined the term ataxic hemiparesis in 1978 (266). No further autopsy cases has been reported, but upper, middle, and lower basis pontis infarcts have been associated with ataxic hemiparesis by CT (18,139,260,267–270) and by MRI (264,271–273). Ataxic hemiparesis with trigeminal weakness has also been described secondary to a small infarct seen on CT in the basis pontis (274). The only case of ataxic tetraparesis was a CT correlation of a small infarct in the basis pontis (275).

The dysarthria–clumsy hand syndrome was reported to be due to a lacunar infarct in the basis pontis by CM Fisher (276). Imaging studies have subsequently confirmed this topography (269,277).

Pure Sensory Stroke

Pure sensory stroke has occasionally been found to be caused by a presumed pontine lacunar infarct on MRI. The sensory disturbance may involve face, arm, trunk, and leg (141,142), or only the lip and hand (140).

Sensorimotor Stroke

A small paramedian pontine infarct can give rise to a sensorimotor stroke (137,260).

Other Lacunar Syndromes

A pontine location is probable if pontine tegmental signs are associated with a classic lacunar syndrome. A pure motorhemiparesis with a crossed sixth nerve palsy (Landry's syndrome) (278) has been reported only three times (65,278,279). A pure motor hemiparesis associated with a one-and-a-half syndrome has been reported at autopsy (1) and with imaging (280,281).

A pontine location is possible when there is a horizontal gaze palsy, horizontal one-and-a-half syndrome (1,65,280,282), or a paramedian pontine reticular formation syndrome characterized by horizontal gaze palsy with the preservation of lateral gaze toward the lesion during the oculocephalic maneuver (283). In unilateral internuclear ophthalmoplegia, the infarct can be located in the medial longitudinal fasciculus of either the pons or the midbrain (284,285). In one patient with an isolated sixth nerve palsy the causative small deep infarct was located in the base of the pons (286).

Some unusual combination of signs can also be related to pontine small infarcts. Fisher reported a patient with a pontine small deep infarct who presented with dysarthria, staggering gait, incoordination, facial weakness, nystagmus, ocular overshoot, ataxia, and dissociated loss of pain and temperature (287). Vermersch et al. reported a patient who had a small deep pontine infarct with hemifacial spasm (288).

Medulla Oblongata

Lacunar syndromes due to medulla oblongata lacunar infarcts are uncommon. However, a medial medullary infarct can produce a proportional pure motor stroke (289). The arm and leg may be more affected than the face, producing the so-called variant pure motor stroke sparing the face (257,290–292). When the infarct affects both pyramidal tracts, it may produce a pure motor quadriparesis (293). Although medial medullary infarcts usually produce complex syndromes, involvement of pyramidal and lemniscal tracts may occasionally give rise to sensorimotor strokes (137,294).

CONCLUSION

The multiplicity of signs and symptoms related to small deep infarcts and lacunar infarcts is impressive. Lacunar infarcts, however, most commonly cause classic lacunar syndromes when they damage strategic anatomical structures. They are, however, often asymptomatic, especially if they are located in the basal ganglia (100). Small deep infarcts seen on imaging studies are often relatively large, and consequently more frequently give rise to miscellaneous syndromes. As shown in Chapter 10, however, lacunar syndromes are not specific for ischemia, and imaging is always needed to confirm their ischemic origin.

REFERENCES

1. Fisher CM, Caplan LR. Basilar artery branch occlusion: a cause of pontine infarction. *Neurology* 1971;21:900–905.
2. Caplan LR. Intracranial branch atheromatous disease: a neglected, understudied, and underused concept. *Neurology* 1989;39:1246–1250.
3. Carpenter MB, Sutin J. *Human neuroanatomy.* 8th ed. Baltimore, Maryland: Williams & Wilkins; 1983.
4. Chamorro A, Sacco RL, Mohr JP, et al. Clinical-computed tomographic correlations of lacunar infarction in the Stroke Data Bank. *Stroke* 1991;22:175–181.
5. Soisson T, Cabanis EA, Iba-Zizen MT, Bousser MG, Laplane D, Castaigne P. Pure motor hemiplegia and computed tomography. *J Neuroradiology* 1982;9:304–322.
6. Donnan GA, Tress BM, Bladin PF. A prospective study of lacunar infarction using computerized tomography. *Neurology* 1982;32:49–56.
7. Ciucci G, Stracciari A, Bissi G, Piscaglia MG, Guidi AR, Rebucci GG. Lacunar infarcts: a personal series of 92 consecutive cases. *Eur Neurol* 1989;29[Suppl 2]:10–12.
8. Boiten J, Lodder J. Discrete lesions in the sensorimotor control system. A clinico-topographical study of lacunar infarcts. *J Neurol Sci* 1991;105:154.
9. Weisberg LA. Computed tomography and pure motor hemiparesis. *Neurology* 1979;29:490–495.
10. Norrving B, Cronqvist S. Clinical and radio-

logic features of lacunar versus nonlacunar minor stroke. *Stroke* 1989;20:59–64.
11. Pitres A. *Recherche sur les lésions du centre ovale des hémisphères cérébraux étudies du point de vue des localisations cérébrales* [Thesis]. Paris, 1877.
12. Cruveilhier J. *Atlas d'anatomie pathologique du corps humain.* Paris: JB Bailliere; 1829–1842.
13. Takamatsu N, Yamanouchi H, Yamada H. Lacune in the white matter revealed by MRI in a case of pure motor monoparesis. *Clin Neurol* 1990;30:898–900.
14. Biller J, Scardigli K. Ataxic hemiparesis from lesions of the corona radiata. *Arch Neurol* 1984;41:136.
15. Magrotti E, Borutti G, Mariani G, Donati E, Faggi L. Ataxic hemiparesis syndrome. Clinical and CT study of 20 new cases. *Funct Neurol* 1990;5:65–71.
16. Donati E, Callea L, Faggi L, Bargnani C. Ataxic hemiparesis: further CT confirmation of an old localizing hypothesis. *Ital J Neurol Sci* 1984;5:275–278.
17. Sage JI, Lepore FE. Ataxic hemiparesis from lesions of the corona radiata. *Arch Neurol* 1983;40:449–450.
18. Colombo A, Crisi G, Guerzoni MC, Panzetti P. Vascular ataxic hemiparesis: a prospective clinical and CT study. *Ital J Neurol Sci* 1986;7:253–256.
19. Huang CY, Lui FS. Ataxic hemiparesis, localisation and clinical features. *Stroke* 1984;15:363–366.
20. Jokelainen M, Pilke A. Ataxic hemiparesis. *Arch Neurol* 1983;40:326.
21. Rosenberg NL, Koller R. Computerized tomography and pure sensory stroke. *Neurology* 1981;31:217–220.
22. Huang CY, Woo E, Chan FL. When is sensorimotor stroke a lacunar syndrome? *J Neurol Neurosurg Psychiatry* 1987;50:720–726.
23. Miyashita K, Naritomi H, Sawada T, et al. Identification of recent lacunar lesions in cases of multiple small infarctions by magnetic resonance imaging. *Stroke* 1988;19:834–839.
24. Ozaki I, Baba M, Narita S, Matsunaga M, Takebe K. Pure dysarthria due to anterior internal capsule and/or corona radiata infarction: a report of five cases. *J Neurol Neurosurg Psychiatry* 1986;49:1435–1437.
25. Fromm D, Holland AL, Swindell CS, Reinmuth OM. Various consequences of subcortical stroke. Prospective study of 16 consecutive cases. *Arch Neurol* 1985;42:943–950.
26. Abadie JLIJ. *Les localisations fonctionnelles de la capsule interne* [Thesis]. Bordeaux, 1900.
27. Kashihara M, Matsumoto K. Acute capsular infarction. Location of the lesions and the clinical feature. *Neuroradiology* 1985;27:248–253.
28. Ross ED. Localization of the pyramidal tract in the internal capsule by whole brain dissection. *Neurology* 1980;30:59–64.
29. Tredici G, Pizzini G, Bogliun G, Tagliabue M. The site of motor corticospinal fibres in the internal capsule in man. A computerised tomographic study of restricted lesions. *J Anat* 1982;134:199–208.
30. Rascol A, Clanet M, Manelfe C, Guiraud B, Bonafé A. Pure motor hemiplegia: CT study of 30 cases. *Stroke* 1982;13:11–17.
31. Mohr JP. Lacunes. *Neurol Clin* 1983;1:201–221.
32. Manelfe C, Clanet M, Gigaud M, Bonafé A, Guiraud B, Rascol A. Internal capsule: normal anatomy and ischemic changes demonstrated by computed tomography. *AJNR* 1981;2:149–155.
33. Moffie D, Ongerboer de Visser BW, Van der Sande JJ. "Pure motor hemiplegia"; de plaatsbepaling van de piramidebaan in de capsula interna. *Ned Tijdschr Geneesk* 1979;123:822–825.
34. Pullicino P, Nelson RF, Kendall BE, Marshall J. Small deep infarcts diagnosed on computed tomography. *Neurology* 1980:30:1090–1096.
35. Rougemont D, Baron JC, Lebrun-Grandie P, Bousser MG, Soisson T, Comar D. Débit sanguin cérébral et extraction d'oxygène dans les hémiplégies lacunaires. Etude semi-quantitative par l'oxygène-15 et la tomographie d'émission. *Pathol Biol (Paris)* 1982;30:295–302.
36. Pitres A. A propos d'un cas de monoplégie persistante du membre inférieur gauche causé par une lésion très limitée de la capsule interne droite. *Arch Clin Bordeaux* 1893;1–14.
37. Huang C, Broe G. Isolated facial palsy: a new lacunar syndrome. *J Neurol Neurosurg Psychiatry* 1984;47:84–86.
38. Benett AH, Campbell CM. Case of brachial monoplegia, with lesion to the internal capsule. *Brain* 1885;8:78–84.
39. Prince M. A case of incipient locomotor ataxia and monoplegia from focal lesion of the internal capsule in the same patient. *J Nerv Ment Dis* 1895:685.
40. Garel J, Dor L. Du centre cortical moteur larynx et du trajet intra-cérébral des fibres qui en manent. *Ann Maladies Oreille Larynx* 1890; 16:209–235.
41. Fisher CM. Bilateral capsular infarcts—the mechanism of recovery from hemiplegia. *J Neuropathol Exp Neurol* 1978;37:613.
42. Michielsen B, Van den Bergh R. Bilateral faciobrachial paresis as a consequence of symmetrical capsular infarcts. *Acta Neurol Belg* 1991;91:280–287.
43. Rosa A, Mizon JP, Betermiez P. Hémiparésie crurale avec ataxie homolatérale. A propos d'un cas avec étude tomodensitométrique. *Rev Otoneuroophtalmol* 1983;55:283–288.
44. De Vries L, Sno HN. Ataktische hemiparese en "dysarthria–clumpsy hand," twee vervante syndromen veroorzaakt door een lacunair herseninfarct. *Ned Tijdschr Geneeskd* 1985;129:1628–1631.
45. Ichikawa K, Tsutsumishita A, Fujioka A. Capsular ataxic hemiparesis. A case report. *Arch Neurol* 1982;39:585–586.
46. Iragui VJ, MacCutchen CB. Capsular ataxic hemiparesis. *Arch Neurol* 1982;39:528–529.

47. Jacome DE. Homolateral ataxia and crural paresis. *Arch Neurol* 1983;40:662–663.
48. Rosa A, Mizon JP. Hémiparésie crurale avec ataxie ipsilatérale. *Rev Neurol* 1984;140: 515–516.
49. Sanguineti I, Tredici G, Beghi E, et al. Ataxic hemiparesis syndrome: clinical and CT study of 20 new cases and review of the literature. *Ital J Neurol Sci* 1986;7:51–59.
50. Tredici G, Bogliun G, Sanguineti I. Capsular ataxic hemiparesis. *Arch Neurol* 1983;40:326.
51. Weisberg LA. Lacunar infarcts. Clinical and computed tomographic correlations. *Arch Neurol* 1982;39:37–40.
52. Helweg-Larsen S, Larsson H, Henriksen O, Sorensen PS. Ataxic hemiparesis: three different locations of lesions studied by MRI. *Neurology* 1988;38:1322–1324.
53. De Renzi E, Nichelli P, Crisi G. Hemiataxia and crural hemiparesis following capsular infarct. *J Neurol Neurosurg Psychiatry* 1983; 46:561–563.
54. Perman GP, Racy A. Homolateral ataxia and crural paresis: case report. *Neurology* 1980; 30:1013–1015.
55. Helgason CM, Wilbur AC. Capsular hypesthetic ataxic hemiparesis. *Stroke* 1990;21:24–33.
56. Nelson RF, Pullicino P, Kendall BE, Marshall J. Computed tomography in patients presenting with lacunar syndromes. *Stroke* 1980;11:256–261.
57. Spertell RB, Ransom BR. Dysarthria–clumsy hand syndrome produced by capsular infarct. *Ann Neurol* 1979;6:263–265.
58. Derouesné C, Yelnik A, Castaigne P. Déficit sensitif isolé par infarctus dans le territoire de l'artère choroïdienne antérieure. *Rev Neurol* 1985;141:311–314.
59. Mohr JP, Kase CS, Meckler RJ, Fisher CM. Sensorimotor stroke due to thalamocapsular ischemia. *Arch Neurol* 1977;34:739–741.
60. Dechambre A. Mémoire sur la curabilité du ramollissement cérébral. *Gaz Med Paris* 1838; 6:305–314.
61. Turck L. Über die Beziehung gewisser Krankheitsherde des grossen Gehirnes zur Anesthesie. Sitzungsberichte der Mathematisch Naturunissenschaftlichen. *Classe Kaiserlichen Akademie Wissenschaften* 1859;36:191–199.
62. Garcin R, Lapresle J. Syndrome sensitif de type thalamique et topographie cheiro-orale par lésion localise du thalamus. *Rev Neurol* 1954; 90:124–129.
63. Robinson RK, Richey ET, Kase CS, Mohr JP. Somatosensory evoked potentials in pure sensory stroke and related conditions. *Stroke* 1985;16:818–823.
64. Mauguière F, Courjon J. The origins of short-latency somatosensory evoked potentials in humans. *Ann Neurol* 1981;9:607–611.
65. Fisher CM. Cerebral ischemia—less familiar types. *Clin Neurosurg* 1971;18:267–336.
66. Scoditti U, Rustichelli P, Calzetti S. Spontaneous hemiballism and disappearance of parkinsonism following contralateral lenticular lacunar infarct. *Ital J Neurol Sci* 1989;10:757–577.
67. Bogousslavsky J, Regli F. Capsular genu syndrome. *Neurology* 1990;40:1499–1502.
68. Yagnik P, Dhopesh V. Unilateral asterixis. *Arch Neurol* 1981;38:601–602.
69. Massey EW, Goodman JC, Stewart C, Brannon WL. Unilateral asterixis: motor integrative dysfunction in focal vascular disease. *Neurology* 1979;29:1188–1190.
70. Mohr JP, Steinke W, Timsit SG, Sacco RL, Tatemichi TK. The anterior choroidal artery does not supply the corona radiata and lateral ventricular wall. *Stroke* 1991;22:1502–1507.
71. Masson M, Decroix JP, Henin D, Dairou R, Graveleau P, Cambier J. Syndrome de l'artère choroïdienne antérieure: étude clinique et tomodensitométrique de 4 cas. *Rev Neurol* 1983; 139:547–552.
72. Helgason C, Caplan LR, Goodwin J, Hedges T. Anterior choroidal artery-territory infarction. Report of cases and review. *Arch Neurol* 1986; 43:681–686.
73. Grochovicki M, Vighetto A. Homonymous horizontal sectoranopia: report of four cases. *Br J Ophthalmol* 1991;75:624–628.
74. Cambier J, Graveleau P, Decroix JP, Elghozi D, Masson M. Le syndrome de l'artère choroïdienne antérieure: étude neuropsychologique de 4 cas. *Rev Neurol* 1983;139:553–559.
75. Hommel M, Dubois F, Pollak P, et al. Syndrome de l'artère choroïdienne antérieure gauche avec troubles du langage et apraxie constructive. *Rev Neurol* 1985;141:137–142.
76. Tanridag O, Kirshner HS. Aphasia and agraphia in the lesions of the posterior internal capsule and putamen. *Neurology* 1985;35:1797–1801.
77. Ferro JM, Kertesz A. Posterior internal capsule infarction associated with neglect. *Arch Neurol* 1984;41:422–424.
78. Ferro JM, Kertesz A, Black SE. Subcortical neglect: quantitation, anatomy, and recovery. *Neurology* 1987;37:1487–1492.
79. Soroker N, Bar-Israel Y, Schechter I, Solzi P. Stuttering as a manifestation of right-hemispheric subcortical stroke. *Eur Neurol* 1990; 30:268–270.
80. Duncan R, Bone I, Melville ID. Essential tremor cured by infarction adjacent to the thalamus. *J Neurol Neurosurg Psychiatry* 1988; 51:591–592.
81. Mendez MF, Adams NL, Lewandowski KS. Neurobehavioral changes associated with caudate lesions. *Neurology* 1989;39:349–354.
82. Habib M, Poncet M. Perte de l'élan vital, de l'intéret, et de l'affectivité (syndrome athymormique) au cours de lésions lacunaires des corps striés. *Rev Neurol* 1988;144:571–577.
83. Trillet M, Croisille B, Tourniaire D, Schott B. Perturbations de l'activité motrice volontaire et lésions des noyaux caudés. *Rev Neurol* 1990; 146:338–344.
84. Caplan LR, Schmahmann JD, Kase CS, Feld-

mann E, Baquis G, Greeberg JP, Gorelick PB, Helgason C, Hier DB. Caudate infarcts. *Arch Neurol* 1990;47:133–143.
85. Saris S. Chorea caused by caudate infarction. *Arch Neurol* 1983;40:590–591.
86. Goldblatt D, Markesbery W, Reeves AG. Recurrent hemichorea following striatal lesions. *Arch Neurol* 1974;31:51–54.
87. Dooling EC, Adams RD. The pathological anatomy of posthemiplegic athetosis. *Brain* 1975;98:29–48.
88. Ikeda M, Tsukagoshi H. Monochorea caused by a striatal lesion. *Eur Neurol* 1991;31:257–258.
89. Kawamura M, Takahashi N, Hirayama K. Hemichorea and its denial in a case of caudate infarction diagnosed by magnetic resonance imaging. *J Neurol Neurosurg Psychiatry* 1988;51:590–591.
90. Austregesilo A, Borges-Forte A. Sur un cas d'hémichorée avec lésion du noyau caudé. (Contribution anatomo-clinique aux localisations du striatum.) *Rev Neurol* 1937;67:477–488.
91. Austregesilo A, Gallotti O. Sur un cas d'hémiparésie et d'hémichorée avec lésion du noyau caudé. *Rev Neurol* 1924:41–43.
92. Davison C, Goodhart SP. Monochorea and somatotopic localization. *Arch Neurol Psychiatry* 1940;43:792–803.
93. Kim JS. Delayed onset hand tremor caused by cerebral infarction. *Stroke* 1992;23:292–294.
94. Goldblatt J, White NW, Wright MGE. Bilateral chorea associated with caudate nuclei lacunar infarcts. *S Afr Med J* 1989;75:443–445.
95. Tabaton M, Mancardi G, Loeb C. Generalized chorea due to bilateral small, deep cerebral infarcts. *Neurology* 1985;35:588–589.
96. Lazzarino LG, Nicolai A, Toppani D. Subacute parkinsonism from a single lacunar infarct in the basal ganglia. *Acta Neurol Napoli* 1990;12:292–295.
97. Boylan KB, Chin JH, DeArmond SJ. Progressive dystonia following resuscitation from cardiac arrest. *Neurology* 1990;40:1458–1461.
98. Demierre B, Rondot P. Dystonia caused by putamino-capsulo-caudate vascular lesions. *J Neurol Neurosurg Psychiatry* 1983;46:404–406.
99. Kase CS, Maulsby GO, deJuan E, Mohr JP. Hemichorea—hemiballism and lacunar infarction in the basal ganglia. *Neurology* 1981;31:452–455.
100. Fisher CM. Lacunes: small, deep cerebral infarct. *Neurology* 1965;15:774–784.
101. Donnan GA, Bladin PF, Berkovic SF, Longley WA, Saling MM. The stroke syndrome of striatocapsular infarction. *Brain* 1991;114:51–70.
102. Bladin PF, Berkovic SF. Striatocapsular infarction: large infarcts in the lenticulostriate artery territory. *Neurology* 1984;34:1423–1430.
103. Naeser MA, Alexander MP, Helm-Estabrooks N, Levine HL, Laughlin SA, Geschwind N. Aphasia with predominantly subcortical lesion sites. Description of three capsular/putaminal aphasia syndromes. *Arch Neurol* 1982;39:2–14.
104. Alexander MP, Naeser MA, Palumbo CL. Correlations of subcortical CT lesion sites and aphasia profiles. *Brain* 1987;110:961–991.
105. Godefroy O, Rousseaux M, Leys D, Destée A, Scheltens P, Pruvo JP. Frontal lobe dysfunction in unilateral lenticulo-striate infarcts: prominent role of cortical lesions. *Arch Neurol* 1992;49:1285–1289.
106. Laplane D, Baulac M, Widlocher D, Dubois B. Pure psychic akinesia with bilateral lesions of basal ganglia. *J Neurol Neurosurg Psychiatry* 1977;47:377–385.
107. Martin R, Bogousslavsky J, Regli F. Striatocapsular infarction and "release" visual hallucinations. *Cerebrovasc Dis* 1992;2:111–113.
108. Shuttleworth EC, Drake ME. Asterixis after lacunar infarctions. *Eur Neurol* 1987;27:62–63.
109. Friedman A, Kang UJ, Tatemichi TK, Burke R. A case of parkinsonism following striatal lacunar infarction. *J Neurol Neurosurg Psychiatry* 1986;49:1087–1088.
110. Tolosa ES, Santamaria J. Parkinsonism and basal ganglia infarcts. *Neurology* 1984;34:1516–1518.
111. Bornstein NM, Reider-Grosswasser I, Korczyn AD. Clinical correlates of lacunar infarcts in the basal ganglia. *Stroke* 1989;20:136.
112. Murrow RW, Schweiger GD, Kepes JJ, Koller WC. Parkinsonism due to a basal ganglia lacunar state: clinicopathologic correlation. *Neurology* 1990;40:897–900.
113. Barré JA, Reys. Syndrome parkinsonien avec signe de Babinski bilatéral. Lésion symétrique des putamens. *Rev Neurol* 1925:968–977.
114. Lhermitte J, Cornil L. Un cas de syndrome parkinsonien: lacunes symétriques dans le globus pallidus. *Rev Neurol* 1921;371:189–191.
115. Folstein S, Abbott M, Moser R, Parhad I, Clark A, Folstein M. A phenocopy of Huntington's disease: lacunar infarcts of the corpus striatum. *Johns Hopkins Med J* 1981;148:104–108.
116. Russo LS. Focal dystonia and lacunar infarction of the basal ganglia. *Arch Neurol* 1983;40:61.
117. Marsden CD, Obeso JA, Zarranz JJ, Lang AE. The anatomical basis of symptomatic hemidystonia. *Brain* 1985;108:463–483.
118. Burton K, Farrel K, Li D, Calne DB. Lesions of the putamen and dystonia: CT and magnetic resonance imaging. *Neurology* 1984;34:962–965.
119. Traub M, Ridley A. Focal dystonia in association with cerebral ischemia. *J Neurol Neurosurg Psychiatry* 1982;45:1073–1074.
120. Grimes JD, Hassan MN, Quarrington AM, D'Alton. Delayed-onset posthemiplegic dystonia: CT demonstration of basal ganglia pathology. *Neurology* 1982;32:1033–1035.
121. Lodder J, Baard WC. Paraballism caused by bilateral hemorrhagic infarction in the basal ganglia. *Neurology* 1981;31:484–486.
122. Mas JL, Launay M, Derouesné C. Hemiballism and CT-documented lacunar infarct in the lenticular nucleus. *J Neurol Neurosurg Psychiatry* 1987;50:104–105.

123. Destée A, Muller JP, Vermersch P, Pruvo JP, Warot P. Hémiballisme hémichorée infarctus striatal. *Rev Neurol* 1990;146:150–152.
124. Mabboux M. Contribution à l'étude de l'hémichoré symtomatique dans les lésions cérébrales. *Rev Med* 1883;10:1054–1063.
125. Bruno A, Rosenberg GA. The spectrum of lacunar infarction in the elderly. *Clin Geriatr Med* 1991;7:443–453.
126. Von Steck H. Zur pathologischen anatomie der echten posthemiplegischen athetose. *Schweiz Arch Neurol* 1926;8:75–85.
127. Purdon Martin J. Hemichorea (hemiballismus) without lesions in the corpus Luysii. *Brain* 1957;80:2–10.
128. Labadie EL, Awerbuch GI, Hamilton RH, Rapcsak SZ. Falling and postural deficits due to acute unilateral basal ganglia lesions. *Arch Neurol* 1989;46:492–996.
129. Fisher CM. Pure sensory stroke involving face, arm and leg. *Neurology* 1965;15:76–80.
130. Fisher CM. Pure sensory stroke and allied conditions. *Stroke* 1982;13:434–447.
131. Fisher CM. Thalamic pure sensory stroke. *Neurology* 1978;28:1141–1144.
132. De Ajuriaguerra J. *La douleur centrale* [Thesis]. Paris, 1937:66–67.
133. Lhermitte J, Fumet. Syndrome hémialgique pur d'origine thalamique chez un lacunaire. *Rev Neurol* 1921;37:468–473.
134. Decroix JP, Graveleau P, Masson M, Cambier J. Infarctus cérébraux et déficit sensitif pur. *Rev Neurol* 1989;145:111–117.
135. Gorsselink EL, Lodder J. Pure sensory stroke with lacunar infarction in the posteroventral thalamus on CT. *Clin Neurol Neurosurg* 1985;87:45–46.
136. Graff-Radford NR, Damasio H, Yamada T, Eslinger PJ, Damasio AR. Nonhemorrhagic thalamic infarction. Clinical, neuropsychological and electrophysiological findings in four anatomical groups defined by computerized tomography. *Brain* 1985;108:485–516.
137. Landi G, Anzalone N, Vaccari V. CT scan evidence of postero-lateral thalamic infarction in pure sensory stroke. *J Neurol Neurosurg Psychiatry* 1984;47:570–571.
138. Rothrock JF, Lyden PD, Hesselink JR, Brown JJ, Healy ME. Brain magnetic resonance imaging in the evaluation of lacunar stroke. *Stroke* 1987;18:781–786.
139. Sacco RL, Bello JA, Traub R, Brust J. Selective proprioceptive loss from a thalamic lacunar stroke. *Stroke* 1987;18:1160–1163.
140. Kappelle LJ, Van Gijn J. Lacunar infarcts. *Clin Neurol Neurosurg* 1986;88:3–17.
141. Kawakami Y, Chikama M, Tanimoto T, Shimamura Y. Radiological studies of the cheirooral syndrome. *J Neurol* 1989;236:177–181.
142. Hommel M, Besson G, Pollak P, Borgel F, Le Bas JF, Perret J. Pure sensory stroke due to a pontine lacune. *Stroke* 1989;20:406–408.
143. Garcin R, Lapresle J. Deuxième observation personnelle de syndrome sensitif de type thalamique et topographie cheiro-orale par lésion localisé du thalamus. *Rev Neurol* 1960;103:474–481.
144. Garcin R. Syndrome cérébello-thalamique par lésion localisé du thalamus avec une digression sur le "signe de la main creuse" et son intéret sémiologique. *Rev Neurol* 1955;93:143–149.
145. Murthy JMK. Ataxic hemiparesis-ventrolateral nucleus of the thalamus: yet another site of lesion. *Stroke* 1988;19:122.
146. Hommel M, Gaio JM, Pollak P, Borgel F, Perret J. Hémiparésie ataxique par lacune thalamique. *Rev Neurol* 1987;143:602–604.
147. Boiten J, Lodder J. Ataxic hemiparesis following thalamic infarction. *Stroke* 1990;21:339–340.
148. Bogousslavsky J, Regli F, Ghika J, Feldmeyer JJ. Painful ataxic hemiparesis. *Arch Neurol* 1984;41:892–893.
149. Lee N, Roh JK, Myung H. Hypesthetic ataxic hemiparesis in a thalamic lacune. *Stroke* 1989;20:819–821.
150. Bogousslavsky J, Regli F, Assal G. The syndrome of unilateral tuberothalamic artery territory infarction. *Stroke* 1986;17:434–441.
151. Graff-Radford NR, Eslinger PJ, Damasio AR, Yamada T. Non-hemorrhagic infarction of the thalamus: behavioral, anatomic, and physiologic correlates. *Neurology* 1984;34:14–23.
152. Biller J, Merchut M, Emanuele MA. Nonhemorrhagic infarction of the thalamus. *Neurology* 1984;34:1269–1270.
153. Austin CP, Lessel S. Horner's syndrome from hypothalamic infarction. *Arch Neurol* 1991;48:332–334.
154. Castaigne P, Lhermitte F, Buge A, Escourolle R, Hauw JJ, Lyon-Caen O. Paramedian thalamic and midbrain infarcts: clinical and neuropathological study. *Ann Neurol* 1981;10:127–148.
155. Friedman JH. Syndrome of diffuse encephalopathy due to nondominant thalamic infarction. *Neurology* 1985;35:1524–1526.
156. Watson RT, Valenstein E, Heilman KM. Thalamic neglect. Possible role of the medial thalamus and nucleus reticularis in behavior. *Arch Neurol* 1981;38:501–506.
157. Davous P, Bianco C, Duval-lota AM, de Recondo J, Vedrenne C, Rondot P. Aphasie par infarctus thalamique paramédian gauche. Observation anatomo-clinique. *Rev Neurol* 1984;140:711–719.
158. Louarn F, Gray F, Degos JD, Meyrignac C, Poirier J. Syndrome de l'hémisphère mineur par infarctus thalamique droit: un cas anatomoclinique. *Rev Neurol* 1986;142:777–782.
159. Laplane D, Escourolle R, Degos JD, Sauron B, Massiou H. La négligence motrice d'origine thalamique. A propos de 2 cas. *Rev Neurol* 1982;138:201–211.
160. Elghozi D, Strube E, Signoret JL, Cambier J, Lhermitte F. Quasi-aphasie lors de lésions du thalamus. Relation du trouble du langage et de l'activation élective de l'hémisphère gauche dans 4 observations de lésions thalamiques

droites et gauches. *Rev Neurol* 1978;134:557–574.
161. Cambier J, Graveleau P. Volume I (45): clinical neuropsychology. Thalamic syndromes. In: Fredericks JMA, ed. *Clinical neurology*. Amsterdam: Elsevier; 1985:87–98.
162. Castaigne P, Buge A, Cambier J, Escourolle R, Brunet P, Degos JD. Démence thalamique d'origine vasculaire par ramollissement bilatéral, limité au territoire du pédicule rétro-mamillaire. A propos de deux observations anatomocliniques. *Rev Neurol* 1966;114:89–107.
163. Guberman A, Stuss D. The syndrome of bilateral paramedian thalamic infarction. *Neurology* 1983;33:540–546.
164. Feldmeyer JJ, Bogousslavsky J, Regli F. Asterixis uni- ou bilateral en cas de lésion thalamique ou pariétale: un trouble moteur afférentiel? *Schweiz Med Wochenschr* 1984;114:167–171.
165. Obeso JA, Martinez-Vila E, Delgado G, Vaamonda J, Maravi E, Martinez-Lage JM. Delayed onset dystonia following hemiplegic migraine. *Headache* 1984;24:266–268.
166. Sunohara N, Mukoyama M, Mano Y, Satoyoshi E. Action-induced rhythmic dystonia: an autopsy case. *Neurology* 1984;34:321–327.
167. Combarros O, Gutirrez A, Pascual J, Berciano J. Oral dyskinesias associated with bilateral thalamo-capsular infarction. *J Neurol Neurosurg Psychiatry* 1990;53:168–169.
168. Dubois B, Pillon F, De Saxe H, Lhermitte F, Agid Y. Disappearance of parkinsonian signs after spontaneous "thalamotomy." *Arch Neurol* 1986;43:815–817.
169. Ho KL. Pure motor hemiplegia due to infarction of the cerebral peduncle. *Arch Neurol* 1982;39:524–526.
170. Fisher M, Smith TW, Jacobs R. Pure motor hemiplegia secondary to a saccular basilar artery aneurysm. *Stroke* 1988;19:104–107.
171. Gaymard B, Saudeau D, de Toffol B, Larmande P, Autret A. Two mesencephalic lacunar infarcts presenting as Claude's syndrome and pure motor hemiparesis. *Eur Neurol* 1991;31:152–155.
172. Bogousslavsky J, Miklossy J, Deruaz JP, Regli F, Assal G. Unilateral left paramedian infarction of thalamus and midbrain: a clinico-pathological study. *J Neurol Neurosurg Psychiatry* 1986;49:686–694.
173. Guberman A, Stuss D. The syndrome of bilateral paramedian thalamic infarction. *Neurology* 1983;33:540–546.
174. Lhermitte J. Syndrome de la calotte du pédoncule cérébral. Les troubles psycho-sensoriels dans les lésions du mésocéphale. *Rev Neurol* 1922;38:1359–1365.
175. Van Bogaert L. Syndrome inférieur du noyau rouge, troubles psycho-sensoriels d'origine mésocéphalique. *Rev Neurol* 1924;40:417–423.
176. McKee AC, Levine DN, Kowall NW, Richardson EP. Peduncular hallucinosis associated with isolated infarction of the substantia nigra pars reticulata. *Ann Neurol* 1990;27:500–504
177. Geller TJ, Bellur SN. Peduncular hallucinosis: magnetic resonance imaging confirmation of mesencephalic infarction during life. *Ann Neurol* 1987;21:602–604.
178. Feinberg WM, Rapcsak SZ. "Peduncular hallucinosis" following paramedian thalamic infarction. *Neurology* 1989;39:1535–1536.
179. Caplan LR. "Top of the basilar" syndrome. *Neurology* 1980;30:72–79.
180. Degos JD, Verroust J, Bouchareine A, Serdaru M, Barbizet J. Asterixis in focal brain lesions. *Arch Neurol* 1979;36:705–707.
181. Bril V, Sharpe JA, Ashby P. Midbrain asterixis. *Ann Neurol* 1979;6:362–364.
182. Jankovic J, Patel SC. Blepharospasm associated with brainstem lesions. *Neurology* 1983;33:1237–1240.
183. Segal R, Sroka H, Sandbank U, Kott E. Hemiballismus with lesion of the subthalamic nucleus and neuroaxonal degeneration of the homolateral substantia nigra. *Ann Neurol* 1977;2:169–172.
184. Salama J, Gray F, Kanaan HY, Delaporte P. Le syndrome du corps de Luys. In: *Encycl Méd Chir*. Paris: Neurologie 17037 G10, 6–1988.
185. Biller J, Graff-Radford NR, Smoker WKR, Adams HP, Johnston P. MR imaging in "lacunar" hemiballismus. *J Comput Assist Tomogr* 1986;10:793–797.
186. Château R, Tommasi M, Groslambert R, Pasqier B, Perret J. Une observation de diballisme. Étude clinique et anatomo-pathologique. *Rev Neurol* 1973;129:257–274.
187. Schuster P. Zur Pathologie der vertikalen Blicklähmung. *Dtsch Z Nervenkrank* 1921;70:97–115.
188. Angelergues R, De Ajuriaguerra J, Hécaen H. Paralysie de la verticalité du regard d'origine vasculaire. Étude anatomo-clinique. *Rev Neurol* 1957;96:301–319.
189. Castaigne P, Buge A, Cambier J, Escourolle R, Brunet P, Degos JD. Démence thalamique d'origine vasculaire par ramollissement bilatéral, limité au territoire du pédicule rétro-mamillaire. A propos de deux observations anatomocliniques. *Rev Neurol* 1966;114:89–107.
190. Segarra JM. Cerebral vascular disease and behaviour. I. The syndrome of the mesencephalic artery (basilar artery bifurcation). *Arch Neurol* 1970;22:408–418.
191. Christoff N. A clinicopathologic study of vertical eye movements. *Arch Neurol* 1974;31:1–8.
192. Reagan TJ, Trautman JC. Combined nuclear and supranuclear defects in ocular motility. A clinicopathologic study. *Arch Neurol* 1978;35:133–137.
193. Pierrot-Deseilligny C, Chain F, Gray F, Serdaru M, Escourolle R, Lhermitte F. Parinaud syndrome. Electro-oculographic and anatomical analyses of six vascular cases with deductions about vertical gaze organization in the premotor structures. *Brain* 1982;105:667–696.
194. Büttner-Ennever JA, Büttner U, Cohen B, Baumgartner G. Vertical gaze paralysis and the rostral interstitial nucleus of the longitudinal fasciculus. *Brain* 1982;1105:125–149.

195. Lepore FE, Gulli V, Miller DC. Neuro-ophthalmological findings with neuropathological correlation in bilateral thalamic-mesencephalic infarction. *J Clin Neuro Ophthalmol* 1985;5:224–228.
196. Lapresle J, Said G. Déviation forcée des yeux vers le bas et en dedans et mouvements oculaires périodiques au cours d'une hémorragie anvérysmale de la calotte mésencéphalique. *Rev Neurol* 1977;133:497–503.
197. Petit H, Rousseaux M, Clarisse J, Delafosse A. Troubles oculo-céphalomoteurs et infarctus thalamo-sous-thalamique bilatéral. *Rev Neurol* 1981;137:709–722.
198. Wall M, Slamowits TL, Weisberg LA, Trufant SA. Vertical gaze ophthalmoplegia from infarction in the area of the posterior thalamo-subthalamic paramedian artery. *Stroke* 1986;17:546–555.
199. Swanson RA, Schmidley JW. Amnestic syndrome and vertical gaze palsy: early detection of bilateral thalamic infarction by CT and NMR. *Stroke* 1985;16:823–827.
200. Dereux J. *Paralysie verticale du regard* [Medical Thesis]. Paris: Arnette, 1926.
201. Garcin R, Bertrand I, Frumusan P. Étude anatomo-clinique d'un cas de syndrome de Parinaud et de myoclonies rythmiques du voile du palais. *Rev Neurol* 1933;40:812–820.
202. Molnàr L. Die lokaldiagnostische Bedeutung der vertikalen Blicklähmung. *Arch Psychiatr Nervenkrank Z Neurol* 1959;198:523–534.
203. Leigh RJ, Zee DS. *The neurology of eye movements*. Philadelphia: FA Davis; 1983.
204. Ranalli PJ, Sharpe JA, Fletcher WA. Palsy of upward and downward saccadic, pursuit, and vestibular movements with a midbrain lesion: pathologic correlations. *Neurology* 1988;38:114–122.
205. Bogousslavsky J, Miklossy J, Regli F, Janzer R. Vertical gaze palsy and selective unilateral infarction of the rostral interstitial nucleus of the medial longitudinal fasciculus (riMLF). *J Neurol Neurosurg Psychiatry* 1990;53:67–71.
206. Hommel M, Bogousslavsky J. The spectrum of vertical gaze palsy following unilateral brainstem stroke. *Neurology* 1991;41:1229–1234.
207. Christoff N, Anderson PJ, Bender MB. A clinicopathologic study of associated vertical eye movements. *Trans Am Neurol Assoc* 1962;87:184–186.
208. Csornai M. Über Störungen der vertikalen Blickwegungen und des Bewusstseins bei Herden des mesodiencephalenübergangsgebietes. *Arch Psychiat Nervenkr* 1974;219:79–88.
209. Freund CS. Zur Klinik und Anatomie der vertikalen Blicklähmungen. *Neurologishes Centralblatt* 1913;32:1215–1229.
210. Balthazar K, Hopf A. Die Freund-Vogtsche Herdbildung bei supranuclearer Heberlähmung der Augen mit Lidretraktion. Zur Würdigung eines Falles von C Freund und C.u.O. Vogt. *Dtsch Z Nervenheilk* 1966;189:275–296.
211. Hatcher MA, Klintworth GK. The sylvian aqueduct syndrome. *Arch Neurol* 1966;15:215–222.
212. Serdaru M, Gray F, Lyon-Caen O, Escourolle R, Lhermitte F. Syndrome de Parinaud et déviation tonique verticale du regard. *Rev Neurol* 1982;138:601–617.
213. Smith MS. Upward gaze paralysis following unilateral pretectal infarction. *Arch Neurol* 1981;38:127–129.
214. Rousseaux M, Petit, Hache JC, Devos P, Dubois F, Warot P. La motricité oculaire et céphalique dans les infarctus de la région thalamique. *Rev Neurol* 1985;141:391–403.
215. Muskens LJJ. La base anatomique des positions forcées des yeux. Soit-disant paralysie du regard. *Rev Neurol* 1933;40:287–296.
216. André-Thomas, Schaeffer H, Bertrand I. Paralysie de l'abaissement du regard, paralysie des inférogyres, hypertonie des supérogyres et des releveurs des paupières. *Rev Neurol* 1933;40:535–542.
217. Jacobs L, Anderson P, Bender M. The lesion producing paralysis of downgaze but not upward gaze. *Arch Neurol* 1973;28:319–323.
218. Cogan DC. Paralysis of down-gaze. *Arch Ophthalmol* 1974;91:192–199.
219. Halmagyi MG, Evans AE, Halliman JM. Failure of downgaze. The site and nature of the lesion. *Arch Neurol* 1978;35:22–26.
220. Trojanovski JQ, Wray SH. Vertical gaze ophthalmoplegia: selective paralysis of downgaze. *Neurology* 1980;30:605–610.
221. Trojanovski JQ, Lafontaine MH. Neuroanatomical correlates of selective downgaze paralysis. *J Neurol Sci* 1981;52:91–101.
222. Jacobs L, Heffner RR, Newman RP. Selective paralysis of downward gaze caused by bilateral lesions of the mesencephalic periaqueductal gray matter. *Neurology* 1985;35:516–521.
223. Larmande P, Larmande A, Jan M, Gouae A. Un nouveau cas de paralysie sélective de l'abaissement des yeux avec déviation conjugué permanente vers le haut. *Rev Neurol* 1981;137:625–633.
224. Goldman S, Cordonnier MJB, Sztencel J. Brainstem ischaemia presenting as a naloxone-reversible coma followed by downward gaze paralysis. *J Neurol Neurosurg Psychiatry* 1984;47:77–78.
225. Vighetto A, Confavreux C, Boisson D, Aimard G, Devic M. Paralysie de l'abaissement du regard et amnésie globale durables par lésion thalamo-sous-thalamique bilatérale. *Rev Neurol* 1986;142:449–455.
226. Ford CS, Schwartze GM, Weaver RG, Troost BT. Monocular elevation paresis caused by an ipsilateral lesion. *Neurology* 1984;34:1264–1267.
227. Bogousslavsky J, Regli F, Ghika J, Hungerbühler JP. Internuclear ophthalmoplegia, prenuclear paresis of contralateral superior rectus, and bilateral ptosis. *J Neurol* 1983;230:197–203.
228. Bogousslavsky J, Regli F. Upgaze palsy and monocular paresis of downward gaze from ip-

silateral thalamo-mesencephalic infarction: a vertical "one-and-a-half" syndrome. *J Neurol* 1984;231:43–45.
229. Deleu D, Buisseret T, Ebinger G. Vertical one-and-a-half syndrome. Supranuclear downgaze paralysis with monocular elevation palsy. *Arch Neurol* 1989;46:1361–1363.
230. Miyashita K, Sawada T, Satomi M. Upgaze palsy and monocular paresis of downgaze caused by ipsilateral thalamomesencephalic hemorrhage: a so-called "one-and-a-half" syndrome. *Clin Neurol (Tokyo)* 1987;27:1407–1411.
231. Mehler MF. The neuro-ophthalmologic spectrum of the rostral basilar artery syndrome. *Arch Neurol* 1988;45:966–971.
232. Pierrot-Deseilligny C, Schaison M, Bousser MG, Brunet P. Syndrome nucléaire du nerf moteur oculaire commun: à propos de deux observations cliniques. *Rev Neurol* 1981;137:217–222.
233. Achard C, Levi L. Paralysie totale et isolée du moteur oculaire commun par foyer de ramollissement pédonculaire. *Rev Neurol* 1901;12:646–648.
234. Collard M, Saint-Val C, Mohr M, Kiesmann M. Paralysie isolée du nerf moteur oculaire commun par infarctus de ses fibres fasciculaires. *Rev Neurol* 1990;146:128–132.
235. Bogousslavsky J, Regli F. Atteinte intra-axiale du nerf moteur oculaire commun dans les infarctus mésencéphaliques. *Rev Neurol* 1984;140:263–270.
236. Breen LA, Hopf HC, Farris BK, Gutman L. Pupil-sparing oculomotor nerve palsy due to midbrain infarction. *Arch Neurol* 1990;48:105–106.
237. Nadeau SE, Trobe JD. Pupil sparing in oculomotor palsy: a brief review. *Ann Neurol* 1983;13:143–148.
238. Claude H. Syndrome pédonculaire de la région du noyau rouge. *Rev Neurol* 1912;4:311–313.
239. Claude H, Loyez. Ramollissement du noyau rouge. *Rev Neurol* 1912;13:49–51.
240. Van Bogaert L. Syndrome inférieur du noyau rouge, troubles psycho-sensoriels d'origine mésocéphalique. *Rev Neurol* 1924;417–423.
241. Kistler JP, Buonanno FS, De Witt LD, Davis KR, Brady TJ, Fisher CM. Vertebral basilar posterior cerebral territory stroke delineation by proton nuclear magnetic resonance. *Stroke* 1984;15:417–426.
242. Iwatsubo T, Iwata M, Inoue K, Mannen T. Imagerie par résonance magnétique dans un cas d'infarctus mésencéphalique paramédian. *Rev Neurol* 1987;143:605–607.
243. Sanguineti I, Tagliabue M, Boglium G, Cavaletti G, Crespi V, Delodovici ML. Correspondance. *Rev Neurol* 1988;144:840–841.
244. Benedikt M. Tremblement avec paralysie croisé du moteur oculaire commun. *Bull Med* 1889;3:547–548.
245. Souques, Crouzon, Bertrand I. Révision du syndrome de Benedikt à propos de l'autopsie d'un cas de ce syndrome trémoro-choro-athétoide et hypertonique du syndrome du noyau rouge. Mémoire original. *Rev Neurol* 1930;11:378–417.
246. Chiray M, Foix C, Nicolesco J. Hémitremblement du type de la sclérose en plaques par lésion rubro-thalamo-sous thalamique. Syndrome de la région supro-externe du noyau rouge avec atteinte silencieusee ou non du thalamus. *Ann Med* 1923;14:173–191.
247. Mayor. Paralysie alterne portant sur le moteur oculaire commun. *Bull Soc Anat* 1877;16:239–240.
248. Marrotte. Observation de ramollissement du pédoncule cérébral gauche, avec lésion du nerf moteur oculaire commun. *Union Med* 1853:407–408.
249. Devic A, Paufique, Girard P, Guinet P. Observations anatomocliniques d'un syndrome de Parinaud (paralysie volontaire et réflexe). Considérations sur le rôle de la région commissurale. *Rev Neurol* 1945;77:37–39.
250. Kobayashi S, Mukuno K, Tazaki Y, Ishikawa S, Okada K. Oculomotor nerve complex syndrome. A case with clinico-pathological correlation. *Neuro-Ophthalmology* 1986;6:55–59.
251. Sieben G, De Reuk J, Vander Eecken H. Thrombosis of the mesencephalic artery. A clinico-pathological study of two cases and its correlation to the arterial vascularisation. *Acta Neurol Belg* 1977;77:151–162.
252. Halmagyi GM, Brandt T, Dietrich M, Curthoys LS, Stark RJ, Hoyt WF. Tonic contraversive ocular tilt reaction due to unilateral meso-diencephalic lesion. *Neurology* 1990;40:1503–1509.
253. Selhorst JB, Hoyt WF, Feinsod M, Hosobuchi Y. Midbrain corectopia. *Arch Neurol* 1976;33:193–195.
254. Biller J, Shapiro R, Evans LS, Haag JR, Fine M. Oculomotor nuclear complex infarction. Clinical and radiological correlation. *Arch Neurol* 1984;41:985–987.
255. Growdon JH, Winkler GF, Wray SH. Midbrain ptosis. A case with clinicopathologic correlation. *Arch Neurol* 1974;30:179–181.
256. Chia LG. Locked-in syndrome with bilateral ventral midbrain infarcts. *Neurology* 1991;41:445–446.
257. Fisher CM, Curry B. Pure motor hemiplegia of vascular origin. *Arch Neurol* 1965;13:30–44.
258. Rafalowska J, Rowinska-Marcinska K. On pure motor hemiplegia (Fisher's syndrome). *Pol Med Sci History Bull* 1975;15:3–8.
259. Besson G, Hommel M, Clavier I, Perret J. Failure of magnetic resonance imaging in the detection of pontine lacune. *Stroke* 1992:1535.
260. Huang CY, Woo E, Yu YL, Chan FL. Lacunar syndromes due to brainstem infarct and haemorrhage. *J Neurol Neurosurg Psychiatry* 1988;51:509–515.
261. Johns DR, Tierney M, Parker SW. Pure motor hemiplegia due to meningovascular neurosyphilis. *Arch Neurol* 1987;44:1062–1065.
262. Paolucci S, Prencipe M, Scalabroni A. "Pure motor hemiparesis (P.M.H.)": a proposito di

due casi di emiparesi F.B.C. con rilievo tomodensitometrico di infarto pontino. *Riv Neurol* 1981;51:157–163.
263. Stiller J, Shanzer S, Yang W. Brainstem lesions with pure motor hemiparesis. Computed tomographic demonstration. *Arch Neurol* 1982; 39:660–661.
264. Biller J, Adams HP, Dunn V, Simmons Z, Jacoby CG. Dichotomy between clinical findings and MR abnormalities in pontine infarction. *J Comput Assist Tomogr* 1986;10:379–385.
265. Hopf HC, Tettenborn B, Kramer G. Pontine supranuclear facial palsy. *Stroke* 1990;21:1754–1757.
266. Fisher CM. Ataxic hemiparesis a pathologic study. *Arch Neurol* 1978;35:126–128.
267. Delgado G, Gallego J, Zubieta JL. High resolution CT-scan in pontine ataxic hemiparesis. *J Neurol Neurosurg Psychiatry* 1985;48:1069.
268. Huang CY, Chan KH. Pontine ataxic hemiparesis, a lateral penetrator syndrome. *J Neurol Neurosurg Psychiatry* 1984;47:1046–1047.
269. Koppel BS, Weinberger G. Pontine infarction producing dysarthria–clumsy hand syndrome and ataxic hemiparesis. *Eur Neurol* 1987;26: 211–215.
270. Van Buggenhout E, Dehaene I, Van Zandijcke M. Pontine ataxic hemiparesis. *Arch Neurol* 1984;41:16.
271. Bogousslavsky J, Fox AJ, Barnett HJM, Hachinski VC, Vinitski S, Carey LS. Clinico-topographic correlation of small vertebrobasilar infarct using magnetic resonance imaging. *Stroke* 1986;17:929–938.
272. Nabatame H, Fukuyama H, Akigushi I, Kameyama M, Nishimura K, Torizuka K. Pontine ataxic hemiparesis studied by high resolution magnetic resonance imaging system. *Ann Neurol* 1987;21:204–207.
273. Perret J, Hommel M, Pollak P, Gaio JM, Lebas JF, Crouzet G. Clinical and radiological correlations in ischemic brainstem infarcts: a magnetic resonance imaging study. In: Gouaze A, Salamon G, eds. *Brain anatomy and magnetic resonance imaging.* Paris: Springer 1988:169–177.
274. Sakai T, Murakami S, Ito K. Ataxic hemiparesis with trigeminal weakness. *Neurology* 1981; 31:635–636.
275. Van Gijn J, Vermeulen M. Ataxic tetraparesis from lacunar infarction in the pons. *J Neurol Neurosurg Psychiatry* 1983;46:669–670.
276. Fisher CM. A lacunar stroke. The dysarthria–clumsy hand syndrome. *Neurology* 1967;17: 614–617.
277. Glass JD, Levey AI, Rothstein JD. The dysarthria–clumsy hand syndrome: a distinct clinical entity related to pontine infarction. *Ann Neurol* 1990;27:487–494.
278. Landry M. *Bull Soc Anat Paris* 1858;33:406–410.
279. Hommel M, Besson G, Tarel V, et al. L'imagerie par résonance magnétique dans les paralysies de l'oculomotricité horizontale par infarctus. *Rev Neurol* 1988;144:18–24.
280. Bogousslavsky J, Regli F. Exotropie pontique paralytique et non paralytique. *Rev Neurol* 1983;139:219–223.
281. De Witt LD, Wray S, Kistler JP, Davis KR, Brady TJ, Buonanno F. Nuclear magnetic resonance in neuro-ophthalmologic syndromes. *Neurology* 1984;34:96–97.
282. Wall M, Wray SH. The one-and-a-half syndrome—a unilateral disorder of the pontine tegmentum: a study of 20 cases and review of the literature. *Neurology* 1983;33:971–980.
283. Pierrot-Deseilligny C, Chain F, Gray F, Escourolle R, Castaigne P. Paralysies supranucléaires de la latéralité d'origine protubérantielle. *Rev Neurol* 1979;135:741–762.
284. Cogan DG, Kubik CS, Smith WL. Unilateral internuclear ophthalmoplegia. *Arch Ophthalmol* 1950;44:783–796.
285. Jenkyn LR, Margolis G, Reeves AG. Reflex vertical gaze and the medial longitudial fasciculus. *J Neurol Neurosurg Psychiatry* 1978; 41:1084–1091.
286. Donaldson D, Rosenberg NL. Infarction of abducens nerve fascicle as a cause of isolated sixth nerve palsy related to hypertension. *Neurology* 1988;38:1654.
287. Fisher CM. Lacunar infarct of the tegmentum of the lower lateral pons. *Arch Neurol* 1989; 46:566–567.
288. Vermersch P, Petit H, Marion MH, Montagne B. Hemifacial spasm due to pontine infarction. *J Neurol Neurosurg Psychiatry* 1991;54:1018.
289. Ho KL, Meyer KR. The medial medullary syndrome. *Arch Neurol* 1981;38:385–387.
290. Chokroverty S, Rubino FA. "Pure" motor hemiplegia. *J Neurol Neurosurg Psychiatry* 1975;38:896–899.
291. Leestma JE, Noronha A. Pure motor hemiplegia, medullary pyramid lesion, and olivary hypertrophy. *J Neurol Neurosurg Psychiatry* 1979;36:877–884.
292. Ropper AH, Fisher CM, Kleinmann GM. Pyramidal infarction in the medulla: a cause of pure motor hemiplegia sparing the face. *Neurology* 1979;29:91–95.
293. Jagiella WM, Sung JH. Bilateral infarction of the medullary pyramids in humans. *Neurology* 1989;39:21–24.
294. Trelles JO, Trelles L, Urquiaca C. Le ramollissement médian du bulbe. A propos de 2 cas anatomo-cliniques. *Rev Neurol* 1973;129:91–104.

9

Clinical Features of Multiple Lacunar and Small Deep Infarcts

Marc Hommel and Gérard Besson

Department of Clinical and Biological Neurosciences, Stroke Unit, Centre Hospitalier Universitaire Régional de Grenoble, 38043 Grenoble, France

Multiple small deep infarcts and lacunar infarcts may occur despite careful risk factor management. The individual effects of small lesions summate and may give rise to different clinical manifestations including *état lacunaire*, pseudobulbar palsy, and even dementia. These cognitive features, which are unusual in individual lacunar strokes, may be explained by a deactivation of the cortex due to the interruption of neuronal connections by multiple subcortical lesions. This is supported by flow and metabolic studies.

ÉTAT LACUNAIRE

The term *état lacunaire* was coined by Pierre Marie in 1901 to describe the anatomopathological findings in some of the brains he studied (1). The terms lacunar state and status lacunaris were also used. A clinical syndrome of progressive neurologic decline often occurring with a stepwise course, and produced by multiple recurrent strokes (usually hemiplegia with incomplete recovery), was later ascribed to *état lacunaire*. This syndrome includes a short-step gait called *marche à petits pas*, unilateral or bilateral Babinski signs, dysarthria but not aphasia, incontinence, pseudobulbar palsy, and some degree of dementia. The *marche à petits pas* was described by Pierre Marie as a slow and short (no more than 15 cm) gait. The knees were bent, and the trunk was flexed, looking rather like a man groping in the darkness (2). It should be stressed that the lacunar clinical state as described above is rare.

The pseudobulbar palsy syndrome is often associated with *état lacunaire* and consists of lower cranial nerve palsies caused by bilateral supranuclear lesions of the corticobulbar and corticopontine pathways. This clinical term was coined by Lépine in 1877 (3) in order to differentiate these palsies from bulbar palsy related to lesions of the bulbar nuclei. Pseudobulbar palsy may develop gradually or acutely (4, 5). Supranuclear bulbar palsy consists of a facio-pharyngo-glosso-masticatory diplegia that may be complete or partial (4). There is no muscular atrophy or fasciculations as in bulbar paralysis. An automatic-voluntary dissociation is present and may be marked during episodes of forced laughing and crying. Neurologic examination shows facial diplegia. The mouth remains open and saliva may dribble. Eye closure may be weak, but the corneal reflexes are present. The masticatory muscles are weak bilaterally. The jaw jerk is brisk, the palate has decreased mobility and sags, and the gag reflex may be absent or hyperactive. The patient is unable to chew or swallow well. Tongue protrusion is very weak and bilateral weakness of sternomastoid and trapezius muscles may be present.

In the early phase of an acute pseudobulbar palsy, the patient is mute (5, 6). Late speech returns but is quite dysphonic and dsyarthric. Lévy studied speech in pseudobulbar palsy and pointed out that there is an abnormality of both rhythm and timbre of speech. Speech is monotonous, explosive, and rapid, with short words (7). The dysarthria is characterized by a difficulty in pronouncing labial and labiodental sounds, and initial vowels are usually preceded by an aspirate (7). Severe dysarthria may progress to anarthria. Palilalia is also seen. This is a speech disturbance characterized by the repetition of single words, or a phrase with increasing rapidity and with a progressive decrease in the length of the phrase (7).

Three clinical subtypes of pseudobulbar palsy were identified by Thurel (8):

1. The cortico-subcortical form consists of a facio-pharyngo-glosso-masticatory diplegia with automatic-voluntary dissociation but unaccompanied by forced laughing and crying (9) or dementia (10). Trismus has rarely been noted in this form (11). The cortico-subcortical form, which is also known as the anterior opercular syndrome or Foix-Chavany-Marie syndrome, is usually caused by bilateral large artery infarcts of the opercular cortex (12,13).

2. The striate form consists of a facio-pharyngo-glosso-masticatory diplegia with automatic-voluntary dissociation associated with extrapyramidal rigidity, forced laughing and crying, and cognitive impairment. This form is usually due to bilateral lacunar infarcts (14).

3. The pontine form is characterized by facio-pharyngo-glosso-masticatory diplegia associated with automatic-voluntary dissociation, with forced laughing and crying, and pyramidal and sometimes cerebellar signs, but without dementia. This form was first described by Lhermitte and Cuel in 1921. It has also been reported secondary to pontine lacunar infarcts in an autopsy study by Raymond and Arthaud (15, 16), but there are very few autopsy confirmations of lacunar infarcts causing this form of pseudobulbar palsy (15, 17, 18).

Nowadays, the lacunar state is encountered infrequently in clinical practice (19, 20). Antihypertensive therapy has altered the natural history of lacunar infarcts and has decreased the incidence of the lacunar state. Fisher has suggested that some of Marie's patients may have suffered from symptomatic normal-pressure hydrocephalus rather than the lacunar state (19), and that normal-pressure hydrocephalus might predispose to lacunar infarction by its compressive effects (19). The association of lacunar infarcts and normal-pressure hydrocephalus has been described (21–24) (see Chapter 11).

LACUNAR DEMENTIA

In 1901, Pierre Marie reported that the lacunar state could be associated with an impairment of cognitive functions, but he did not report severe dementia (1). In 1965, Fisher stated that in lacunar infarcts "dementia if present at all, was mild" (25). In 1982, Fisher included dementia caused by a thalamic lacunar infarct as one of the lacunar syndromes (19). Dementia in patients with lacunar or small deep infarcts can thus be caused by (a) multiple lacunar infarcts scattered in the brain and sometimes associated with white matter disease, or (b) by a strategically located lacunar infarct, particularly in the thalamus.

Multiple Lacunar Infarcts in the Lacunar State or in Binswanger's Encephalopathy

The introduction of efficient antihypertensive medications has prevented the development of the lacunar state in many patients. The prevalence of the lacunar state appears to have decreased in comparison with the early literature (19). For this reason, it is difficult to collect large series of patients with the lacunar state. The presence of dementia in the lacunar state is still disputed. Hughes et al. reported that dementia could be present, but might not occur even in severe cases (26). Fisher later criticized the concept of dementia in the lacunar state, suggesting that at least some of Pierre Marie's patients could have had normal-pressure hydrocephalus (19, 21, 22). In these cases, the cognitive dysfunctions attributed by Pierre Marie and others to the lacunar state could have been related to the hydrocephalus. Such cases have been reported and have even been found to respond to shunting (21,22).

There is probably a link between the lacunar state and Binswanger's encephalopathy. Lacunar or small deep infarcts are often found in Binswanger's encephalopathy, and dementia is one of the clinical features (see Chapter 11). Hypertension is the main vascular risk factor both for Binswanger's disease and for the lacunar state, and lacunar infarcts are present in both conditions. Ishii et al. (27) reported the autopsy findings in patients with vascular dementia and the lacunar state. Clinical features in these patients included grasp reflexes and incontinence, and in the terminal stages they became bedridden with flexion contractures. The cognitive and behavioral symptoms consisted of acute, often nocturnal, confusion; mood lability with outbursts of rage; laughing or crying; and depression. All showed lack of initiative or spontaneity, or profound slowing of psychomotor activity. Preservation of personality was sometimes observed. At autopsy, there were lacunar infarcts and incomplete infarctions or softenings, predominating in the periventricular white matter around the anterior horn of the lateral ventricle, the head of the caudate nucleus, and the putamen. The authors attributed the predominantly frontal symptoms to the frontal topography of many of the lesions. They suggested that the white matter infarcts were probably important in the genesis of the dementia. The study of Fukuda et al. supported this hypothesis. They reported a correlation between the severity of mental deterioration and the severity of white matter abnormal signals with magnetic resonance imaging in patients with dementia related to lacunar infarctions (28). Wolfe et al. reported neuropsychological signs of frontal dysfunction in a study of cognitive impairment in patients with multiple lacunar infarcts. These patients had deficits in shifting mental set, response inhibition, and executive function. They were also more apathetic than normal controls (29). Part of the disagreement about the existence of lacunar dementia probably centers on the criteria used for the diagnosis of dementia: Most patients with multiple lacunar infarcts have impairments, but only about 30% of these patients meet strict clinical criteria for the diagnosis of dementia (30).

Strategically Located Lacunar or Small Deep Infarcts Causing Cognitive Impairment or Dementia

Mendez et al. reported a patient who had acute confusion and subsequent residual dementia due to bilateral caudate infarcts (31). Caudate infarcts are often characterized by the sudden onset of minor and often transient motor deficit. Confusion and behavioral changes often lead to the patient being referred to general medical or to psychiatric institutions. The cognitive abnormalities are characterized by apathy with decreased spontaneous verbal and motor activities and a lack of initiative. The attention span is limited. There is an impairment in problem-solving ability, and in immediate and delayed recall memory. Recognition memory is, however, preserved (see Chapter 8).

Unilateral infarcts of the anterior thalamus (tuberothalamic artery territory infarction) can produce a dementia-like clinical picture (32) (see Chapter 8). Neuropsychological features predominate and are characterized by apathy, a fluctuating level of attention, perseverations and disorientation, personality changes, euphoria, and lack of insight. In left-sided infarcts, transcortical aphasia may be seen with reduction of spontaneous speech, naming impairment, reduced fluency, paraphasias, and moderate impairments in comprehension, but preservation of repetition. In addition there are verbal and visual memory impairments, acalculia, and a reduction of vocal volume. In some cases the changes are compatible with dementia (32).

Unilateral or bilateral paramedian thalamic infarcts (occlusion of the paramedian thalamic and mesencephalic arteries) can cause a thalamic dementia. Four of 28 autopsy-proven cases reported by Castaigne et al. (33) had unilateral small deep infarcts. Clinically, mood and behavioral changes were prominent in these patients. In addition, the patients were disoriented, and agitation and aggression alternated with apathy and prostration. Five patients with bilateral paramedian thalamic small deep infarcts presented with disturbances of consciousness, including deep coma or hypersomnia, and had disturbances of behavior, apathy, akinetic mutism, dysphoria, and amnesia. These features were associated with a vertical gaze palsy. Three paramedian thalamic small deep infarcts reported by Graff-Radford et al. (34) had similar clinical features. Friedman reported a patient with a thalamic infarct who presented with a diffuse encephalopathy (35). Bilateral thalamic infarcts may lead to a dementia syndrome characterized by a loss of initiative, perseverations, and severe attention and memory deficits (36–39).

CEREBRAL BLOOD FLOW IN MULTIPLE SUBCORTICAL INFARCT STATE

Cerebral blood flow and cerebral metabolism are normally closely coupled, but this is not true in patients with acute diseases such as stroke. Some reports suggest that small deep lesions located in the white matter or deep nuclei (thalamus, basal ganglia) can interrupt the connections between these deep structures and the cerebral or cerebellar cortex, causing a remote metabolic deactivation and a reduction in blood flow in the related cortex (40–42). Clinical neuropsychological disturbances associated with small deep infarcts could be the consequences of this metabolic deactivation (40,43). Rougemont et al. did not, however, find abnormal blood flow and metabolism in patients with pure motor hemiplegia (44). Perani et al. reported a crossed cerebellar diaschisis in patients with ataxic hemiparesis (45). Metter et al. (42) reported the autopsy findings of a patient with multiple small deep and lacunar infarcts studied with computed tomography (CT) and positron emission tomography (PET). PET showed a global decrease in cortical metabolism as compared to normal controls, and there was a focal area of reduced metabolism in the frontal lobes, whose area was larger than that of the infarcts. At autopsy a lacunar infarct was found in the genu of the internal capsule, interrupting connections with the frontal lobes. In addition, microinfarcts that had not been seen on CT were found in the thalamus at autopsy. However, PET had demonstrated a reduced metabolic rate in this structure. The metabolic findings in this patient are typical of those reported both in patients with Binswanger's encephalopathy and in patients with multiple deep infarcts and dementia. There is usually a global reduction in flow and metabolism, associated with an even more pronounced focal decrease in flow and metabolism in the deep nuclei and white matter, as well as in the connected areas of the cortex (46–49). The focal areas of decreased metabolism observed in vascular dementia may help to differentiate vascular dementia patients from degenerative dementia patients who also have a global reduction of flow and metabolism (50).

CONCLUSION

An isolated lacunar infarct is usually asymptomatic or causes only slight residual disability. An increasingly significant clinical deficit occurs, however, with an increasing number of recurrent infarcts. *État lacunaire*, pseudobulbar palsy, multilacunar dementia, and Binswanger's encephalopathy can all be the result. The management of risk factors, and of hypertension, is, therefore, important. When microangiopathy is established, an abrupt drop of blood pressure can result in a distal field ischemia and clinical deterioration. The history, clinical examination, imaging, and blood flow studies may all be important in deciding on the optimal level of blood pressure for any individual patient.

REFERENCES

1. Marie P. Les lacunaires. Foyers de désintégration et différents autres états cavitaires du cerveau. *Rev Med* 1901;21:281–298.
2. Déjerine J. *Sémiologie des affections du système nerveux*. Paris: Masson; 1914.
3. Lépine R. Note sur la paralysie glosso-labiée cérébrale à forme pseudo-bulbaire. *Rev Mens Med Chir* 1877;1:909–922.
4. Besson G, Bogousslavsky J, Regli F, Meader P. Acute pseudobulbar or suprabulbar palsy. *Arch Neurol* 1991;48:501–507.
5. Helgason C, Wilbur A, Weiss A, Redmond KJ, Kingsbury NA. Acute pseudobulbar mutism due to discrete bilateral capsular infarction in the territory of the anterior choroidal artery. *Brain* 1988;111:507–524.
6. Langworthy OR, Hesser FH. Syndrome of pseudobulbar palsy. An anatomic and physiologic analysis. *Arch Intern Med* 1940;65:106–121.
7. Lévy G. Les troubles de la parole au cours des états pseudo-bulbaires. *Rev Neurol* 1932:289–328.
8. Thurel R. *Les pseudo-bulbaires. Étude clinique et anatomo-pathologique* [Thesis]. Paris, 1929.
9. Emile J. *Contribution à l'étude des paralysies pseudo-bulbaires corticales (diplégie facio-linguo-masticatrice)* [Thesis]. Paris, 1965.
10. Château R, Fau R, Groslambert R, Perret J, Boucharlat J, Châtelain R. A propos de trois observations de diplégie linguo-facio-masticatrice d'origine corticale: la forme de l'adulte et celle de l'enfant. *Rev Neurol* 1966;114:390–395.
11. Schott B, Boulliat G, Cotte L, Vauterin C. Le syndrome operculaire bilatéral et unilatéral. *Lyon Med* 1961;261:365–377.
12. Foix C, Chavany JA, Marie J. Diplégie facio-linguo-masticatrice d'origine cortico sous-corticale. *Rev Neurol* 1926;33:214–219.
13. Mao CC, Coull BM, Golper LAC, Rau MT. Anterior operculum syndrome. *Neurology* 1989;39:1169–1172.
14. Loeb C, Gandolfo C, Caponnetto C, Del Sette M. Pseudobulbar palsy: a clinical computed tomography study. *Eur Neurol* 1990;30:42–46.
15. Raymond F, Artaud G. Contribution à l'étude des localisations cérébrales (trajet intra-cérébral de l'hypoglosse). *Arch Neurol* (Paris) 1884;7:296–307.
16. Lhermitte J, Cuel J. Forme ponto-cérébelleuse de la paralysie pseudo-bulbaire. *Rev Neurol* 1921:364–367.
17. Van Bogaert L, Bertrand I. La rigidité tardive dans les formes ponto-cérébelleuses de la paralysie pseudo-bulbaire. *Rev Neurol* 1930:617–631.
18. Claude H, Cuel J. La meïopragie cérébrale par angiosclérose précoce sans ischémie en foyer (forme de démence présénile artério-scléreuse). *L'Encéphale* 1927:161–171.
19. Fisher CM. Lacunar strokes and infarcts: a review. *Neurology* 1982;32:871–876.
20. Mohr JP. Lacunes. In: Barnett H, Stein B, Mohr J, Yatsu F, eds. *Stroke pathophysiology, diagnosis and management*. New York: Churchill Livingstone; 1988:475–496.
21. Earnest MP, Fahn S, Karp JH, Rowland LP. Normal pressure hydrocephalus and hypertensive cerebrovascular disease. *Arch Neurol* 1974;31:262–266.
22. Koto A, Rosenberg G, Kingesser LH, Horoupian D, Katzman R. Syndrome of normal pressure hydrocephalus possible relation to hypertensive and arteriosclerotic vasculopathy. *J Neurol Neurosurg Psychiatry* 1977;40:73–79.
23. Lorenzo AV, Bresnan MJ, Barlow CF. Cerebrospinal fluid absorption deficit in normal pressure hydrocephalus. *Arch Neurol* 1974;30:387–393.
24. Vessal K, Sperber EE, James AE. Chronic communicating hydrocephalus with normal CSF pressures: a cisternographic-pathologic correlation. *Ann Radiol* 1974;17:785–793.
25. Fisher CM. Lacunes: small, deep cerebral infarcts. *Neurology* 1965;15:774–784.
26. Hughes WH, Dodgson MCH, MacLennan DC. Chronic cerebral hypertensive disease. *Lancet* 1954;2:770–774.
27. Ishii N, Nishihara Y, Imamura T. Why do frontal lobe symptoms predominate in vascular dementia with lacunes? *Neurology* 1986;36:340–345.
28. Fukuda H, Kobayashi S, Okada K, Tsunematsu T. Frontal white matter lesions and dementia in lacunar infarction. *Stroke* 1990;21:1143–1149.
29. Wolfe N, Linn R, Babikian VL, Knoeffel JE, Al-

bert ML. Frontal system impairment following multiple lacunar infarcts. *Arch Neurol* 1990; 47:129–132.
30. Babikian VL, Wolfe N, Linn R, Knoefel JE, Albert ML. Cognitive changes in patients with multiple cerebral infarcts. *Stroke* 1990;21:1013–1018.
31. Mendez MF, Adams NL, Lewandowski KS. Neurobehavioral changes associated with caudate lesions. *Neurology* 1989;39:349–354.
32. Bogousslavsky J, Regli F, Assal G. The syndrome of unilateral tuberothalamic artery territory infarction. *Stroke* 1986;17:434–441.
33. Castaigne P, Lhermitte F, Buge A, Escourolle R, Hauw JJ, Lyon-Caen O. Paramedian thalamic and midbrain infarcts: clinical and neuropathological study. *Ann Neurol* 1981;10:127–148.
34. Graff-Radford NR, Damasio H, Yamada T, Eslinger PJ, Damasio AR. Nonhemorrhagic thalamic infarction. Clinical, neuropsychological and electrophysiological findings in four anatomical groups defined by computerized tomography. *Brain* 1985;108:485–516.
35. Friedman JH. Syndrome of diffuse encephalopathy due to nondominant thalamic infarction. *Neurology* 1985;35:1524–1526.
36. Cambier J, Graveleau P. Volume 1 (45): clinical neuropsychology. Thalamic syndromes. In: Fredericks JMA, ed. *Clinical neurology*. Amsterdam: Elsevier; 1985:87–98.
37. Castaigne P, Buge A. Cambier J, Escourolle R, Brunet P, Degos JD. Démence thalamique d'origine vasculaire par ramollissement bilatéral, limité au territoire du pédicule rétro-mamillaire. A propos de deux observations anatomo-cliniques. *Rev Neurol* 1966;114:89–107.
38. Guberman A, Stuss D. The syndrome of bilateral thalamic infarction. *Neurology* 1983;33:540–546.
39. Bogousslavsky J, Regli F, Uske A. Thalamic infarcts: clinical syndromes, etiology, and prognosis. *Neurology* 1988;38:837–848.
40. Pappata S, Mazoyer B, Tran Dinh S, Cambon H, Levasseur M, Baron JC. Effects of capsular or thalamic stroke on metabolism in the cerebral cortex and cerebellum: a positron tomography study. *Stroke* 21:519–524.
41. Baron JC, d'Antona R, Pantano P, Serdaru M, Samson Y, Bousser MG. Effects of thalamic stroke on energy metabolism of the cerebral cortex. *Brain* 1986;109:1234–1259.
42. Metter EJ, Mazziotta JC, Itabashi HA, Mankovitc NJ, Phelps ME, Kuhl DE. Comparison of glucose metabolism, X-ray CT, and post-mortem data in a patient with multiple cerebral infarcts. *Neurology* 1985;35:1695–1701.
43. Olsen TS, Bruhn P, Öberg RGE. Cortical hypoperfusions a possible cause of subcortical aphasia. *Brain* 1986;109:393–410.
44. Rougemont D, Baron JC, Lebrun-Grandie P, Bousser MG, Cabanis E, Laplane D. Débit sanguin cérébral et extraction d'oxygène dans les hémiplégies lacunaires. *Rev Neurol* 1983;139:277–282.
45. Perani D, Lucignani G, Pantano P, Grundini P, Lenzi GL, Fazio F. Cerebellar diaschisis in pontine ischemia. A case report with single-photon emission computerized tomography. *J Cereb Blood Flow Metab* 1987;7:127–131.
46. Szelies B, Herholz K, Pawlik G, Karbe H, Hebold I, Heiss W-D. Widespread functional effects of discrete thalamic infarction. *Arch Neurol* 1991;48:178–182.
47. Yao H, Sadoshima S, Kuwabara Y, Ichiya Y, Fujishima M. Cerebral blood flow and oxygen metabolism in patients with vascular dementia of the Binswanger type. *Stroke* 1990;21:1694–1699.
48. Toso V. Single photon emission tomography findings in lacunar lesions. *Eur Neurol* 1989; 29[Suppl 2]:36–38.
49. Loizou LA, Kendall BE, Marshall J. Subcortical arteriosclerotic encephalopathy: a clinical and radiological investigation. *J Neurol Neurosurg Psychiatry* 1981;44:294–304.
50. Benson DF, Kuhl DE, Hawkins RA, Phelps ME, Cummings JL, Tsai SY. The fluorodeoxyglucose ^{18}F scan in Alzheimer's disease and multi-infarct dementia. *Arch Neurol* 1983;40:711–714.

10

Lacunar Syndromes Due to Non-Ischemic Small Deep Lesions

Gérard Besson and Marc Hommel

Department of Clinical and Biological Neurosciences, Stroke Unit, Centre Hospitalier Universitaire Régional de Grenoble, 38043 Grenoble, France

When they were first described, lacunar syndromes were associated only with lacunar infarcts (i.e., small deep infarcts due to the occlusion of a single perforating artery) (see Chapters 1 and 7). Radiological studies have since shown that lacunar syndromes may also be caused by non-ischemic lesions (1). A lacunar syndrome is due to a non-ischemic cause in about 9.3% to 9.7% of patients (2,3). Non-Ischemic small lesions causing lacunar syndromes may be divided into intracerebral hemorrhages and other non-ischemic lesions. We report here the non-ischemic causes of only the classic lacunar syndromes.

INTRACEREBRAL HEMORRHAGES

Intracerebral hemorrhages are the most common non-ischemic small lesions producing lacunar syndromes. Lacunar syndromes represent 8.7% (4) to 10.9% (5) of the clinical presentations of patients with intracerebral hemorrhages. The clinical findings of the four main studies of small cerebral hemorrhages are summarized in Table 1.

Pure Motor Stroke

The onset of pure motor hemorrhagic stroke is often sudden, with a maximal neurologic deficit at the onset (6–8). However, it may be gradual, over several hours (9), or rarely over several days (10). Transient motor deficit has been noted (7), occurring a few days before the stroke (7). Headache, nausea, and vomiting, which are signs associated with larger hemorrhages, are rare (5). Although the motor weakness usually involves the face, arm, and leg (4–7), it may involve only the face (11, 12), or the arm and the leg (10). Pure motor quadriplegia sparing the face has also been reported due to two symmetrical internal capsule hemorrhages (13).

Israelowitz reported a case of probable pure motor hemiplegia due to a hemorrhage in the internal capsule, but no detailed neurological examination was reported (14). In 1880 Ballet reported a patient with a brachiofacial deficit (15). At autopsy, he found a small hemorrhage of the lower part of the precentral gyrus. Two cases of isolated lower facial palsy have been reported, which at autopsy were found to be due to deep hematomas involving the posterior (11) and the anterior limbs of the internal capsule (12). Only one case of lower facial palsy due to a hemorrhage in the genu of the internal capsule has been reported (16). This patient also had dysphagia and dysarthria.

Imaging studies have shown deep hemorrhages causing pure motor stroke in the

TABLE 1. Summary of clinical features

Authors	M/F	Mean age (yr)	PMH	AHP DCH	PSS	SMS	Others
Lee et al. (6)	12/7	62.7	3	2	3	7	4
Mori et al. (5)	10/9	60.6	4	8	0	7	0
Iwasaki et al. (4)	10/0	58.2	3	1	1	5	0
Weisberg et al. (7)	7/3	63.9	7	0	0	3	0
	39/19		17	11	4	22	4

PMH, pure motor hemiparesis; AHP, ataxic hemiparesis; DCH, dysarthria–clumsy hand syndrome; PSS, pure sensory stroke; SMS, sensorimotor stroke.

internal capsule (1, 4, 6, 7, 17, 18) involving the caudate nucleus (19), the putamen (5, 8, 20) (Fig. 1), the cerebral peduncle (6), or the pons (21).

Ataxic Hemiparesis and Dysarthria–Clumsy hand Syndrome

Despite recognition that ataxic hemiparesis and the dysarthria–clumsy hand syndrome may be caused by a hemorrhage, no systematic studies have been carried out and few data are available. The onset is often sudden (22–29), but rarely progressive (29). Headache is frequent (22, 23, 25, 28), while nausea is rare (25). The hematoma may be located in the internal capsule (5, 24, 26, 30) (Fig. 2) or may involve the lenticular nucleus (31), the thalamus (27), and the pons (4, 6, 25, 28).

Ataxic hemiparesis with contralateral trigeminal nerve impairment has been reported secondary to a hematoma in the lateral half of the rostral basis pontis (22). Hypesthetic ataxic hemiparesis has been caused by a thalamic hematoma (23, 29).

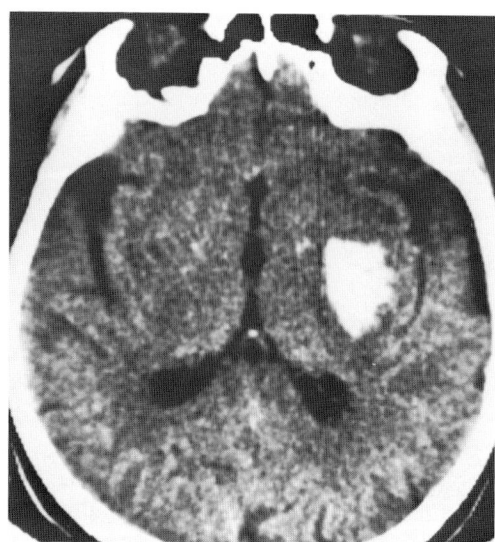

FIG. 1. Pure motor hemiplegia. Capsulolenticular hemorrhage on computed tomography.

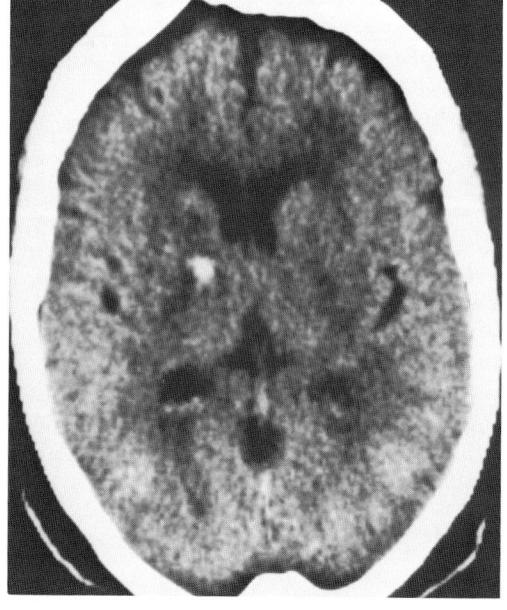

FIG. 2. Ataxic hemiparesis. Capsular hemorrhage on computed tomography.

Hematomas can also give rise to the dysarthria–clumsy hand syndrome when located in the internal capsule (6), the putamen (5), the cerebellum (32) and in the pons (33).

Pure Sensory Stroke

Pure sensory stroke due to a hematoma can affect the face, arm, and leg (34–38), the arm and leg (39), the corner of the mouth and the palm of the hand (cheiro-oral syndrome) (40–43) (Fig. 3), or the face alone (44, 45). Hematomas may produce a selective impairment of lemniscal (36) or spinothalamic sensory modalities (35, 38), or both (46).

Groothuis et al. reported a single autopsy case of pure sensory stroke due to a hematoma in the posterior limb of the internal capsule that minimally involved the thalamus (37). Imaging studies have shown pure sensory stroke to be caused by a deep hemorrhage either in the thalamus (6, 41, 46–48) in the internal capsule interrupting the thalamocortical pathways (37), in the midbrain (35, 39, 43), or in the pons (34, 36, 38, 40, 42, 44, 45).

Sensorimotor Stroke

Deep hematomas have long been known to produce a sensorimotor stroke. Case 12 in Veyssière's thesis (49), case 7 in Lépine's thesis (50), and a case report of Lhermitte (51) can all be considered to be sensorimotor strokes due to capsulothalamic or putaminocapsular hemorrhages. Imaging studies have shown sensorimotor stroke to be associated with deep hemorrhages in the thalamocapsular area (5, 6, 52–54), the putaminocapsular area (5,52) (Fig. 4), the thalamus (4, 6), the internal capsule (4, 6, 52), and in the pons (5).

Nonvascular Causes of Lacunar Syndromes

Lacunar syndromes may be produced by a wide variety of pathologic processes, including demyelinating diseases and space-occupying lesions (subdural hematoma, tumor, abscess).

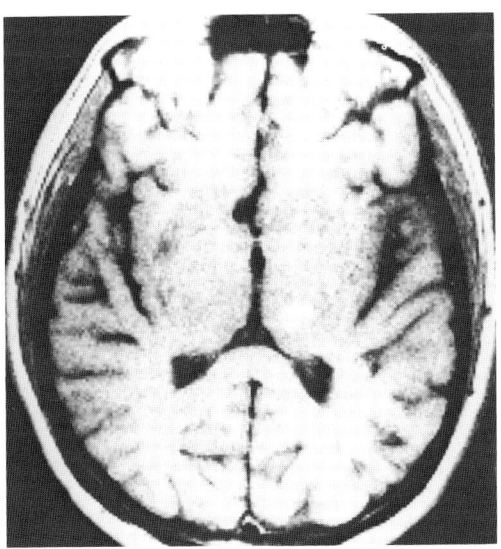

FIG. 3. Sensory cheiro-oral syndrome. Thalamic hemorrhage on magnetic resonance imaging (T1).

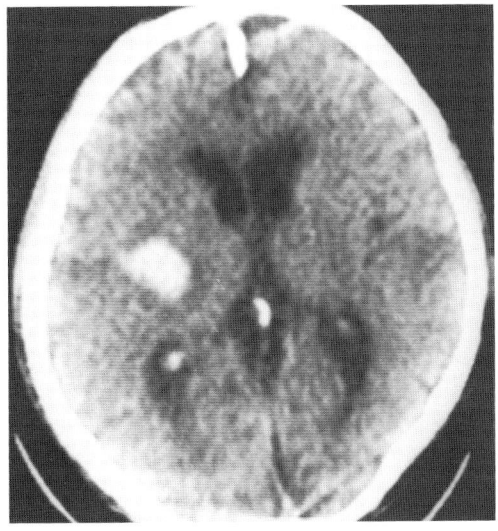

FIG. 4. Sensorimotor deficit. Capsulolenticular hemorrhage on computed tomography.

Pure Motor Hemiparesis

Pure motor hemiparesis is a syndrome that can be caused by any pathological processes that affect the pyramidal motor pathway, either at a supratentorial or at an infratentorial level. Thus, pure motor hemiparesis may result from demyelinating disease (1), nocardial brain abscess (55), brainstem (56, 57) and supratentorial glioma (58), supratentorial metastasis (1, 59), and subdural hematomas (1). An inflammatory arteriopathy such as that induced by syphilis (60) or cysticercosis (61) may cause a pure motor hemiparesis. The clinical deficit in these cases, however, is due to infarction secondary to occlusion of small arteries by endarteritis.

Pure motor monoparesis has been reported secondary to a supratentorial metastasis (62) or a supratentorial abscess (62).

Ataxic Hemiparesis

Nonvascular causes of ataxic hemiparesis were known even before it was reported that ataxic hemiparesis could be caused by lacunar infarction. In 1916, Claude and Lhermitte described "cerebello-spasmodic paraplegia" (63). This syndrome corresponds with bilateral ataxic hemiparesis and was due to bilateral paracentral cortical injuries secondary to gunshots occurring during the first world war. A few years later, Foix and Thévenard described a case of ataxic hemiparesis due to a tuberculoma located in the paracentral area (64). More recently, ataxic hemiparesis has been reported to be caused by demyelinating disease (65,66), brainstem and thalamocapsular glioma (31,67), supratentorial metastasis (31), leukemic infiltrate of the midbrain (68), lymphoma of the corona radiata (69), meningioma of the falx cerebri (70), and subdural hematoma (71). Neurocysticercosis may also produce ataxic hemiparesis (72).

Pure Sensory Deficit

Nonvascular causes of pure sensory deficit are rare, and the topography of the sensory deficit was usually cheiro-oral. Two cases of thalamic tumor (73, 74), one of which was a glioblastoma, have been found at autopsy in patients with cheiro-oral sensory loss. A cholesteatoma of the parietal bone infiltrating the parietal lobe and a subdural hematoma were other reported causes of sensory cheiro-oral syndrome (75). Surgical procedures such as stereotactic thalamotomy may also induce a cheiro-oral sensory deficit (76, 77).

Sensorimotor Deficit

No nonvascular causes of sensorimotor deficit have been reported. However, since deep lesions in the thalamocapsular region can produce a sensorimotor deficit, a nonvascular cause of sensorimotor stroke is probably not uncommon.

CONCLUSION

All the classic lacunar syndromes may be caused by non-ischemic pathologies. In a patient presenting with a lacunar syndrome, therefore, an early computed tomography scan is absolutely necessary to exclude a non-ischemic cause. Magnetic resonance imaging may be useful to exclude the presence of a large artery infarct and may also confirm the diagnosis of a presumed lacunar infarct (78).

REFERENCES

1. Weisberg LA. Computed tomography and pure motor hemiparesis. *Neurology* 1979;29:490–495.
2. Anzalone N, Landi G. Non ischaemic causes of lacunar syndromes: prevalence and clinical findings. *J Neurol Neurosurg Psychiatry* 1989;52: 1188–1190.
3. Loeb C. The lacunar syndromes. *Eur Neurol* 1989;29[Suppl 2]:2–7.

4. Iwasaki Y, Kinoshita M. Lacunar syndrome and intracerebral hemorrhage: clinico-computed tomographic correlations. *Comput Med Imag Graphics* 1988;12:359–363.
5. Mori E, Tabuchi M, Yamadori A. Lacunar syndrome due to intracerebral hemorrhage. *Stroke* 1985;16:454–459.
6. Lee KY, Lie SK, Chiang TR, Hung TP. Small intracerebral hemorrhage clinically simulating lacunar infarction. *J Formosan Med Assoc* 1983;82:993–1000.
7. Weisberg LA, Wall M. Small capsular hemorrhages. Clinical-computed tomographic correlations. *Arch Neurol* 1984;41:1255–1257.
8. Jain S, Maheswari MC, Dhamija RM, Mishra NK. Pure motor hemiparesis due to hypertensive putaminal haemorrhage. *Eur Neurol* 1985;24:205–207.
9. Tapia JF, Kase CS, Sawyer RH, Mohr JP. Hypertensive putaminal hemorrhage presenting as pure motor hemiparesis. *Stroke* 1983;14:505–506.
10. Gobernardo JM, Fernandez De Molina A, Gimeno A. Pure motor hemiplegia due to hemorrhage in the lower pons. *Arch Neurol* 1980;37:393.
11. Parisot P. Monoplégie faciale par lésion limitée de la capsule interne. *Rev Med Est* 1893;25:175–178.
12. Etienne G. Monoplégie faciale et déviation conjuguée de la face et des yeux d'origine capsulaire. *Presse Med* 1896:657–658.
13. Obeso JA, Marti-Masso JF, Carrera N, Astudillo W. Pure motor quadriplegia secondary to bilateral capsular hematomas. *Arch Neurol* 1980;37:248.
14. Israelowitz S. Un cas d'hémorragie linéaire dans la capsule interne. *Rev Neurol* 1908:573–574.
15. Ballet G. Nouveau fait relatif aux localisations cérébrales. Du centre psycho-moteur de la face. *Prog Med* 1880:762–763.
16. Daland J. A case of dysphagia and dysphasia resulting from a lesion in the internal capsule. *J Nerv Ment Dis* 1897:614–619.
17. Rascol A, Clanet M, Manelfe C, Guiraud B, Bonafé A. Pure motor hemiplegia: CT study of 30 cases. *Stroke* 1982;13:11–17.
18. Soisson T, Cabanis EA, Iba-Zizen MT, Bousser MG, Laplane D, Castaigne P. Pure motor hemiplegia and computed tomography. *J Neuroradiol* 1982;9:304–322.
19. Stein RW, Kase CS, Hier DB, Caplan LR, Mohr JP, Hemmati M, Henderson K. Caudate hemorrhage. *Neurology* 1984;34:1549–1554.
20. Tapia JF, Kase CS, Sawyer RH, Mohr JP. Hypertensive putaminal hemorrhage presenting as pure motor hemiparesis. *Stroke* 1983:14:505–506.
21. Gobernardo JM, Fernandez De Molina A, Gimeno A. Pure motor hemiplegia due to hemorrhage in the lower pons. *Arch Neurol* 1980;37:393.
22. Ambrosetto P. Ataxic hemiparesis with contralateral trigeminal nerve impairment due to pontine hemorrhage. *Stroke* 1987;18:244–245.
23. Dobato JL, Villanueva JA, Giménez-Roldan S. Sensory ataxic hemiparesis in thalamic hemorrhage. *Stroke* 1990;21:1749–1753.
24. Elcano Luquin J, Arboix Damunt A, Kulisewsky Borjaski J, Marti-Vilalta JL. Sindrome hemiparesia ataxica por hemorragia capsular. *Med Clin* 1989;92:479.
25. Kobatake K, Shinohara Y. Ataxic hemiparesis in patients with primary pontine hemorrhage. *Stroke* 1983;14:762–764.
26. Mori E, Yamadori A, Kudo Y, Tabuchi M. Ataxic hemiparesis from small capsular hemorrhage. Computed tomography and somato-sensory evoked potentials. *Arch Neurol* 1984;41:1050–1053.
27. Schleimer J, Galasko D, Stern BJ. Ataxic hemiparesis with intact sensory modalities. *Arch Neurol* 1986;43:8.
28. Schnapper RA. Pontine hemorrhage presenting as ataxic hemiparesis. *Stroke* 1982;13:518–519.
29. Verma AK, Maheshwari MC. Hypesthetic-ataxic-hemiparesis in thalamic hemorrhage. *Stroke* 1986;17:49–51.
30. Colombo A, Crisi G, Guerzoni MC, Panzetti P. Vascular ataxic hemiparesis: a prospective clinical and CT study. *Ital J Neurol Sci* 1986;7:253–256.
31. Sanguineti I, Tredici G, Beghi E, et al. Ataxic hemiparesis syndrome: clinical and CT study of 20 new cases and review of the literature. *Ital J Neurol Sci* 1986;7:51–59.
32. Tougeron A, Samson Y, Schaison M, Artigou JY, Bousser MG. Syndrome dysarthrie-main malhabile par infarctus cérébelleux. *Rev Neurol* 1988;144:596–597.
33. Tuhrim S, Yang WC, Rubinowitz H, Weinberger J. Primary pontine hemorrhage and the dysarthria clumsy hand syndrome. *Neurology* 1982;32:1027–1028.
34. Araga S, Fukada M, Kagimoto H, Takahashi K. Pure sensory stroke due to pontine hemorrhage. *J Neurol* 1987;235:116–117.
35. Azouvi P, Tougeron A, Hussonois C, Schouman-Claeys E, Bussel B, Held JP. Pure sensory stroke due to midbrain haemorrhage limited to the spinothalamic pathways. *J Neurol Neurosurg Psychiatry* 1989;52:1427–1428.
36. Graveleau P, Decroix JP, Samson Y, Masson M, Cambier J. Déficit sensitif isolé d'un hémicorps par hématome du pont. *Rev Neurol* 1986;142:788–790.
37. Groothuis DR, Duncan GW, Fisher CM. The human thalamo-cortical sensory pathway in the internal capsule: evidence from a small capsular hemorrhage causing a pure sensory stroke. *Ann Neurol* 1977;2:328–331.
38. Kim JS, Jo KD. Pure lemniscal sensory deficit caused by pontine hemorrhage. *Stroke* 1992;23:300–301.
39. Tuttle PV, Reinmuth OM. Midbrain hemorrhage producing pure sensory stroke. *Arch Neurol* 1984;41:794–795.
40. Iwasaki Y, Kinoshita M, Ikeda K, Takamiya K, Shiojima T. Pure sensory stroke and cheiro-oral syndrome. *J Neurol* 1989;236:186–187.

41. Kawakami Y, Chikama M, Tanimoto T, Shimamura Y. Radiological studies of the cheiro-oral syndrome. *J Neurol* 1989;236:177–181.
42. Matsumoto S, Kaku S, Yamasaki M, Imai T, Nabatame H, Kameyama M. Cheiro-oral syndrome with bilateral oral involvement: a study of pontine lesions by high-resolution magnetic resonance imaging. *J Neurol Neurosurg Psychiatry* 1989;52:792–794.
43. Ono S, Inoue K. Cheiro-oral syndrome following midbrain haemorrhage. *J Neurol* 1985;232:304–306.
44. Holtzmann R, Zablozki V, Yang W, Leeds N. Lateral pontine tegmental hemorrhage presenting as isolated trigeminal sensory neuropathy. *Neurology* 1987;37:704–706.
45. Berlit P. Trigeminal neuropathy in pontine hemorrhage. *Eur Neurol* 1989;29:169–170.
46. Rosenberg NL, Koller R. Computerized tomography and pure sensory stroke. *Neurology* 1981;31:217–220.
47. Azouvi P, Papatta S, Baron P, Bousser MG, Laplane D. Attaque sensitive pure par hématome thalamique. *Rev Neurol* 1988;144:212–214.
48. Fisher CM. Pure sensory stroke and allied conditions. *Stroke* 1982;13:434–447.
49. Veyssière R. *Recherches cliniques et expérimentales sur l'hémianesthésie de cause cérébrale* [Thesis]. Paris, 1874.
50. Lépine R. *De la localisation dans les maladies cérébrales* [Thesis]. Paris, 1875.
51. Lhermitte J. Les syndromes thalamiques dissociés. Les formes analgiques et hémialgiques. *Ann Med* 1925;17:488–501.
52. Huang CY, Woo E, Chan FL. When is sensorimotor stroke a lacunar syndrome? *J Neurol Neurosurg Psychiatry* 1987;50:720–726.
53. Mauguière F, Courjon J. The origins of short-latency somatosensory evoked potentials in humans. *Ann Neurol* 1981;9:607–611.
54. Kawahara N, Sato K, Muraki M, Tanaka K, Kaneko M, Uemura K. CT classification of small thalamic hemorrhages and their clinical implications. *Neurology* 1986;36:165–172.
55. Weintraub MI, Glaser GH. Nocardial brain abscess and pure motor hemiplegia. *NY State J Med* 1970;70:2717–2721.
56. Levitt LP, Selkoe DJ, Frankenfield B, Schoene W. Pure motor hemiplegia secondary to brainstem tumor. *J Neurol Neurosurg Psychiatry* 1975;38:1240–1243.
57. Rothman SJ, Olanow CW. Brain stem glioma in childhood: acute hemiplegic onset. *J Can Sci Neurol* 1981;8:263–264.
58. Fisher M, Recht LD. Brain tumor presenting as an acute pure motor hemiparesis. *Stroke* 1989;20:288–291.
59. Chokroverty S, Rubino FA. "Pure" motor hemiplegia. *J Neurol Neurosurg Psychiatry* 1975;38:896–899.
60. Johns DR, Tierney M, Parker SW. Pure motor hemiplegia due to meningovascular neurosyphilis. *Arch Neurol* 1987;44:1062–1065.
61. Barinagarrementeria F, Del Brutto OH. Neurocysticercosis and pure motor hemiparesis. *Stroke* 1988;19:1156–1158.
62. Ashizawa T, Rolak LA, Hines M. Spastic pure motor monoparesis. *Ann Neurol* 1986;20:638–641.
63. Claude H, Lhermitte J. Les paraplégies cérébello-spasmodiques et ataxo-cérébello-spasmodiques consécutives aux lésions bilatérales des lobules paracentraux par projectiles de guerre. *Bull Soc Med Hop Paris* 1916;40:796–804.
64. Foix C, Thévenard B. Symptomes pseudo-cérébelleux d'origine cérébrale, tubercule de la région paracentrale postérieure. *Rev Neurol* 1922;1502–1504.
65. Jabbari B, Gunderson CH, MacBurney JW. Improvement of ataxic hemiparesis with trihexyphenidyl. *Neurology* 1983;33:1627–1628.
66. Helweg-Larsen S, Larsson H, Henriksen O, Soelberg Sorensen P. Ataxic hemiparesis: three different locations of lesions studied by MRI. *Neurology* 1988;38:1322–1324.
67. Radhakrishnan K, Malhotra AK, Shridharan R, Chopra JS, Banerjee AK. Original articles: ataxic hemiparesis clinical, electrophysiologic, radiologic and pathologic observations. *Clin Neurol Neurosurg* 1982;84:91–100.
68. Bendheim PE, Berg BO. Ataxic hemiparesis from a midbrain mass. *Ann Neurol* 1981;9:405–407.
69. Biller J, Scardigli K. Ataxic hemiparesis from lesions of the corona radiata. *Arch Neurol* 1984;41:136.
70. Mizon JP, Rosa A. Hémiparésie à prédominance crurale et ataxie ipsilatérale par méningiome de la faux du cerveau. *Rev Neurol* 1986;142:68–69.
71. Gaymard B, Autret A, Lamisse F, Larmande P. Chronic subdural hematoma presenting as ataxic hemiparesis. *Eur Neurol* 1989;29:77–79.
72. Barinagarrementeria F, Del Brutto OH, Otero E. Ataxic hemiparesis from cysticercosis. *Arch Neurol* 1988;45:246.
73. Adler A. Zur Topik des Verlaufes der Geschmackssinnsfasern und anderer afferenter Bahnen im Thalamus. *Z Ges Neurol Psychiat* 1934;149:208–220.
74. Bouttier H, Bertrand I, Marie AP. Sur un cas anatomo-clinique de syndrome thalamique dissociée. *Rev Neurol* 1922:1492–1502.
75. Haguenau MD. *Contribution à l'étude des syndromes sensitifs chéiro-oraux* [Thesis]. Paris, 1965.
76. Hassler R, Riechert T. Klinische und anatomische Befunde bei stereotaktischen Schmerzoperationen im Thalamus. *Arch Psychiat Z Ges Neurol* 1959;200:93–122.
77. Mark VH, Ervin FR, Yakovlev PI. The treatment of pain by stereotactic methods. *Conf Neurol* 1962;22:238–245.
78. Hommel M, Besson G, Le Bas JF, et al. Prospective study of lacunar infarcts using magnetic resonance imaging. *Stroke* 1990;21:546–554.

11
Binswanger's Disease

John C. van Swieten and Louis R. Caplan*

*Dijkzigt Hospital, Erasmus University Rotterdam, The Netherlands; and *Department of Neurology, Tufts New England Medical Center, Boston, Massachusetts 02111*

Knowledge of the relationship between tissue ischemia and occlusive vascular disease evolved after the pioneering studies of Virchow. Since Virchow, the traditional concept has been that occlusion of an artery causes a discrete, well-circumscribed infarct in the center of the zone of the arterial supply. Foix applied this pathophysiological concept to the brain, showing the relationship of brain infarcts (then called ramollisements or softenings) to blockage of arteries proximal to the infarcts. Foix, Marie, and later Fisher described brains with multiple lacunar infarcts (état lacunaire) due to changes in the penetrating brain arteries (microangiopathy) (1–3). Although pathological descriptions of Binswanger's disease showed lacunar infarcts and small artery disease similar to that seen in *état lacunaire*, these brains in addition showed extensive demyelination, atrophy of the white matter, and dilated ventricles (4–7). This diffuse white matter abnormality was difficult to explain on the basis of Virchow's traditional concept of ischemia. More recently, it was found that computed tomography (CT) scans often revealed periventricular white matter low attenuation (WMLA) in the elderly. This white matter abnormality was found to be the radiological equivalent of Binswanger's disease. Two major questions arose, however. Firstly, whereas Binswanger's disease was considered to be rare and was always associated with dementia and minor strokes, the imaging counterpart was found commonly in the elderly who were often asymptomatic. Secondly, it was difficult to understand why patients with apparently identical small artery disease could show either only multiple small deep infarcts or only diffuse white matter disease. Clinicians and radiologists began to see a spectrum of findings on CT ranging from multiple small deep infarcts alone to WMLA alone. Most patients, however, had both.

This chapter reviews the clinical and pathological findings of Binswanger's disease, and reviews the pathologically proven cases of Binswanger's disease with WMLA on CT or periventricular white matter hyperintensity (WMHI) on T2-weighted magnetic resonance (MR). We also discuss the incidence and the clinical significance of WMLA on CT or WMHI on MR, and we discuss the conditions associated with WMLA.

CLASSICAL DESCRIPTION

Diffuse demyelination of the white matter in the brains of elderly patients is the hallmark of so-called Binswanger's disease. In 1894 Binswanger described grossly visible atrophy of the cerebral white matter in the brains of patients with severe dementia during life (4); he considered this clinicopathological combination to be a separate entity, distinct from general paralysis (syphilis). Although he did not describe the microscopic features, he suggested that the white matter atrophy was caused by deficient blood supply, resulting from arteriolosclerosis. Alzheimer confirmed the observations of Binswanger, and described the microscopic features in detail (5).

Olszewski, Caplan and Schoene, and later Ropper and Babikian successively analyzed the clinical findings in patients with Binswanger changes in the white matter (6–8). Dementia can be the initial symptom in Binswanger's disease, or may appear later, after one or more strokes (6,7). The clinical picture of dementia and recurrent strokes usually begins after 50 years of age. Patients are usually hypertensive but occasional patients with normal blood pressure, such as one of Caplan and Schoene's cases, are reported (7). The features of dementia vary considerably. Memory problems, confusion, loss of initiative and interest, and slowing of thought are the most prominent features, while focal cortical deficits such as apraxia, neglect, and aphasia are noted in some other patients (7,8). Neurological examination shows disorientation, poor recall of recent events, and slow answering, sometimes with nonfluent, spontaneous speech. Most patients have one or more strokes early in the course of the illness, some at a later stage, and a few had no strokes at all (6). Focal neurological deficits, pseudobulbar palsy, and uni- or bilateral pyramidal signs in the limbs are often present (6–8). Symptoms usually attributed to cerebral cortex disease, such as visual field defects, speech difficulties, and seizures, occur in only a minority of these patients. On angiography, severe stenosis is not found in either the carotid or vertebral arteries. Electroencephalography is normal or shows diffuse nonspecific changes, such as delta and theta waves (7).

Pathological examination shows diffuse demyelination of the white matter with sparing of the subcortical U-fibers (9). The pattern of demyelination can be homogeneous or patchy (10), mostly symmetrical, but occasionally asymmetrical. Mikol (11) described a number of *formes apparentés*: one patient had demyelination restricted to the occipital white matter, another had asymmetrical demyelination, while the demyelination was spotty in a third patient. The lateral ventricles were always enlarged in the original description by Binswanger (4), but several cases with a normal ventricular system have since been reported (9,12).

The accompanying pathological features consist of numerous infarcts, varying from a few millimeters to a centimeter in size, frequently scattered throughout the white matter (6). These small infarcts are not an essential feature of Binswanger's disease, and consist of old cystic spaces with dense gliosis, or recent necrotic foci containing necrotic debris and macrophages. Cortical infarcts were found in only a few patients (13). Severe microangiopathy of the small arteries and arterioles of the white matter and basal ganglia was found in all reported cases (6–12,14). The arteriolosclerosis consisted of hypertrophy and hyalinization of the tunica media, fibrous intimal proliferation, and degeneration of the internal elastic lamina. These changes are similar to those labelled lipohyalinosis by Fisher, found in patients with lacunar infarcts. Dilatation of perivascular spaces (*état criblé*), as usually found around arteriosclerotic arterioles in brains of hypertensive patients (15), was mentioned in a few postmortem studies of Binswanger's disease (9–12).

In summary, Binswanger's disease is a condition usually seen in hypertensives and typically beginning after the age of 50 years, and characterized clinically by a slowly progressive dementia, often with one or more minor strokes occurring during the course of the illness. Microscopically, extensive demyelination of the white matter and arteriolosclerosis are characteristically present, often in association with multiple lacunar infarcts and dilated perivascular spaces throughout the basal ganglia and white matter.

CT AND MR IN PATHOLOGICALLY PROVEN CASES OF BINSWANGER'S DISEASE

The number of well-documented cases of Binswanger's disease with WMLA on CT is sparse. Rosenberg et al. (16) reported for the first time that the diffuse demyelination of Binswanger's disease was visible as diffuse areas of low attenuation in the white matter on CT. He described in detail a 64-year-old man with uncontrolled hypertension, episodes of focal neurological deficit, and a progressive mental deterioration over 6 years. The patient had subsequent slowing of gait, frequency of micturition, and seizures. The neuropathological findings were consistent with Binswanger's disease (16). Goto et al. (17) described ten patients with dementia and extensive white matter involvement. Six patients had a CT scan, which showed decreased attenuation extending from the periventricular white matter to the subcortical areas; small deep infarcts in basal ganglia were found in four patients. The dementia mostly had a fluctuating course, with marked memory disturbance, labile emotions and confusion. Seven patients had urinary incontinence. Sudden focal neurological deficits, particularly motor signs due to strokes, occurred in most patients. Hypertension was common, although two patients had normal blood pressure, and some patients had epileptic seizures. Lacunar infarcts in the basal ganglia and the deep white matter were found at pathological examination in most patients. The ventricles were moderately to severely dilated (17). There was no significant evidence of Alzheimer's disease, neurofibrillary tangles, or senile plaques. Gupta et al. (18) reported similar pathological findings in three patients with WMLA on CT, and also mentioned the presence of dilated perivascular spaces in three brains.

MR imaging showed that the counterpart of WMLA on CT consisted of diffuse lesions of increased signal intensity on T2-weighted images involving most of the white matter (WMHI) (19,20). Kinkel et al. (19) described a 62-year-old man with severe dementia and stroke with pathologically proven Binswanger's disease. The MR scan in this patient showed extensive WMHI, but a normal ventricular system. Multiple lacunar infarcts were found at necropsy in several patients with Binswanger's disease who had only one episode of minor stroke during life (17,18,19). The association of diffuse demyelination of the white matter with cortical infarcts is reported in other cases (21,22). A cortical infarct in the territory of the posterior cerebral artery was found in two cases of Binswanger's disease described by DeWitt et al. and by Leiffer et al. (21,22).

The CT in normotensive patients with pathologically proven Binswanger's disease does not differ noticeably from that in hypertensive patients. Loizou et al. (23) described a 49-year-old normotensive man with multiple strokes and slowly progressive dementia over 23 years. The CT showed extensive WMLA that was identical to those seen in hypertensive Binswanger's disease. Fibrohyalinosis of arterioles and perforating arteries, diffuse demyelination of the white matter, and a number of cortical infarcts were found at postmortem. Fredriksson et al. (24,25) recently reported the clinicopathological findings in 14 patients with necropsy-proven Binswanger's disease, of whom 4 were normotensive. Five of these patients had CT scans, some early in their course. CT showed WMLA in 2 patients and enlargement of the third and lateral ventricles in 4 patients. In 1 patient, CT was normal. The clinical picture and pathological findings had strong similarities with the lacunar state (*état lacunaire*).

BINSWANGER-LIKE WMLA ON CT

WMLA denotes bilateral, diffuse areas of low attenuation predominantly in the periventricular cerebral white matter, with a gray-white matter difference of more than 10 Hounsfield units (17,26). Patients with this CT abnormality sometimes have only nonspecific complaints (17,19,27), so WMLA on CT is not synonymous with Binswanger's disease. The severity of WMLA may vary from being confined to the periventricular region to involving the whole white matter. Bogousslavsky (28) studied only severe WMLA with extension into the centrum semiovale, whereas in another study WMLA was graded according to a severity rating scale (29). A few investigators subdivided WMLA into frontal, occipital, or diffuse types (17,30). Rezek (31) studied the severity in more than 15 regions to give a summed score up to 180. Van Swieten et al. have described a simple 3-point scale for frontal and parieto-occipital white matter separately that combines the severity and distribution of lesions (32).

Incidence

The incidence of WMLA is dependent upon the selection of the patient population, and on the quality of the CT scanner (and thus indirectly on the year of the study). There are only a few studies of the incidence of WMLA in a large series of patients (17,28,30). WMLA of the white matter was found in 1.6% of 1,700 patients who also had cerebral atrophy on CT scan (30). The frequency of WMLA was higher in patients with stroke (3%), particularly in patients with deep infarcts (8%) (28), in elderly patients with mental deterioration (8%) (17), and in patients with intracerebral hemorrhage (18%) (33). Moderate and severe WMLA was present in 11% of patients with transient ischemic attacks or minor ischemic strokes in the Dutch TIA trial (34). The incidence of WMLA also gradually increases from a few percent in the age group 50–59 years to 30% in the age group 70–79 years (17,29).

Clinical Findings

Patients with WMLA on CT had a mean age between 65 and 70 years in several studies (17,18,27,28,30). A history of hypertension was a common finding (about 80%) in several series of patients with WMLA (18,19,28). Higher diastolic blood pressures in these patients were found in one study (30), whereas the average systolic blood pressure was significantly higher than in patients without WMLA in other studies (28,31,35). Blood pressure monitoring during 24 hours in patients with presumed lacunar stroke and WMLA showed significantly greater 24-hour mean systolic blood pressure (with sustained nighttime elevation), and greater variations in systolic blood pressure than in controls (36). Patients with WMLA in the Dutch TIA trial of patients with transient ischemic attacks or minor ischemic strokes were 7 years older and more often had hypertension than patients with normal white matter (34). Acute strokes had often occurred in patients with WMLA (17,27). In a logistic regression analysis, WMLA correlated with a higher age, a history of hypertension or a higher systolic blood pressure, and a history of stroke (25,35).

Dementia was frequently present in patients with WMLA. In some patients, dementia occurred as the only presenting symptom (18,19). In large series of patients, mental deterioration was present in 30 to 60% (17,19,30). Symptoms of impairment of memory and other intellectual functions were found in 20% of stroke patients with WMLA, and an even higher percentage of patients had cognitive impairment on neuropsychological evaluation (28). The cognitive changes had features of subcortical dementia, with decreased attention and concentration, memory problems, and slowness in responding (18,37). Steingart (38) found significantly lower scores in elderly subjects with WMLA, but only a trend toward lower scores in demented subjects with WMLA (39). Urinary incontinence was frequently reported in these patients (17,30).

Focal neurological deficits due to strokes were often present in patients with WMLA (17,18). Unilateral or bilateral weakness, hyperreflexia, Babinski signs, and pseudobulbar palsy were also frequently found (17,18,27). Disturbance of gait is another common feature in these patients. The abnormal gait was pyramidal (17,18), extrapyramidal (27,30), or ataxic (27,30). Conversely, elderly patients with impaired gait and balance showed WMLA more frequently in a case-control study (40). Epileptic seizures were occasionally mentioned in series of patients with WMLA (17,24). However, some patients had no neurological deficits at all or only nonspecific complaints (17,19).

The risk for stroke has been shown to be higher in patients with WMLA. In the Dutch TIA trial, patients with WMLA have nearly twice the frequency of stroke during follow-up (15%) than the patients with normal white matter (8%) (34). After adjustment for differences in age and other clinical features between the two groups, the risk for stroke remained higher for patients with WMLA [hazard ratio 1.6; 95% confidence interval (CI) 1.2–2.2)]. Patients younger than 70 years were even more at risk for stroke (34).

Investigations

Small deep infarcts are common on CT in patients with WMLA (Fig. 1), and their frequency ranges from 40% (34,41) to 90% (27,28,37). Cortical infarcts were much less often found (41) in these patients (27,34). The lateral ventricles were slightly enlarged in two studies (18,30), or markedly enlarged in others (18,27,37,41).

Electroencephalography has shown only nonspecific bilateral moderate to marked slow-wave activity in most patients with WMLA (27). Electrocardiographic abnor-

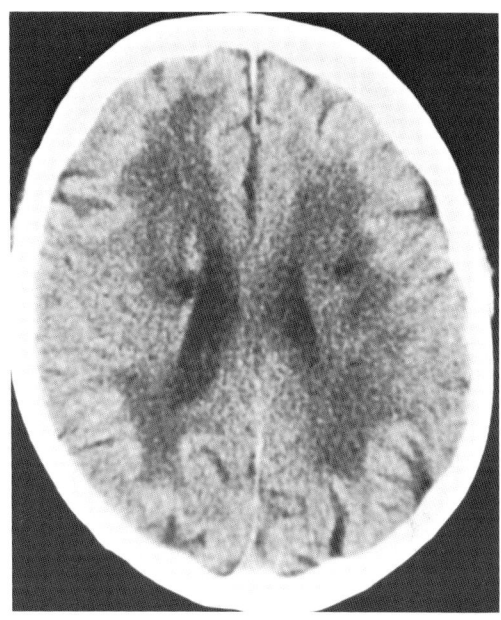

FIG. 1. CT scan: low attenuation in the frontal and parieto-occipital white matter, and two (left and right) lacunar infarcts in the basal ganglia.

malities have been reported in some patients (left ventricle hypertrophy, ischemic changes, or arrythmias) (27), and P-terminal force > 0.03 and S-T depression were significantly more frequent in stroke patients with WMLA (27,34). Schneider et al. (42) studied hemorrheological variables in 21 patients with the clinical features of Binswanger's disease and WMLA, 40 patients with lacunar infarcts, and 275 control subjects, and found that the first two groups had a raised erythrocyte concentration, raised plasma viscosity, and elevated fibrinogen concentration compared with those of controls. Plasma viscosity in patients with WMLA was significantly higher than in patients with presumed lacunar infarcts (42). The extracranial arteries in stroke patients with WMLA did not show more stenosis than those with normal white matter (28).

A few investigators studied the pattern of cerebral blood flow of different cerebral regions in patients with WMLA. In a study of

35 patients with multi-infarct dementia, Kawamara (43) found that decreased local cerebral blood flow in putamen and thalamus measured by xenon-enhanced CT correlated with the severity of WMLA in the frontal white matter. The cerebral blood flow and the cerebral metabolism rate of oxygen, measured by positron emission tomography, was decreased in five other patients with hypertension, dementia, lacunar stroke, and WMLA to 54 to 84% of that of controls, particularly in the frontal white matter (44). Patients with dementia showed a reduction of regional blood flow and oxygen metabolism not only in the white matter, but also in the frontal, parietal, and temporal cortex (44,45).

ABNORMAL WMHI ON MR

MR imaging shows more definite, and often more extensive, abnormalities of the white matter than CT (19,46). WMLA on CT corresponds to areas of increased signal intensity on T2-weighted MR images (WMHI), and to areas of decreased signal intensity on inversion recovery (IR; prolonged T1) images (19).

Heterogeneity of WMHI

A wide spectrum of WMHI is seen on MR in the elderly with variable extent, anatomical distribution, and shape. When the white matter is only partially involved, WMHI in the periventricular white matter can easily be distinguished from focal WMHI that are separate from the ventricles. WMHI has been graded according to their extent ranging from punctate lesions to thick caps around the frontal and occipital horns (47). Periventricular and focal WMHI have usually been taken together to express the severity of WMHI (48–50). The most commonly used classification of WMHI is one that distinguishes small, punctate WMHI and large confluent WMHI, irrespective of their site (periventricular or subcortical), and their anatomical region (5,19,32,48). A more objective method is to measure the thickness of periventricular caps (51), or to count the number of punctate WMHI (52,53). The different patterns, however, might have different pathological and clinical significance (see Chapter 4). Recently, the anatomical distribution of periventricular WMHI has been analyzed separately from that of subcortical WMHI (50,52,54,55).

Incidence

WMHI on MRI occurs more often with increasing age (20,48,54). Confluent WMHI was found in 30% of an unselected group of patients over the age of 60 years (head trauma, craniotomy, and multiple sclerosis excluded), and in only 5% in the age group of 41–60 years (48). Five to nine percent of healthy elderly persons over the age of 60 or 70 showed confluent WMHI (50,56). In a study of the general population, the prevalence of severe WMHI was 9% ranging from 3% in the age group 65–69 years to 27% in the age group 80–84 years (57). Twenty percent of patients with hypertension over the age of 50 years had confluent WMHI (48), as did 30% of patients with TIA or stroke (48,49). Similar results were found in a case-control study of elderly patients with chronic hypertension, in which confluent WMHI was present in 24% (55). In a study of periventricular WMHI, this was severe in approximately 25% of patients older than 50 years (54), and less severe in nearly half (47).

Clinical Findings

Kinkel et al. reported a series of 23 patients with predominantly moderate or severe WMHI on MR (19). Fifteen patients presented with stroke or slowly progressive dementia and gait disturbance or dementia alone, whereas eight patients had only nonspecific, vague complaints. Most patients in this series were hypertensive, and also had small deep infarcts (19). A history of myocardial infarction or stroke occurred significantly more often in subjects with WMHI (57). In other studies as well, confluent WMHI was associated with risk factors for stroke (hypertension, diabetes mellitus, and cardiac disease) or with actual stroke (47,53). A significant correlation between blood pressure [particularly diastolic (51,58)] and severity of WMHI has been found in patients with lacunar infarcts (51), as well as in the general population (57). In other studies there was only a trend with higher values of diastolic as well as systolic blood pressure (55). A multiple regression analysis showed that hypertension and stroke were independently associated with WMHI, although less strongly than age (48).

Dementia and focal neurological deficits were most often found in patients with confluent or extensive WMHI (Fig. 2) (52,58). Patients with lacunar stroke and dementia (according to the DSM-III criteria and an additional neuropsychological examination) showed more extensive WMHI than nondemented patients (58). Frontal WMHI was particularly associated with dementia in patients with presumed lacunar infarcts (51). In a case-control study of patients with hypertension, those patients with confluent WMHI performed worse in some neuropsychological subtests than hypertensive patients and controls with normal white matter, or with only small focal WMHI (55). Small focal or punctate WMHI were not correlated with cognitive impairment, or there was only a trend toward lower neuropsychological test scores in elderly with WMHI (50).

Investigations

Ventriculomegaly was found to be associated with both extensive periventricular WMHI and focal WMHI (19,54). In one study of patients with WMHI, ventricular enlargement was the only feature more commonly seen in demented than in nondemented patients with stroke (49). Elevated plasma fibrinogen has been associated with confluent WMHI in the general population (57). De Cristofaro (59) studied patients with periventricular caps or patchy WMHI by single photon emission computed tomography (SPECT), and found reduced perfusion in supra- and periventricular white matter. Positron emission tomography in 20 patients, of which 8 had confluent WMHI, showed that cerebral blood flow was significantly lower in a hemisphere with confluent WMHI than in other hemispheres. Focal cerebral blood flow was also reduced in the cortical areas overlying such confluent WMHI (60).

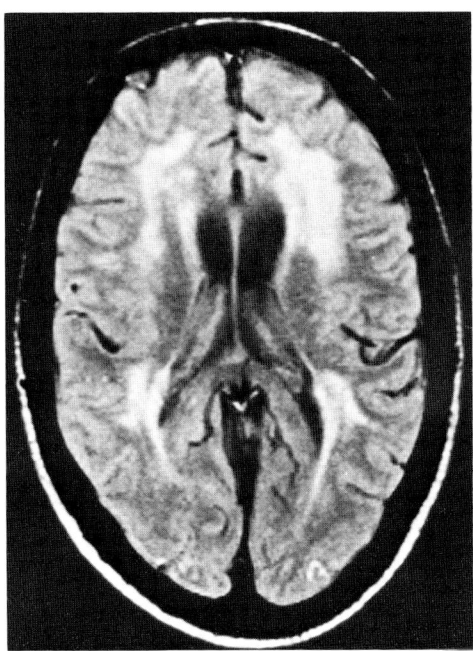

FIG. 2. MR scan: extensive white matter hyperintensity in the frontal white matter and centra semiovalia on lightly weighted T2 images (TR 2250; TE 30 milliseconds).

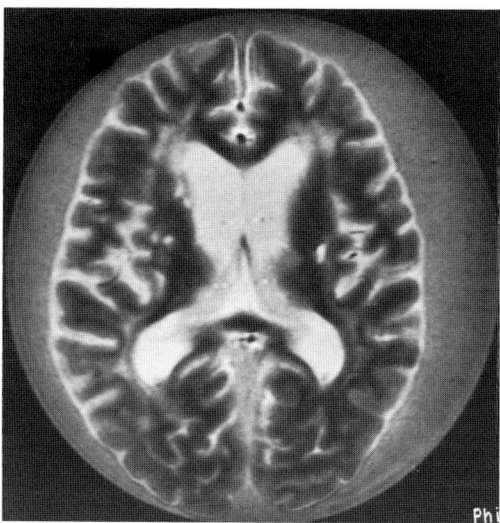

FIG. 3. Postmortem *in vitro* T2-weighted MR scan of a formalin-fixed brain specimen (**a**) periventricular hyperintensity in the frontal white matter.

PATHOLOGICAL CORRELATION OF CT AND MR LESIONS

Lotz et al. (61) studied brains of 18 patients with mild to moderate periventricular WMLA. All patients had a history of hypertension, or evidence of long-standing hypertension at autopsy. Seven patients had dementia (two had Alzheimer's disease), but there was no correlation between the presence of dementia and the severity of WMLA. The pathological findings were similar to those of Binswanger's disease, although of a lesser degree: demyelination, loss of axons, and fibrous thickening of small arteries. Most brains also showed lacunar infarcts in basal ganglia or white matter (61), and some had cortical infarcts (61). In another series of 20 brains with ischemic white matter changes at autopsy, the vascular changes of medullary arteries were expressed as a sclerotic rate (percentage of wall thickness over external diameter) and compared with those in brains from patients with Alzheimer's disease (62). Eleven of these 20 patients had premortem CT showing WMLA and large ventricles. The sclerotic rate correlated significantly with the degree of white matter changes seen at autopsy (62). Fibrohyaline thickening of walls corresponded with proliferation of collagen fibers, accumulation of cell debris, and deposition of amorphous material in the subaventitia on electron microscopy (62).

Leiffer et al. (22) studied the pathology of periventricular WMHI and found a zone of finely textured myelin and subependymal gliosis (22). Moderate and severe periventricular WMHI on postmortem MR images in brains of elderly patients (Fig. 3) also showed grossly visible myelin pallor of the white matter on coronal whole-brain slices (Fig. 4) (63,64). Microscopically, the demyelination was associated with arteriolosclerosis (Fig. 5a), astrocytic gliosis, and a variable degree of axonal loss. Lacunar infarcts (Fig. 5b) were nearly always found in the basal ganglia and the white matter. Dilated perivascular spaces (Fig. 5c) were present in most brains with severe demyelination (63,64). These spaces probably reflect brain atrophy, since they correlated strongly with lower brain weight, corrected for age and sex (64).

Electron microscopical examination of seven brains with diffuse myelin pallor showed a decreased number of nerve fibers, particularly in the deep white matter and anterior part of the corpus callosum (65,66). The diameter of nerve fibers and their myelin width were also smaller, although not significantly, than in brains of age-matched controls (65,66).

PATHOGENESIS OF BINSWANGER'S DISEASE

Most studies support the hypothesis that hypertension plays an important role in the development of Binswanger's disease or subcortical arteriosclerotic encephalopathy (SAE). Long-standing hypertension correlates with the presence of both WMLA on CT, and confluent or severe WMHI, al-

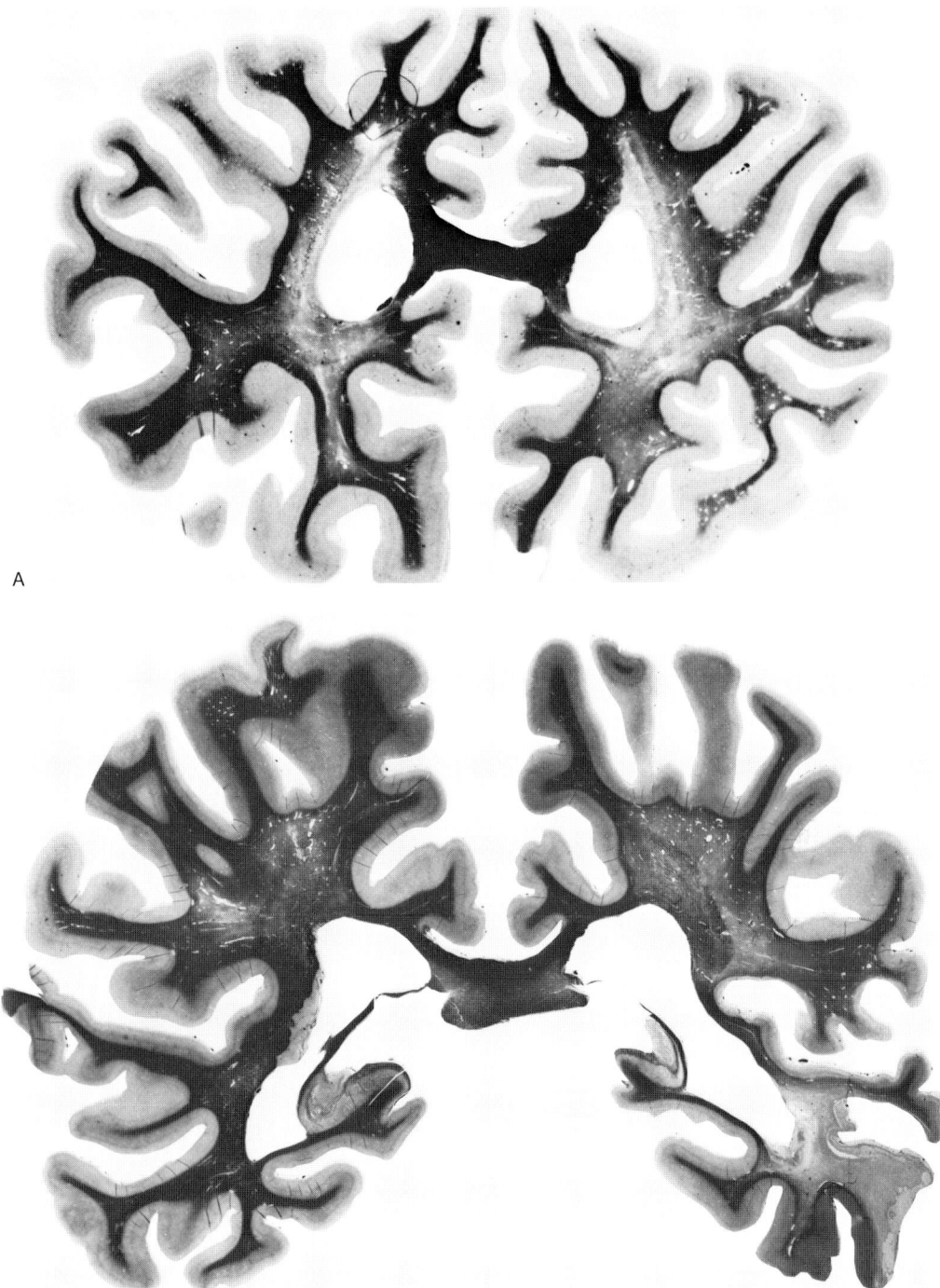

FIG. 4. Coronal whole brain specimens through (**A**) the frontal horns (**B**) the occipital horns: extensive demyelination of the white matter with sparing of the U-fibers.

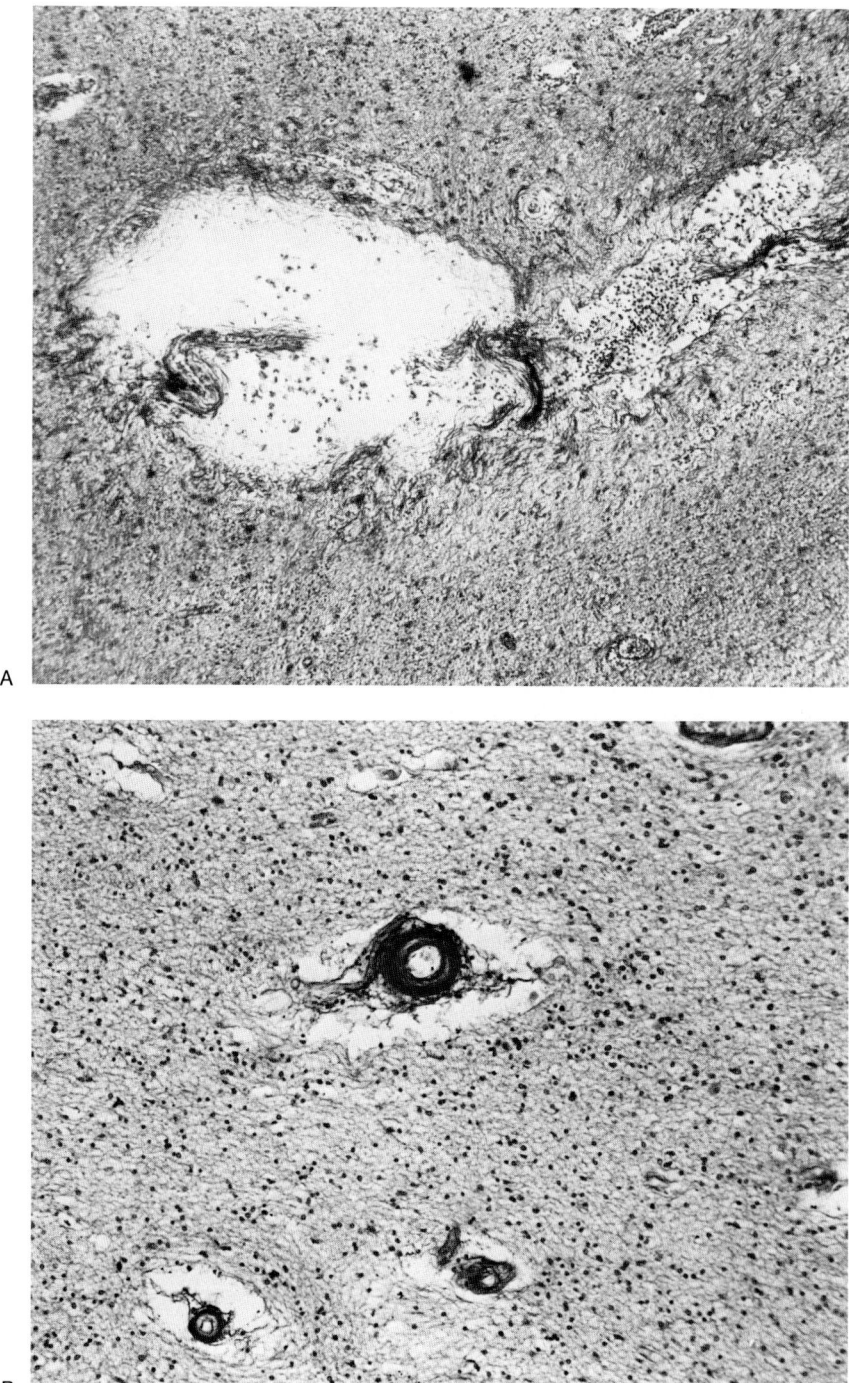

FIG. 5. (**A**) Fibrohyaline thickening of arteriolar walls (elastica van Gieson); (**B**) Small lacunar infarct with irregular borders and surrounding gliosis, with an occluded arteriole containing lipid-loaded macrophages (PTAH stain).

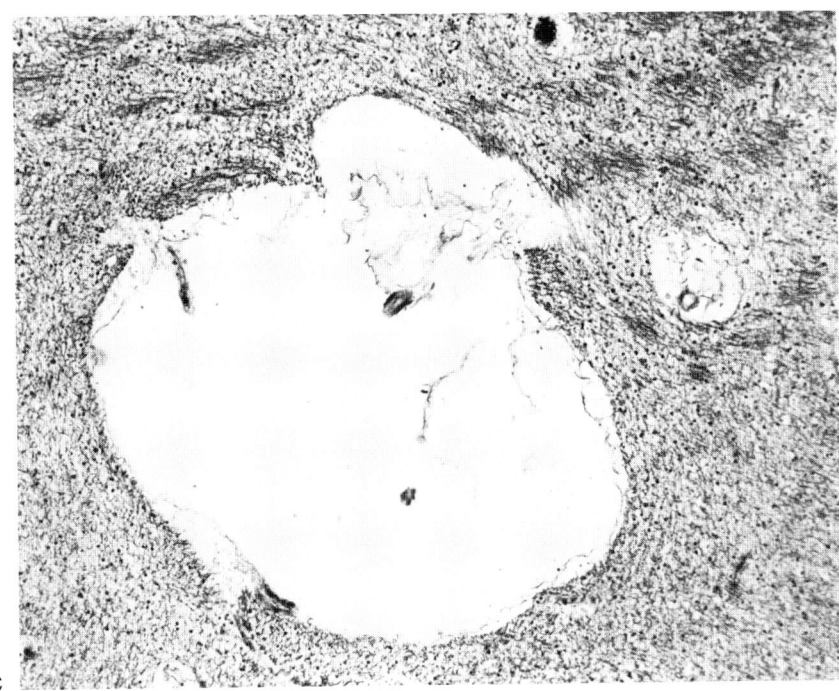

FIG. 5. Continued. **(C)** dilated perivascular space showing regular borders without gliosis (PTAH stain).

though diastolic blood pressure seems to be more closely related to WMLA and WMHI than the systolic pressure. Arteriolosclerosis, universally accepted to be caused by hypertension, is found in most patients with extensive SAE. The severity of WMLA has been correlated significantly with an elevated blood pressure (31,51), although the duration of hypertension in patients with WMLA or WMHI was not found to be different from those without (51,64). A correlation has also been found between the presence of white matter lesions seen at autopsy and the rate of sclerosis of medullary arteries in the frontal white matter (62). Hypertrophy of the medial layer of small arteries was also found more prominently in brains with diffuse SAE than in brains with hypertensive encephalopathy or hemorrhage (67).

There are several explanations for the occurrence of white matter lesions in hypertensive patients. Virchow related an infarct to decreased flow secondary to a stenosis or occlusion in the distribution of a single artery. But what if multiple segments of different arteries are involved? This might lead to a less severe ischemia over a wider zone. Alternatively, the white matter might respond differently to ischemia than the cortex and basal ganglia. The hypothesis most often supported for diffuse injury to the white matter is still that originally proposed by Binswanger, which postulates a diffuse and chronic ischemia of the white matter, secondary to arteriolosclerosis (4). This chronic hypoperfusion would lead to diffuse demyelination and corresponding lesions on CT or MR. This is soon followed by loss of axons, and later by dilatation of perivascular spaces.

In several reports, additional factors have been proposed to explain diffuse white matter injury. Transient episodes of cardiac failure, cardiac rhythm disorders or systemic hypotension might cause a relative hypoperfusion of the white matter (14,36,61,68). However, marked variations in casual blood pressure and repeated hypotension could not be confirmed on closer investigations in a group of aged hypertensives (66). Another explanation could be an impairment of autoregulation, with lower cerebral blood flow values in some white matter regions (19,60).

Increased blood viscosity caused by altered blood rheological factors might also contribute to a diffuse decrease in brain perfusion in patients with narrowed small arteries. Schneider et al. evaluated patients with Binswanger's disease, patients with lacunar infarcts and healthy controls for hemorrheological abnormalities (42). Patients with Binswanger's disease had a high frequency of increased erythrocyte aggregation, and of raised plasma viscosity (19 of 21 patients) and of raised fibrinogen concentrations. The abnormalities were present to a lesser degree in patients with small deep infarcts but not in controls (42). The most important determinants of whole blood viscosity are hematocrit and fibrinogen level (57). Occasionally, hyperglobulinemia, especially with macroglobulinemia, and severe hyperlipidemia also alter viscosity and flow. This hypothesis has not been well tested. If true, effective reduction of viscosity might reduce the likelihood of further white matter damage.

A few investigators have suggested that SAE in the elderly might be a late effect of antecedent edema (69), instead of ischemia or hypoxia. In this view, the leakage of fluid from the vascular system into the extracellular space might be a cause of interstitial damage. This leakage might occur particularly in the borderzones (66,70). The diffuse damage in SAE could thus be a late effect of cerebral edema, initiated by hypertension (69). Another suggestion is that the development of edema could be attributed to back pressure due to disturbances in the venous drainage (70).

OTHER CONDITIONS WITH BINSWANGER-LIKE WHITE MATTER LOW ATTENUATION ON CT

Alzheimer's Disease

Conflicting results have been published with respect to the frequency of white matter abnormalities in patients with Alzheimer's disease. George et al. (29) found WMLA on CT in 30% of a population of 151 patients with Alzheimer's disease, and this was significantly higher than in control subjects. In another study (38), WMLA was present in 31.9% of Alzheimer's patients, but only 10% had severe WMLA. Rezek (31) studied the severity of WMLA, and found more severe WMLA in patients with Alzheimer's disease than in age-matched controls, although the frequency was similar in both groups. Kertesz et al. (71) found moderate to severe WMHI in a higher frequency of Alzheimer's patients. In other studies, confluent or severe periventricular WMHI were found in only 10% of Alzheimer's patients, the proportion of which did not differ from that found in age-matched controls (72) or in healthy elderly subjects (50).

Brun and Englund (68) studied microscopical changes of the white matter in brains of 48 patients with dementia of Alzheimer type. Severe changes, present in 10 brains, appeared as pale areas on myelin stains extending from the periventricular region toward the cortex. These changes consisted of partial loss of axons, myelin sheaths and oligodendrocytes, with reactive astrocytic gliosis. White matter changes did not correlate topographically with Alzheimer's changes in the cortex (68). Fibrohyalinosis was found in the smallest arterioles of the white matter, but there was no evidence of hypertensive angiopathy. In contrast to this, brains from patients with multi-infarct dementia showed hypertensive angiopathy, and multiple infarcts in gray and white matter (68). Two CT studies have shown pallor of the white matter on myelin stains in brains of Alzheimer's patients with WMLA (31,73). The hypothesis that demyelination of the white matter is part of the process of Wallerian degeneration, secondary to Alzheimer's changes in the cortex of patients with dementia, is not very likely (22,43): firstly, demyelination is not more pronounced in white matter adjacent to cortical areas with a high number of senile plaques and neurofibrillary tangles (68); secondly, biochemical analysis of samples of demyelinated areas showed predominantly a reduction of cerebrosides, which is against a secondary, Wallerian-type of degeneration (74). Brun and Englund (68) proposed that the demyelination probably represented incomplete infarction as a result of small-vessel changes in deeper regions of the white matter.

Amyloid Angiopathy

Cerebral amyloid angiopathy (CAA) has also been associated with an SAE-like picture. Gray et al. (75) reported a series of 12 patients, 8 of whom had severe changes, and 7 of these 8 patients had a slowly progressive dementia and focal neurological deficits. Strokelike episodes were present in five patients, and CT scan showed bilateral WMLA in three patients. Pathological examination showed a diffuse hemorrhagic CAA, small cortical infarcts, and one or more lobar hematomas, predominantly in the occipital lobe, in all cases (10,75). Amyloid deposits were found in arterioles and capillaries of the leptomeninges and cerebral cortex, whereas the small arteries of the white matter showed only mild fibrohyalinosis. There was a homogenous or spotty myelin pallor of the centrum semiovale with sparing of the U-fibers (10), the lesions of the white matter being present in eight cases. WMHI on MR were recently reported in a series of patients with cerebral hemorrhage from hereditary amyloid angiopathy. The white matter lesions corresponded with incomplete infarction and demyelination on neuropathological examination (76). Amyloid angiopathy has thus been implicated as another cause of chronic hypoperfusion, particularly in the border zone between cortical medullary arteries and the long perforating arteries to the white matter (75,76).

A Familial Disorder with Leukoencephalopathy

A familial, autosomal-dominant occurrence of SAE has recently been reported (77–79). The patients were of middle age, and had episodes of sudden focal neurological deficits and dementia. Migraine attacks with headache, one-sided paresthesia, or blurring of vision were mentioned in a few members (77,79). Hypertension was uncommon in these families. Neurological examination showed bilateral pyramidal signs. Asymptomatic but affected patients within the family also had WMLA and WMHI with diffuse lesions of the white matter and focal lesions in the basal ganglia (79). Extensive cardiovascular and appropriate genetic investigations did not reveal an underlying cause (79). Some members of one family had a benign monoclonal gammopathy, and muscle biopsy showed sudanophilic lipids in muscle fibers, together with type I predominance and type II atrophy (77).

On pathological examination of the brain, vascular changes consisted of thickening and splitting of internal lamina, and fibrous proliferation of the vessel wall (78).

A nonamyloid eosinophilic deposit was found in the media of the thickened medullary arteries (80).

SAE and Vascular Dementia

There is a strong association between SAE and multiple infarcts. Patients with previous infarcts very often have WMLA and, conversely, brains of patients with Binswanger's disease usually show multiple infarcts in the white matter and basal ganglia. Cortical infarcts are occasionally reported in well-documented cases of Binswanger's disease. Huang (13) described seven cases with one or more cortical infarcts, and in these cases the white matter damage was separate from these infarcts. Patients with WMLA on CT also have an increased frequency of small deep or cortical infarcts. In the CT-postmortem study of Lotz et al. (61), cortical infarcts were found in 10 of 18 brains with mild to severe white matter changes (61). In a study of stroke patients with WMLA, van Swieten et al. found that patients with WMLA often had multiple infarcts (40%), but had fewer cortical infarcts (25%) (34). Both SAE and lacunar infarcts are expressions of a disease of small penetrating vessels. The presence of cortical infarcts may be explained by the coexistence of extracranial and intracranial large artery occlusive disease. Hypertension predisposes to both large artery atherosclerosis and microangiopathy, and some patients have both patterns of disease.

Multiple sequential infarcts tend to have a cumulative effect on cognitive function, which may lead to dementia. Tomlinson et al. (97) have related dementia to infarcts with a total volume exceeding 50 ml (81). Hachinski (98) introduced the term multi-infarct dementia in the 1970's and developed an ischemic score to distinguish this condition from Alzheimer's dementia. We believe, however, that multi-infarct dementia may not relate solely to infarct volume. We prefer to divide multi-infarct dementia into two groups: (a) a macroangiopathic group (large cortical and subcortical infarcts and/or hemorrhages) due to thrombosis, embolism, or intracerebral hemorrhage arising from disease of large extracranial and intracranial arteries; and (b) a microangiopathic group in which arteriolosclerosis gives rise to poor perfusion of the deep regions of the gray and white matter (lacunar infarcts and SAE).

Tatemichi (82) found dementia in 16% of stroke patients. An estimated 40% of this demented population had stroke as the most likely cause of dementia. In macroangiopathic multi-infarct dementia, there is little doubt that the infarct volume and number of infarcts are important factors in the development of dementia after stroke, although most patients with dementia have less than 50 ml volume of infarct (82–84). Dementia appears to be more frequent among patients with one or more cortical infarcts, particularly in the posterior part of the brain than in patients with lacunar infarcts in the basal ganglia, or infarcts in the cerebellum (82,85,86).

In macroangiopathic multi-infarct dementia, Loeb et al. have shown that small deep infarcts, particularly in the thalamus, increase the frequency of dementia in patients with cortical infarcts (83). The microangiopathic group includes patients with only multiple lacunar infarcts in the basal ganglia and white matter (*état lacunaire*). Some of these patients have cognitive impairment but without true dementia (86). In an autopsy study, patients with lacunar infarcts in the frontal white matter usually had small-stepped gait, dysarthria, urinary incontinence, loss of spontaneity, and mood changes (85). In another study of 40 brains with vascular lesions, lacunar state was a significant predictor of dementia (87).

Diffuse softening and demyelination of the periventricular white matter are always found in these patients with multiple lacunar infarcts (85), and appears to have an independent effect on cognitive functioning. In a discriminant analysis of 53 stroke patients (24 with and 29 without dementia), Liu et al. (84) found that total infarct area and total area of white matter lesions correlated independently with dementia.

The results of these studies imply that both lacunar state and diffuse white matter lesions contribute to microangiopathic multi-infarct dementia. Binswanger's disease and the lacunar state have similar clinical features, and the two conditions often coexist (85). It seems likely therefore that in the past, due to an infrequent use of whole brain slices stained for myelin (25), the two entities have frequently not been distinguished from each other.

Normal Pressure Hydrocephalus

Normal pressure hydrocephalus (NPH) is a condition characterized by dementia, gait ataxia, and urinary incontinence. Periventricular lucencies are frequently found on CT in patients with NPH (88). Improvement of the clinical picture secondary to shunting was correlated with a known cause (meningitis, subarachnoid hemorrhage), a short history, and the presence of periventricular lucencies. In a large retrospective multicenter study, Vanneste et al. (89) found that the idiopathic type of NPH (without a known cause) responded to shunting in only 15%. Shunting also had no or only a transient effect in a few patients with idiopathic NPH associated with hypertensive cerebrovascular disease (90,91). Pathological examination in these patients showed multiple lacunar infarcts in basal ganglia and cerebral white matter, and hypertensive vascular changes of the small arteries (90–92). This association of NPH and cerebrovascular disease is also supported by the study of Graff-Radford and Godersky, who showed a higher frequency of hypertension in patients with the idiopathic type of NPH compared with both a control group with dementia and the U.S. population of the same age (93).

In addition, ventriculomegaly is also strongly associated with Binswanger's disease. Enlarged ventricles and multiple lacunar infarcts were already reported in the original description and in most subsequent case reports of patients with Binswanger's disease. Several series of WMLA on CT and WMHI on MR showed ventriculomegaly (18,19,27,54). Bradley et al. (94) found a significant association between WMHI and clinically and radiologically confirmed NPH. Some patients with WMHI on MRI had not only enlarged ventricles, but also an increased cerebrospinal fluid (CSF) flow void in the cerebral aqueduct. Bradley et al. concluded that the two diseases were probably not independent processes, and showed a considerable overlap between WMHI and patients with NPH (94). Bradley et al. hypothesized that an increased flow void may help to select patients with NPH that will respond to shunting. The explanation most often proposed for ventriculomegaly in pathological and radiological studies of Binswanger's disease is that of an *ex vacuo* phenomenon caused by loss of tissue from lacunar infarction and diffuse demyelination. However, it has been suggested that an increase in the interstitial pressure in the brain due to NPH might lead to ischemia in the periventricular white matter, which, being a watershed area, would already be marginally supplied in the elderly (99). It is uncertain whether the increased flow void is the cause or the result of ventricular enlargement. If the former is the case, hypertension may cause increased CSF flow void and high pulsatile pressures within the ventricles, resulting in periventricular damage of the white matter. In addition, it may give rise to arteriolosclerosis, lacunar infarcts, dilated perivascular spaces, and demyelination. Studies of CSF flow void within the aqueduct in patients with hypertension and with normal blood pressure may elucidate this issue.

Hypertensive Encephalopathy

SAE in the elderly patients differs in several aspects from hypertensive encephalopathy (95,96). Episodes of malignant hypertension are not typically associated with SAE and have been mentioned in only one series of patients with WMLA (30). Secondly, white matter lesions in hypertensive encephalopathy usually disappear after regulation of blood pressure (96), whereas in SAE they are permanent. Finally, the lesions on CT or MR in hypertensive encephalopathy have been explained by a breakdown of autoregulation and extravasation of plasma into the white matter (95). This is in contrast with the idea of chronic ischemia in SAE in the elderly.

CONCLUSION

In conclusion, the recognition of WMLA and WMHI after the introduction of CT and MR has resulted in renewed interest in Binswanger's disease, which was until then considered a rare type of vascular dementia. Elderly patients frequently show WMLA on CT or WMHI on MR imaging of varying severity and extent. Advanced age, a history of hypertension, and one or more strokes are strongly associated with this imaging abnormality. Cognitive impairment often accompanies the white matter changes. There are strong similarities between the pathological features of SAE and multiple lacunar infarcts. SAE and the lacunar state may thus represent different types of a microangiopathic process that gives rise to insidious dementia. They frequently coexist, they are both associated with hypertensive disease of small arteries, and they have a similar clinical picture.

REFERENCES

1. Foix C, Hillemand P. Contributions a l'étude des ramollisements protuberentiels. *Rev Med* 1926;43:287–305.
2. Marie P. Des foyers lacunaires de desintégration et des differents autres états cavitaires du cerveau. *Rev Med (Paris)* 1901;21:281.
3. Fisher CM. Lacunes, small deep cerebral infarcts. *Neurology* 1965;15:774–784.
4. Binswanger O. Die Abgrenzung der allgemeinen progressiven Paralyse. *Berl Klin Wochenschr* 1894;49:1103–1105; 50:1137–1139; 52:1180–1186.
5. Alzheimer A. Neuere Arbeiten über die Dementia senilis und die auf atheromatoser Gefasserkrankung basierenden Gehirnerkrankungen. *Monatsschrift Psychiat Neur* 1898;3:101–115.
6. Olszewski J. Subcortical arteriosclerotic encephalopathy. *World Neurol* 1965;3:359–373.
7. Caplan LR, Schoene WC. Clinical features of subcortical arteriosclerotic encephalopathy (Binswanger disease). *Neurology* 1978;28:1206–1215.
8. Babikian V, Ropper AH. Binswanger's disease: a review. *Stroke* 1987;18:2–12.
9. Garcin R, Lapresle J, Lyon G. Encephalopathie sous-corticale chronique de Binswanger. Étude anatomique de trois observations. *Rev Neurol* 1960;102:423–439.
10. Dubas F, Gray F, Roullet E, Escourolle R. Leucoencéphalopathies artériopathiques. *Rev Neurol* 1985;41:93–108.
11. Mikol J. Maladie de Binswanger et formes apparantés. Contribution a l'étude des leucoencéphalopathies arteriosclereuses. *Rev Neurol* 1968;118:11–132.
12. Nissl F. Zr Kasuistik der arteriosklerotischen Demenz (Ein Fall von sog. "Encephalitis subcorticalis"). *Z Gesamten Neurol Psychiatr* 1920;19:438–443.
13. Huang K, Wu L, Luo Y. Binswanger's disease: progressive subcortical encephalopathy or multi-infarct dementia? *Can J Neurol Sci* 1985;12:88–94.
14. DeReuck J, Crevits L, Coster WD, Sieben G, VanderEecken HV. Pathogenesis of Binswanger chronic progressive subcortical encephalopathy. *Neurology* 1980;30:920–928.
15. Cole FM, Yates PO. Intracerebral microaneurysms and small cerebrovascular lesions. *Brain* 1968;90:759–769.
16. Rosenberg GA, Kornfeld M, Stovring J, Bicknell JM. Subcortical arteriosclerotic encephalopathy (Binswanger): computerized tomography. *Neurology* 1979;29:1102–1106.
17. Goto K, Ishii N, Fukasawa H. Diffuse white matter disease in geriatric population. *Radiology* 1981;141:39–48.
18. Gupta SR, Naheedy MH, Young JC, Ghobrial M, Rubino FA, Hindo W. Periventricular white matter changes and dementia. Clinical, neuropsychological, radiological and pathological correlation. *Arch Neurol* 1988;45:637–641.
19. Kinkel WR, Jacobs L, Polachini I, Bates V, Heffner RR. Subcortical arteriosclerotic encephalopathy (Binswanger's disease). CT, NMR and clinical correlations. *Arch Neurol* 1985;42:951–959.
20. George AE, de Leon MJ, Gentes CI, Miller, London E, Budzilovich. Leukoencephalopathy in normal and pathologic aging: 2. MRI of brain lucencies. *AJNR* 1986;7:567–570.
21. DeWitt LD, Kistler PH, Miller DC, Richardson EP, Buonanno FS. NMR-neuropathologic correlation in stroke. *Stroke* 1987;18:342–351.
22. Leiffer D, Buonanno FS, Richardson EP Jr. Clinicopathologic correlations of cranial magnetic resonance imaging of periventricular white matter. *Neurology* 1990;40:911–918.

23. Loizou LA, Jefferson JM, Smith WTH. Subcortical arteriosclerotic encephalopathy (Binswanger's type) and cortical infarcts in a young normotensive patient. *J Neurol Neurosurg Psychiatry* 1982;45:409–417.
24. Frederiksson K, Brun A, Gustafson L. Pure subcortical arteriosclerotic encephalopathy (Binswanger's disease). A clinicopathologic study. Part 1 clinical features. *Cerebrovasc Dis* 1992;2:82–86.
25. Brun A, Fredriksson K, Gustafson L. Pure subcortical arteriosclerotic encephalopathy (Binswanger's disease). A clinicopathologic study. Part 2 pathologic features. *Cerebrovasc Dis* 1992;2:87–92.
26. Zeumer H, Schonsky B, Sturm KW. Predominant white matter involvement in subcortical arteriosclerotic encephalopathy (Binswanger disease). *J Comput Assist Tomogr* 1980;4:14–19.
27. Loizou LA, Kendall BE, Marshall J. Subcortical arteriosclerotic encephalopathy: a clinical and radiological investigation. *J Neurol Neurosurg Psychiatry* 1981;44:294–304.
28. Bogousslavsky J, Regli F, Uske A. Leukoencephalopathy in patients with ischemic stroke. *Stroke* 1987;18:896–899.
29. George AE, de Leon MJ, Gentes CI, et al. Leukoencephalopathy in normal and pathological aging 1. CT of brain lucencies. *AJNR* 1986;7:561–566.
30. Valentine AR, Moseley IF, Kendall BE. White matter abnormality in cerebral atrophy: clinicoradiological correlations. *J Neurol Neurosurg Psychiatry* 1980;43:139–142.
31. Rezek DL, Morris JC, Fullnig KH, Gado MH. Periventricular white matter lucencies in senile dementia of Alzheimer type and in normal aging. *Neurology* 1987;37:1365–1368.
32. van Swieten JC, Hijdra A, Koudstaal PJ, van Gijn J. Grading white matter lesions on CT or MRI: a simple scale. *J Neurol Neurosurg Psychiatry* 1990;19:604–607.
33. Inzitari D, Giordano GP, Ancona AL, Pracucci G, Mascalchi M, Amaducci L. Leukoaraiosis, intracerebral hemorrhage and arterial hypertension. *Stroke* 1990;21:1419–1423.
34. van Swieten JC, Kappelle LJ, Algra A, van Latum JC, Koudstaal PJ, van Gijn J. Hypodensity of the cerebral white matter on CT in patients with TIA or minor stroke: influence on the rate of subsequent stroke. *Ann Neurol* 1992;32:177–183.
35. Inzitari D, Diaz F, Fox A, et al. Vascular risk factors and leuko-araiosis. *Arch Neurol* 1987;44:42–47.
36. Toghi H, Chiba K, Kimura M. Twenty-four-hour variation of blood pressure in vascular dementia of the Binswanger type. *Stroke* 1991;22:603–608.
37. Derix MMA, Hijdra A, Verbeeten BWJ. Mental changes in subcortical arteriosclerotic encephalopathy. *Clin Neurol Neurosurg* 1987;89:71–78.
38. Steingart A, Hachinski VC, Lau C, Fox AJ, Fox H, Lee D. Cognitive and neurologic findings in demented patients with white matter lucencies on computed tomographic scan (Leuko-araiosis). *Arch Neurol* 1987;44:36–39.
39. Steingart A, Hachinski VC, Lau C, Fox AJ, Diaz F, Cape R. Cognitive and neurologic findings in subjects with diffuse white matter lucencies on computed tomographic scan (Leuko-araiosis). *Arch Neurol* 1987;44:32–35.
40. Masdeu JC, Wolfson L, Lantos G, Tobin JN, Grober E, Whipple R, Amerman P. Brain whitematter changes in the elderly prone to falling. *Arch Neurol* 1989;46:1292–1296.
41. Hijdra A, Verbeeten B, Verhulst JAPM. Relation of leukoaraiosis to lesion type in stroke patients. *Stroke* 1990;21:890–894.
42. Schneider R, Ringelstein EB, Zeumer H, Kiesewetter H, Jung F. The role of plasma hyperviscosity in subcortical arteriosclerotic encephalopathy (Binswanger's disease). *J Neurol* 1987;234:67–73.
43. Kawamura J, Meyer JS, Terayama Y, Weathers S. Leukoaraiosis correlates with cerebral hypoperfusion in vascular dementia. *Stroke* 1991;22:609–614.
44. Yao H, Sadoshima S, Kuwabara Y, Ichiya Y, Fujishima M. Cerebral blood flow and oxygen metabolism in patients with vascular dementia of the Binswanger type. *Stroke* 1990;21:1694–1699.
45. DeReuck J, Van Aken J, Decoo D, Strijckmans K, Lemahieu I. Cerebral blood flow and oxygen metabolism in leuko-araiosis. *Cerebrovasc Dis* 1991;1:25–30.
46. Erkinjuntti T, Ketonen L, Sulkava R. Do white matter changes on MRI differentiate vascular dementia from Alzheimer's disease? *J Neurol Neurosurg Psychiatry* 1987;50:37–42.
47. Gerard G, Weisberg LA. MRI periventricular lesions in adults. *Neurology* 1986;36:998–1001.
48. Awad IA, Spetzler RF, Hodak JA, Awad CA, Carey R. Incidental subcortical lesions identified on magnetic resonance imaging in the elderly. 1. Correlation with age and cerebrovascular risk factors. *Stroke* 1986;17:1084–1089.
49. Hershey LA, Modic MT, Greenough PG, Jaffe DF. Magnetic resonance imaging in vascular dementia. *Neurology* 1987;37:29–36.
50. Hunt AL, Orrison WW, Yeo RA, et al. Clinical significance of MRI white matter lesions in the elderly. *Neurology* 1989;39:1470–1474.
51. Fukuda H, Kobayashi S, Okada K, Tsunematsu T. Frontal white matter lesions and dementia in lacunar infarction. *Stroke* 1990;21:1143–1149.
52. Jungue C, Pujol J, Vendrell P, et al. Leukoaraiosis on magnetic resonance imaging and speed of mental processing. *Arch Neurol* 1990;47:151–156.
53. Lechner H, Schmidt R, Bertha G, Justich E, Offenbacher H, Schneider G. Nuclear magnetic resonance imaging: white matter lesions and risk factors for stroke in normal individuals. *Stroke* 1988;19:263–265.
54. Kertesz A, Black SE, Tokar G, Benke TH, Carr T, Nicholson L. Periventricular and subcortical hyperintensities on magnetic resonance imag-

ing. Rims, caps and unidentified bright objects. *Arch Neurol* 1988;45:404–408.
55. van Swieten JC, Geyskes GG, Derix MMA, Ramos LMP, van Latum JC, van Gijn J. Hypertension in the elderly is associated with diffuse lesions of the cerebral white matter and with cognitive decline. *Ann Neurol* 1991;30:825–830.
56. Fazekas F, Niederkorn K, Schmidt R, et al. White matter signal abnormalities in normal individuals: correlation with carotid ultrasonography, cerebral blood flow measurements, and cerebrovascular risk factors. *Stroke* 1988;19:1285–1288.
57. Breteler MMB, van Swieten JC, Bots ML, et al. Cerebral white matter lesions, vascular risk factors and cognitive function: the Rotterdam Elderly Study. (submitted for publication).
58. Tanaka Y, Tanaka O, Mizuno Y, Yoshida M. A radiologic study of dynamic processes in lacunar dementia. *Stroke* 1989;20:1488–1493.
59. De Cristofaro MR, Mascalchi M, Pupi A, et al. Subcortical arteriosclerotic encephalopathy: single photon emission computed tomography-magnetic resonance imaging correlation. *Am J Phys Imaging* 1990;5:68–74.
60. Kobari M, Meyer JS, Ichijo M. Leuko-araiosis, cerebral atrophy, and cerebral perfusion in normal aging. *Arch Neurol* 1990;47:161–165.
61. Lotz PR, Ballinger WE, Quisling RG. Subcortical arteriosclerotic encephalopathy: CT spectrum and correlation. *Am J Neuroradiol* 1986;7:817–822.
62. Furuta A, Ishii N, Nishihara Y, Horie A. Medullary arteries in aging and dementia. *Stroke* 1991;22:442–446.
63. Revész T, Hawkins CP, Du Boulay EPGH, Barnard RO, McDonald WI. Pathological findings correlated with magnetic resonance imaging in subcortical arteriosclerotic encephalopathy (Binswanger's disease). *J Neurol Neurosurg Psychiatry* 1989;52:1337–1344.
64. van Swieten JC, van den Hout JHW, van Ketel BA, Hijdra A, Wokke JHJ, van Gijn J. Periventricular lesions in the white matter on magnetic resonance imaging in the elderly. *Brain* 1991;114:761–774.
65. Yamanouchi H, Sugiara S, Tomonaga M. Decrease in nerve fibres in cerebral white matter in progressive subcortical vascular encephalopathy of Binswanger type. *J Neurol* 1989; 236:382–387.
66. Yamanouchi H, Sugiura S, Shimada H. Loss of nerve fibres in the corpus callosum of progressive subcortical vascular encephalopathy. *J Neurol* 1990;237:39–41.
67. Okeda R. Morphometrische Vergleichunsuntersuchungen an Hirnarterien bei Binswangerscher Encephalopathie und Hochdruckencephalopathie. *Acta Neuropathologica* 1973;26:23–43.
68. Brun A, Englund E. A white matter disorder in dementia of the Alzheimer type: a pathoanatomical study. *Ann Neurol* 1986;19:253–262.
69. Feigin I, Popoff N. Neuropathological changes late in cerebral edemea: the relationship to trauma, hypertensive disease, and Binswanger's encephalopathy. *J Neuropathol Exp Neurol* 1963;22:500–511.
70. Poppe W, Tennstedt A. Ein Beitrag zur Encephalopathia subcorticalis Binswanger. *Psychiat Neurol* 1963;145:27–35.
71. Kertesz A, Polk M, Carr T. Cognition and white matter changes on magnetic resonance imaging in dementia. *Arch Neurol* 1990;47:387–391.
72. Kozachuk WE, DeCarli CH, Schapiro MB, Wagner EE, Rapoport SI, Horwitz B. White matter hyperintensities in dementia of Alzheimer's type and in healthy subjects without cerebrovascular risk factors. *Arch Neurol* 1990;47:1306–1310.
73. Janota I, Mirsen THR, Hachinski VC, Lee DH, Merskey H. Neuropathologic correlates of leuko-araiosis. *Arch Neurol* 1989;46:1124–1128.
74. Englund E, Brun A, Alling C. White matter changes in dementia of Alzheimer's type. *Brain* 1988;111:1425–1439.
75. Gray F, Roullet E, Escourolle R. Leukoencephalopathy in diffuse hemorrhagic cerebral amyloid angiopathy. *Ann Neurol* 1985;18:54–59.
76. Haan J, Roos RAC, Algra PR, Lanser JBK, Bots GTAM, Vegter-Van der Vlis M. Hereditary cerebral hemorrhage with amyloidosis-Dutch type. Magnetic resonance imaging in 7 cases. *Brain* 1990;113:1251–1268.
77. Tournier-Lasserve E, Iba-Zizen M-Th, Romero N, Bousser M-G. Autosomal dominant syndrome with strokelike episodes and leukoencephalopathy. *Stroke* 1991;22:1297–1302.
78. Davous P, Fallet-Bianco C. Démence sous-corticale familiale avec leucoencéphalopathie. Observation clinico-pathologique. *Rev Neurol* 1991;147:376–384.
79. Mas JL, Dilouya A, de Recondo J. A familial disorder with subcortical ischemic strokes, dementia, and leukoencephalopathy. *Neurology* 1992;42:1015–1019.
80. Baudrimont M, Tournier-Lasserve E, Dubas F, Bousser M-G. Mendelian ischemic stroke and leukencephalopathy: pathologic data. *Cerebrovasc Dis* 1992;2:195.
81. Tomlinson BE, Blessed G, Roth M. Observation on the brains of demented old people. *J Neurol Sci* 1970;11:205–242.
82. Tatemichi THK, Foulkes MA, Mohr JP, et al. Dementia in stroke survivors in the Stroke Data Bank cohort. Prevalence, incidence, risk factors, and computed tomographic findings. *Stroke* 1990;21:858–866.
83. Loeb C, Gandolfo C, Bino G. Intellectual impairment and cerebral lesions in multiple cerebral infarcts. A clinical-computed tomography study. *Stroke* 1988;19:560–565.
84. Liu CK, Miller BL, Cummings JL, et al. A quantitative MRI study of vascular dementia. *Neurology* 1992;42:138–143.
85. Ishii N, Nishihara Y, Imamura T. Why do frontal lobe symptoms predominate in vascular dementia with lacunes? *Neurology* 1986;36:340–345.
86. Babikian VL, Wolfe N, Linn R, Knoefel JE, Al-

bert ML. Cognitive changes in patients with multiple cerebral infarcts. *Stroke* 1990;21:1013–1018.
87. del Ser T, Bermejo F, Portera A, Arredondo JM, Bouras C, Constantinidis J. Vascular dementia. *J Neurol Sci* 1990;96;1–17.
88. Thomsen AM, Borgesen SE, Bruhn P, Gjerris F. Prognosis of dementia in normal-pressure hydrocephalus after a shunt procedure. *Ann Neurol* 1986;20:304–310.
89. Vanneste J, Augustijn P, Dirven C, Tan WF, Goedhart ZD. Shunting normal-pressure hydrocephalus: do the benefits outweigh the risks? *Neurology* 1992;42:54–59.
90. Earnest MP, Fahn S, Karp JH, Rowland LP. Normal pressure hydrocephalus and hypertensive cerebrovascular disease. *Arch Neurol* 1974;31:262–266.
91. Koto A, Rosenberg G, Zingeser LH, Horoupian D, Katzman R. Syndrome of normal pressure hydrocephalus: a possible relation to hypertensive and arteriosclerotic vasculopathy. *J Neurol Neurosurg Psychiatr* 1977;40:73–79.
92. Shukla D, Singh B, Strobos RJ. Hypertensive cerebrovascular disease and normal pressure hydrocephalus. *Neurology* 1980;30:998–1000.
93. Graff-Radford NR, Godersky JC. Idiopathic normal pressure hydrocephalus and systemic hypertension. *Neurology* 1987;37:868–871.
94. Bradley WG, Whittemore AR, Watanabe AS, Davis SJ, Teresi LM, Homyak M. Association of deep white matter infarction with chronic communicating hydrocephalus: implications regarding the possible origin of normal-pressure hydrocephalus. *AJNR* 191;12:31–39.
95. Chester EM, Agamanolis DP, Banker BQ, Victor M. Hypertensive encephalopathy: a clinicopathologic study of 20 cases. *Neurology* 1978;28:928–939.
96. Hauser RA, Lacey M, Knight MR. Hypertensive encephalopathy. Magnetic resonance imaging demonstration of reversible cortical and white matter lesions. *Arch Neurol* 1988;45:1078–1083.
97. Fisher CM. Dementia in cerebrovascular disease. In: Toole JG, Siekert R, Whisnant J, eds. *Cerebral vascular disease. Sixth Princeton Conference.* New York: Grune & Stratton; 1968:232–236.
98. Hachinski VC. Multi-infarct dementia. A cause of mental deterioration in the elderly. *Lancet* 1974;1:207–209.
99. Román GC. White matter lesions and normal-pressure hydrocephalus: Binswanger disease or Hakim procedure? *AJNR* 1991;12:40–41.

12

Incidence, Natural History, and Risk Factors in Lacunar Infarction

Jan Lodder and Jelis Boiten

Department of Neurology, University Hospital Maastricht, NL-6202 AZ Maastricht, The Netherlands

Despite the fact that lacunar infarcts make up approximately 20–25% of all ischemic strokes (1–6), a discussion of epidemiology is lacking in most reviews. This reflects the paucity of adequate data (7–10). Malmgren et al. (11) found that only 9 of 63 stroke epidemiological studies met at least five basic epidemiological criteria. Only one of these studies classified stroke into subtypes: infarction, primary intracerebral hemorrhage, and subarachnoid hemorrhage. Further subdivision of cerebral infarcts was only pursued in one study, the Oxfordshire Community Stroke Project, from which emerged the first natural history study of lacunar stroke (4). After clinical researchers became more aware of the importance of distinguishing lacunar infarcts from other brain infarcts, several incidence and natural history studies were initiated. However, only a few of these studies meet strict epidemiological criteria (4,6). The other studies suffered from referral bias because they were hospital based (2, 5,12–14). Although the Rochester stroke study was selected by Malmgren et al. from among studies that met basic methodological criteria (11), the change that occurred in the definition of lacunar infarction adversely affected this partially retrospective study on lacunar infarcts.

Apart from the above-mentioned methodological difficulties, the variability of the definition of a lacunar infarct makes comparison of different studies difficult. Ideally, only first-ever lacunar infarcts should be included in epidemiological studies because recurrent strokes have different characteristics (15). In addition, for epidemiological purposes, lacunar infarct patients should not be selected by the presence of a small deep lesion on computed tomography (CT) because this will underestimate the rate of lacunar infarction. [Approximately 40% of scans remain negative in patients with lacunar infarcts (16).] Although magnetic resonance imaging (MRI) is likely to improve detection of lacunar infarcts, it also often detects multiple small lesions that may be difficult to differentiate from lacunar infarcts (17,18). In addition, MRI is not yet available for the routine study of all stroke patients. For these reasons, patient selection for epidemiological purposes should be based on clinical rather than radiological parameters. This means that the signs and symptoms should match one of the classical lacunar syndromes: pure motor stroke, sensorimotor stroke, pure sensory stroke, dysarthria–clumsy hand syndrome, or ataxic hemiparesis. CT or MR findings should be compatible with lacunar infarction (4,19).

Patient inclusion by clinical presentation is justified because lacunar syndromes accurately predict lacunar infarction. Clinical features alone give a positive predictive value of approximately 90% (4,19,20), and a negative predictive value of 97% (17). This means that a patient presenting with a lacunar syndrome has a 90% chance of having a lacunar infarct, whereas without such a syndrome there is a 97% chance that the symptoms are caused by something other than a lacunar infarct. Pure motor monoparesis should not be included as a lacunar syndrome, because it is more likely to be associated with a small cortical lesion (21). The exclusion of patients from lacunar infarct series because they have a cardioembolic source or a high-grade carotid stenosis seems unjustified (5,13). Such features are uncommon causes of lacunar infarcts (see below) and might merely be fortuitous findings reflecting more generalized atherosclerosis (22).

Most studies on lacunar infarct incidence rates suffer from one of the above described methodological shortcomings. Only two studies presenting lacunar infarct incidence rates were population based, with a high rate of case ascertainment, used the above described clinical criteria for patient inclusion, and did not exclude CT-negative cases or those with a potential cardiac or carotid source of embolism. These studies are the Oxfordshire Community Stroke Project (OCSP) (4,23,24) and the Italian SEPIVAC study (6). The OCSP found a crude annual incidence rate of lacunar infarction of 33/100,000 and of 160/100,000 for all types of first-ever strokes (21%). The SEPIVAC study found an annual incidence rate of 52.8/100,000, this being 24% of the annual first-ever stroke incidence of 220/100,000. Both OCSP and SEPIVAC figures for lacunar infarction are higher than the age- and sex-adjusted average annual incidence rate of lacunar infarction of 13.4/100,000 infarction in the Mayo Clinic series, which accounted for only 12% of all first brain infarcts (25). This difference reflects the above-mentioned exclusion of CT-negative cases in the study of Sacco et al., and the inclusion of patients with sensorimotor stroke only during the latter part of the study (25).

NATURAL HISTORY OF LACUNAR INFARCTS

It is generally assumed that the prognosis of a lacunar infarct is more favorable than that of cortical infarcts. If this is true, this would suggest that lacunar infarcts have a different natural history and would suggest a need to tailor measures to prevent stroke recurrences differently. A study of the natural history of lacunar infarcts is therefore important. It would establish the relative contribution of different factors to the risk of lacunar stroke. It could also facilitate specific preventive strategies and might increase our insight into the underlying pathophysiology of lacunar infarction and help determine whether small and large vessel vasculopathy are different entities. It is also important to study the type of a recurrent stroke to see whether recurrent strokes are of the same subtype as the initial stroke.

Natural history studies are scarce, and in virtually all of them patients received treatment. It might thus be more appropriate to speak of prognosis rather than natural history. Moreover, few studies meet basic methodological criteria for studying lacunar infarct series as described in the foregoing section. Table 1 shows the percentage of patients with recurrent stroke, the percentage surviving up to 1 year, and the percentage functionally independent at 1 year estimated from the literature. Differences between the studies may be accounted for by differences in patient selection, and in the proportion of patients that were followed up to 1 year.

During their 1975–1984 study period, Sacco et al. (25) found a cumulative probability of recurrent stroke in patients with lacunar infarcts of 4% at 1 month, and 10% at 1 year. For nonlacunar infarcts, the rates

TABLE 1. *Percentage of recurrent stroke, patients surviving, and those independent after lacunar (LACI) or cortical (CORTI) infarct.*

Study	% recurrent stroke				% surviving				% independent at one year	
	LACI		CORTI		LACI		CORTI			
	30 d	1 yr	30 d	1 yr	30 d	1 yr	30 d	1 yr	LACI	CORTI
Sacco (25)	4	10	2	8	100	97	86	72		
Hier (26)	2	12[b]	4	12[b]						
Bamford (4,23,24)	1	12	4	16	99	90	87	73	66	46
Boiten (30)	0	5	0	2	98	85	88	72	83[c]	46[c]
Landi (29)		8		11	100	91[a]	85	66[a]		
Norrving (27)					99	90				
Jamrozik (28)					100					

[a], survival at 2 years; [b], recurrent stroke at 2 years; [c], independent at 3–6 months

were 2% and 8%, which was not significantly different. The 5-year actuarial survival, free of stroke recurrence was 26% for lacunar and 27% for nonlacunar infarcts. Survival after a lacunar infarct was 100% at 30 days, 97% at 1 year, and 75% at 5 years, whereas these figures were 86%, 72%, and 45% for nonlacunar infarcts. The differences in late survival were thus partially due to a worse early survival in the nonlacunar stroke group. These data however, should be interpreted with caution, because of problems with the definition of a lacunar infarct in this study. The same problems of definition apply to the study of Hier et al., who found a similar 2-year cumulative stroke recurrence rate for both lacunar and nonlacunar infarcts in the Stroke Data Bank (26). Hier et al. (26) found most of the recurrent strokes to be of the same subtype as the index stroke, suggesting different, underlying types of vascular pathology.

Others have also found a lower early mortality rate in lacunar stroke patients (4,27–30). The OCSP provided data on both early (30 days) and late (1 year) survival and handicap (4). The case fatality rate was 2% at 1 month and 11% at 1 year for lacunar infarcts. These figures were more favorable than for nonlacunar infarcts, although there were significant differences among different subgroups in the latter stroke type (24). The same applies to the degree of handicap in the OCSP: 62% of the lacunar stroke patients were independent at day 30, and 60% at 1 year. No attempt was made in this study to identify the type of recurrent stroke.

Boiten and Lodder, in a hospital-based series, compared 103 lacunar infarct patients with 94 patients with cortical infarcts most likely due to large vessel thromboembolism, and found a 1-month case fatality rate of 2% in the lacunar and 12% in the cortical group (30). The more favorable 1-year survival in the lacunar group of 85% compared with 72% in the cortical group, was related to the worse 30-day survival in the latter group. The 1-year cumulative risk of recurrent stroke was 5% in the lacunar and 2% in the cortical infarct groups. This favorable recurrent stroke risk in the cortical group compared with other series is most likely due to the exclusion of patients with a cardioembolic type of brain infarct in the cortical group. Six of the seven recurrences in the lacunar stroke group were lacunar again. This concurs with the findings of Hier et al. (26) and argues in favor of a small vessel vasculopathy, which is distinct from large vessel disease, to be the cause of lacunar infarction. After approximately 6 months, 83% of the lacunar stroke survivors in the study of Boiten and Lodder were functionally independent, which was higher than in the cortical group (46%) (30).

Because of the low number of recurrent strokes, our study did not aim to identify independent predictors of either stroke recurrence, degree of handicap, or death.

Using a proportional hazards survival model, Brainin et al. found that age and diabetes increased the risk of death in lacunar infarct patients (31). Landi et al. found a zero 1-month cumulative case fatality rate in 88 lacunar infarcts compared with a rate of 15% in 103 nonlacunar infarcts (29). After a mean follow-up of 28 months, these figures increased to 9% and 34%, or 9% and 20% if deaths only later than 1 month were considered. This difference with the data of Boiten and Lodder (30) might be due to the exclusion of cardioembolic stroke in the latter study. The 1-year probability of stroke recurrence in the study of Landi et al. was 7.9% for lacunar and 11.4% for nonlacunar stroke (29). In a multivariate regression analysis, age, prior transient ischemic attacks (TIA), and nonlacunar stroke were found to be independent risk factors for major vascular events such as stroke or myocardial infarction (29).

In summary, most studies have shown a more favorable early and late stroke recurrence rate in lacunar compared with nonlacunar stroke, and the same is true for survival, although this is less consistent between studies, probably due to differences in study design. Besides, comparison with nonlacunar brain infarcts is difficult because these infarcts constitute a heterogeneous group containing distinct prognostic subgroups.

Future follow-up studies on lacunar infarcts should try to identify independent predictors of different measures of stroke outcome, such as degree of handicap, recurrent stroke, and cause of vascular or other death. It is also important to identify the type of recurrent stroke. Point estimates should be made at least at 1 month and at 1 year after stroke. Nonlacunar stroke control groups need to be uniformly characterized to allow comparison between different studies. Only if these requirements are met will we be able to assess the response to the management of different risk factors or to carotid endarterectomy or anticoagulant treatment of lacunar stroke patients.

RISK FACTORS FOR LACUNAR INFARCTION INTRODUCTION

Comparison of risk factor profiles between lacunar and other infarct subtypes could provide insight into differences in the underlying vascular pathology and might lead to more rational stroke treatment and prevention. It could also aid in the prevention of lacunar stroke–related cognitive decline. Some risk factors for stroke are more definitely established (e.g., hypertension, diabetes mellitus, cigarette smoking, TIA) than others (e.g., increased serum lipids, obesity) (32,33). The known risk factors account for only a part of the risk of stroke, because some stroke victims do not have any risk factors. Future studies should aim to identify new vascular risk factors. There are several studies on risk factors in lacunar

TABLE 2. *Risk factors for lacunar infarction*

Established
Age and sex
Hypertension
Diabetes mellitus
Ischemic heart disease
Transient ischemic attack
Cigarette smoking
Unlikely
Emboligenic cardiac disease
Carotid stenosis
Possible
Hyperlipidemia
Alcohol abuse
Elevated fibrinogen level
Increased hematocrit
Lower limb claudication
Of further interest
Heredo-familial
Race
Environment
Life-style
Diet
Unknown

infarction but many are rather small or retrospective. Here we will discuss only the larger, well-defined studies, particularly those that compared lacunar with nonlacunar infarct patients. We also indicate which factors might be worthwhile studying in the future (Table 2).

ESTABLISHED RISK FACTORS FOR LACUNAR INFARCTION

Age and Sex

Age is an important risk factor for lacunar infarction. The mean age of patients suffering from lacunar infarction ranged widely from 58 to 72 years in various studies (4,12,16,20,25,27,34–37), but a population-based study showed that the incidence rate of lacunar infarction increases with age (4). In most studies men were more often affected than women (16,20,27,34–38), but not in all (4,12,16,39).

Hypertension

Hypertension has often been considered as a specific risk factor for lacunar infarction, but recently its role has been called into question (Table 3). In Fisher's study all but three of 114 cases with one or more lacunar infarcts at autopsy had documented hypertension (40). As a result of this, Fisher concluded that lacunar infarcts were directly related to hypertension. Recently, he assessed that 80 to 90% of lacunar infarcts were associated with hypertension (7,41). However, in a retrospective study of 2,859 autopsies, Tuszynski et al. found that 169 (6%) had lacunar infarctions, and 64% of these had a history of hypertension (42). Fisher's series showed a much higher frequency of hypertension (97%) (40). The difference between this and Fisher's pathological series relates to differences in the definition of hypertension. Fisher's definition of hypertension was a blood pressure greater than 140/90 mm Hg (7,40,41), and Tuszynski et al.'s was greater than 160/95 mm Hg (42). Another autopsy study of 1,086 cases, of which 532 (49%) had one or more lacunes, showed that cases that were hypertensive (>160/95 mm Hg) or borderline hypertensive (>140/90 and <160/95 mm Hg) had more lacunar infarcts than normotensive ones. Diastolic hypertension was more strongly related to the number of lacunar infarcts than systolic hypertension (43).

A substantial number of clinical studies addressed the issue of hypertension in la-

TABLE 3. *Clinical studies comparing the frequency of hypertension between lacunar and nonlacunar infarcts.*

		Lacunar infarct			Nonlacunar infarct					
			Hypertension			Hypertension				
	Definition	N	No	(%)	N	No	(%)	OR;	95% CI	p-value
Tegeler (59)	?	55	33	(60)	54	30	(56)	1.20;	0.56–2.57	NS
Loeb (53)	a	154	116	(75)	111	66	(59)	2.08;	1.22–3.53	<0.01
					*154	54	(35)	5.65;	3.45–9.26	<0.001
Boiten (16)	b,c	103	51	(50)	94	35	(37)	1.65;	0.94–2.91	NS
Lodder (44)	c	102	45	(44)	202	95	(47)	0.89;	0.55–1.43	NS
Gandolfo (34)	b,c	108	70	(65)	*216	63	(30)	4.47;	2.74–7.32	<0.001
Norrving (35)	b,c	61	32	(53)	61	27	(44)	1.39;	0.68–2.83	NS
Pullicino (82)	?	42	24	(57)	122	52	(43)	1.80;	0.88–3.65	NS

*Control subjects without cerebral infarction.
Definition of hypertension: a, > 160/95 mm Hg; b, antihypertensive treatment; c, > 160/90 mm Hg.
OR, odds ratio; CI, confidence interval.

cunar infarction. However, many of these studies differ in study design and in the definition of hypertension. In studying the relationship of hypertension to lacunar infarction, it is important both to look for interactions between hypertension and other risk factors, as well as to make comparison with nonlacunar brain infarcts. In order to make inferences about the underlying vascular pathology, lacunar infarcts should preferably be compared with infarcts related to large vessel disease, whereas cortical infarcts caused by cardiogenic embolism should be excluded, as was done in the study of Boiten and Lodder (16).

Data from different studies of lacunar and small deep infarcts in hypertension are shown in Table 3. Comparison between lacunar and nonlacunar brain infarct groups showed no significant differences in the frequency of hypertension in the majority of studies. Several parameters of hypertension were studied by Lodder et al. in the OCSP study: the maximum systolic and diastolic blood pressure prior to stroke, the last family doctor's blood pressure measurement prior to stroke, the blood pressure at stroke onset and the presence of left ventricular hypertrophy. None of these parameters differed between lacunar and cortical infarcts (44). In summary, hypertension is an important risk factor for lacunar infarction, but many patients with lacunar infarction do not have hypertension. There is also no evidence that it is a specific risk factor for lacunar stroke. This conclusion is derived both from population-based (44) and from hospital-based (16) studies.

We have recently suggested (45) that the different frequencies of hypertension in various pathological and clinical studies of lacunar infarction may be due to different numbers of patients with lipohyalinosis and with microatheroma as a cause of their infarcts. These are two different pathological causes of lacunar stroke that were distinguished by Fisher (7,46,47). Hypertension is a risk factor for both of these pathologies, but lipohyalinosis is mainly found in hypertensive patients with small, multiple, and usually asymptomatic lacunar infarcts, and microatheroma mainly gives rise to larger, usually single, symptomatic lacunar infarcts. About 80% of the lacunar infarcts in the pathological study of Fisher (40) were asymptomatic and were probably caused by lipohyalinosis and consequently strongly related to hypertension. The symptomatic lacunar infarcts in clinical studies are more likely to be related to microatheroma, which, like large vessel atherosclerosis, is less strongly related to hypertension. Blood pressure values in patients with lipohyalinosis may be higher but may be diluted by patients with other causes of lacunar infarct. Further studies are needed to confirm or reject this hypothesis.

In conclusion, hypertension is an important and treatable, but rather nonspecific, risk factor for lacunar infarction. It may well be a highly specific risk factor for lacunar infarcts caused by lipohyalinosis. The risk of lacunar infarction may be related to the height of the blood pressure levels as has been found with all types of infarctions combined (48,49). It is thus important to treat hypertension, especially marked hypertension, in patients with lacunar infarcts. This should not only prevent recurrent stroke but is also likely to slow development and progression of subcortical arteriosclerotic encephalopathy (see Chapter 11).

Diabetes Mellitus

Diabetes mellitus is a major risk factor for stroke. It can cause small vessel arteriopathy, especially in the retina and kidney, and might therefore be a risk factor for cerebral small vessel disease and lacunar infarction (Table 4).

Fisher found diabetes mellitus in only 11% of his pathological cases. The number of lacunar infarcts was approximately the same in diabetic as in nondiabetic persons

TABLE 4. Clinical studies comparing the frequency of diabetes mellitus between lacunar and nonlacunar infarcts.

		Lacunar infarct			Nonlacunar infarct					
			Diabetes			Diabetes				
	Definition	N	No	(%)	N	No	(%)	OR;	95% CI	p-value
Tegeler (59)	?	55	19	(35)	54	16	(30)	1.25;	0.56–2.81	NS
Loeb (53)	?	154	38	(25)	111	28	(25)	1.01;	0.57–1.76	NS
					*154	20	(13)	2.27;	1.26–4.12	<0.01
Boiten (16)	a,b	103	28	(27)	94	25	(26)	1.03;	0.55–1.93	NS
Lodder (44)	?	102	13	(13)	202	19	(9)	1.41;	0.66–2.98	NS
Gandolfo (34)	a,c	108	23	(21)	*216	24	(11)	2.17;	1.16–4.05	<0.025
Norrving (35)	?	61	5	(8)	61	6	(10)	0.82;	0.24–2.84	NS
Pullicino (82)	?	42	1	(2)	122	7	(6)	0.40;	0.05–3.36	NS

*Control subjects without cerebral infarction.
Definition of diabetes mellitus: a, treated with diet or medication, or both; b, two or more fasting serum glucose levels ≥ 6 mmol/l; c, two glucose levels ± 110 mg%.
OR, odds ratio; CI, confidence interval.

(40). This led Fisher to conclude that cerebral small vessel disease is usually not related to diabetes mellitus. However, in the autopsy study of Tuszynski et al., 34% of the cases had diabetes mellitus, suggesting that diabetes could be a risk factor for lacunar infarcts (42). Table 4 shows the incidence of diabetes mellitus in various clinical CT studies comparing lacunar and small deep infarcts with nonlacunar infarcts. The definition of diabetes varied, and was not stated in some studies. In two prospective clinical studies, one of which was population based, the incidence of diabetes mellitus did not differ between patients with lacunar and nonlacunar infarction (16,44). Since diabetes mellitus is an important risk factor for cerebral infarction in general, it is likely to be a risk factor for lacunar infarction as well. Diabetes is commonly associated with other risk factors, particularly hypertension (32). Due to possible interactions between diabetes and other risk factors, the risk associated with a combination of two factors may be more significant than that associated with diabetes alone (50). The association of hypertension and diabetes mellitus has been reported in 20% of lacunar infarct patients, but no comparison was made with nonlacunar infarcts (37).

Fifteen percent of the lacunar infarct patients in our study had diabetes mellitus associated with hypertension, which, however, did not differ from the incidence in nonlacunar infarction [10%, odds ratio (OR) 1.61; 95% confidence interval (CI) 0.67–3.87] (16). Pullicino et al. did not find a synergistic effect between hypertension and diabetes on the incidence of small deep infarcts (51).

Ischemic Heart Disease

Ischemic (coronary) heart disease is a risk factor for stroke (32,52), and a major cause of death among stroke survivors (32). Eight to forty-seven percent of lacunar infarct patients have a history of ischemic heart disease (Table 5). A history of ischemic heart disease was more frequent among patients with lacunar infarction than control subjects without cerebral infarction (34,53). However, no difference was found on comparison between lacunar and nonlacunar infarct patients in two prospective studies, suggesting that ischemic heart disease is a risk factor for lacunar infarction in the same way as for other types of cerebral infarction (16,44).

TABLE 5. *The frequency of different types of vascular risk factors in lacunar infarct patients.*

	Number of patients	Ischemic heart disease		Previous TIA		Smoking	
		No	(%)	No	(%)	No	(%)
Mohr (1)	131			30	(23)		
Foulkes (39)	337	67	(20)[a]	44	(13)		
Norrving (27)	180	31	(17)[a]	29	(16)	51	(28)
Tegeler (59)	55			4	(7)	21	(38)
Ghika (36)	100					33	(33)
Arboix (37)	227	58	(26)[b]	40	(18)		
Loeb (53)	154	25	(16)	52	(34)[c]		
Boiten (16)	103	27	(26)				
Lodder (44)	102	40	(39)	18	(18)	69	(68)
Gandolfo (34)	108	31	(29)[d]	37	(34)	59	(55)
Norrving (35)	61	5	(8)[a]	15	(25)	31	(51)
Anzalone (20)	88			20	(23)	30	(34)

[a] Percentages with myocardial infarction and angina together.
[b] Heart disease also including dysrhythmia.
[c] RIA: reversible ischemic attack.
[d] Ischemic ECG abnormalities.

TIA

A TIA may be the clinical manifestation of a small stroke (32). However, the occurrence of TIA allows us to identify patients with a high risk of stroke and as such TIA is a risk factor for stroke, although it is a factor that is dependent on other risk factors (32). In clinical studies, 7 to 34% of lacunar stroke patients experienced previous TIAs (Table 5). Compared with control subjects without cerebral infarctions, lacunar stroke patients had a previous TIA significantly more frequently (34% versus 3%), with a relative risk of 35 (95% CI 14–87) (34). In a population-based, prospective study, however, the incidence of previous TIA did not differ significantly between patients with lacunar and those with cortical infarction (18% versus 18%) (44). The majority of TIAs appear to be due to transient ischemia in penetrating arteries rather than in cortical arteries (54,55). Since symptomatic penetrating artery disease presents more frequently as TIA than symptomatic disease in cortical artery territories, this suggests that lacunar TIAs are less frequently followed by infarction than cortical TIAs. This concurs with the lower rate of recurrent stroke after lacunar infarction (see above, natural history). From the available clinical data, however, TIA does appear to be a risk factor for lacunar infarction as it is for ischemic stroke in general.

Cigarette Smoking

A meta-analysis of 32 separate studies provided strong evidence of an excess risk of stroke among cigarette smokers, with an overall relative risk of 1.5 (95% CI 1.4–1.6) (56). The relative risk for cerebral infarction was 1.9. A dose response relationship was found between the number of cigarettes smoked and the relative risk for stroke. In the Framingham study, after a follow-up of 26 years, cigarette smoking was a significant independent risk factor for stroke and specifically for brain infarction (57). After cessation of smoking, stroke risk decreased significantly in 2 years and reached the level of nonsmokers after 5 years. This rapid reduction in risk after cessation suggests that smoking plays a role in precipitating a stroke, possibly by increasing the fibrinogen level and promoting platelet aggregation (57).

Twenty-eight to sixty-eight percent of the lacunar stroke patients were found to be cigarette smokers in different studies (Table 5). In the study of Gandolfo et al., an associated relative risk of lacunar infarction of 2.3 was found, which was statistically significant (34). In the OCSP study, the incidence of smoking was similar in patients with lacunar infarction and in those with cortical infarction (68% versus 69%; OR 0.94; 95% CI 0.57–1.58) (44).

In conclusion, smoking seems to be a nonspecific risk factor for lacunar infarction.

UNPROVEN RISK FACTORS FOR LACUNAR INFARCTION

Emboligenic Cardiac Disease

Cardiac disease increased the risk for ischemic stroke more than twice in the Framingham study, an effect independent of blood pressure (58). Emboligenic cardiac disease or, in other words, a potential cardioembolic source, was found in up to 17% of patients with lacunar infarction (Table 6). Prospective clinical studies have demonstrated that a potential cardioembolic source was significantly less frequent in patients with lacunar than in those with nonlacunar infarction (16,44). In a case-control study, patients with lacunar infarction had a similar frequency of atrial fibrillation as control subjects without cerebral infarction (34). The frequency of atrial fibrillation did not differ between patients with lacunar stroke and those with primary intracerebral hemorrhage (22). These studies suggest that emboligenic cardiac disease is merely a marker for generalized atherosclerosis. Although individual lacunar infarcts may be caused by cardiogenic embolism, there is as yet no convincing statistical evidence to connect emboligenic cardiac disease and lacunar infarction.

Carotid Stenosis

Artery-to-artery embolism from the internal carotid artery (ICA) is considered to be one of the main causes of brain infarction. Up to 13% of lacunar infarct patients had a significant stenosis (>50% or >75%) of the ipsilateral ICA, diagnosed either noninvasively or by angiography (Table 7). The study of Ghika et al. (36) also included patients with only ulceration on angiography. In comparison with patients with nonlacunar infarcts, those with a lacunar infarct had an ICA stenosis significantly less frequently (16,35,59). Considering that carotid stenosis also occurs in neurologically asymptomatic patients or healthy people (59,60–62), and that many lacunar infarct patients also had a significant stenosis of the contralateral ACE, these studies do not support embolism from the carotid as a cause of lacunar infarction. As with emboligenic cardiac disease, carotid stenosis might merely be an indicator of generalized atherosclerosis and may not be directly related to the cause of the stroke in most lacunar infarct patients. Although there is no convincing statistical connection between carotid or other arterial disease and lacunar stroke, a patient that suffered lacunar infarction during life was shown to have multiple cholesterol emboli of probable aortic origin occluding small arteries around the lacunar infarcts on neuropathological examination (63). In addition, pure motor hemiplegia has developed during cardiac or aortic arch angiography in two cases, suggesting an arteriogenic embolic cause (64).

POSSIBLE RISK FACTORS FOR LACUNAR INFARCTION

Some more (e.g., fibrinogen and increased hematocrit) or less (e.g., hyperlipidemia) established risk factors for stroke have not as yet been established as risk factors for lacunar infarction, and may warrant future investigation.

Hyperlipidemia

Although elevated blood lipids and cholesterol are strongly related to coronary heart disease, their association with stroke is unclear (32). The Framingham study

TABLE 6. *Clinical studies comparing the frequency of potential cardioembolic sources.*

		Lacunar infarct			Nonlacunar infarct					
	Definition	N	Cardio-embolic sources No	(%)	N	Cardio-embolic sources No	(%)	OR;	95% CI	p-value
Loeb (53)	b	154	13	(8)	111	32	(30)	0.23;	0.11– 0.46	<0.001
Boiten (16)	a	103	15	(15)	*154	4	(3)	3.46;	1.10–10.85	<0.05
	b	103	10	(10)	144	50	(35)	0.32;	0.17– 0.61	<0.001
Lodder (44)	b	102	10	(10)	144	43	(30)	0.25;	0.12– 0.53	<0.001
	c	102	2	(2)	202	44	(22)	0.39;	0.19– 0.81	<0.025
	d	102	9	(9)	202	17	(8)	0.22;	0.05– 0.96	<0.025
Gandolfo (34)	b	108	9	(8)	202	22	(11)	0.79;	0.35– 1.79	NS
Pullicino (82)	a	42	5	(12)	*202	9	(4)	1.95;	0.75– 5.07	NS
					122	20	(17)	0.69;	0.24– 1.97	NS
Sacco (25)	a	78	9	(12)	±600	±168	(28)	0.34;	0.17– 0.70	<0.01

*Control subjects without cerebral infarction.
Definition of potential cardioembolic sources: a, all potential cardioembolic sources; b, non-rheumatic atrial fibrillation; c, recent myocardial infarction (≤ 6 weeks); d, valvular heart disease alone.
OR, odds ratio; CI, confidence interval.

TABLE 7. *Frequency of significant carotid stenosis.*

| | | Lacunar infarct | | | Nonlacunar infarct | | | | | |
| | | | Carotid sten. | | | Carotid sten. | | | | |
	Definition	N	No	(%)	N	No	(%)	OR;	95% CI	p-value
Boiten (16)*	a	86	11	(13)	75	28	(37)	0.35;	0.16–0.76	<0.001
Ghika (36)†	b,c	100	28	(28)						
Tegeler (59)*	a	55	7	(13)	4	22	(41)	0.21;	0.08–0.56	<0.005
Kappelle (83)†	a	45	6	(13)						
Norrving (35)†	a	61	2	(3)	53	35	(66)	0.02;	0.00–0.08	<0.001
Olsen (84)†	b	15	1	(7)	45	12	(27)	0.20;	0.02–1.66	NS

*non-invasive; †angiographic study.
Definition of carotid stenosis: a, stenosis ≥ 50% of ipsilateral ICA; b, stenosis ≥ 75% of ipsilateral ICA; c, also including carotid ulceration on angiography.
OR, odds ratio; CI, confidence interval.

showed that hyperlipidemia probably contributed a small risk of stroke for men under age 55 (65). Hyperlipidemia has been found in 16 to 44% of lacunar stroke patients (20,34–36), but in a case-control study, lacunar stroke was not associated with hypercholesterolemia or hypertriglyceridemia (34). Adams et al. (66) showed that patients with lacunar infarction had higher concentrations of high-density lipoprotein (HDL) cholesterol than patients with cortical stroke. No differences were observed in the concentrations of total cholesterol, triglycerides, low-density lipoprotein cholesterol, very low density lipoprotein cholesterol, or apolipoproteins A1 and B. More studies are needed to investigate hyperlipidemia as a possible risk factor for lacunar infarction.

Alcohol Consumption

Recent evidence suggests that excess alcohol consumption is a risk factor for both ischemic and hemorrhagic cerebrovascular disease, whereas moderate alcohol consumption may exert a protective effect similar to that proposed in coronary artery disease (67). Based on an extensive review of 62 epidemiologic studies on the relation between moderate alcohol consumption and risk of stroke, Camargo (68) described a J-shaped association between moderate drinking and ischemic stroke in predominantly white populations. Little if any association was found among the Japanese. There are no clear data available about alcohol consumption as a risk factor for ischemic stroke subgroups like lacunar infarction.

Fibrinogen

Two prospective studies showed that raised blood fibrinogen level was an independent risk factor for stroke, especially in men (69,70). The fibrinogen level was also found to be a risk factor that is related to other vascular risk factors like hypertension and cigarette smoking. Data on fibrinogen as a risk factor for lacunar infarction as a subgroup are lacking.

Increased Hematocrit (Erythrocytosis)

The Framingham study showed increased hematocrit to be a risk factor for cerebral infarction only when associated with elevated blood pressure and cigarette smoking (71). In a population-based study, LaRue et al. (72) showed that patients with lacunar stroke tended to have a higher hematocrit than patients with thrombotic or embolic stroke, the difference being significant only when systolic hypertension was also present. The authors suggested that patients with high hematocrit may be at increased risk for lacunar infarction. In a case-control study, however, elevated hematocrit was not associated with lacunar stroke (34). More studies are needed to assess a raised hematocrit as a possible risk factor for lacunar infarction.

Lower Limb Claudication

Four to eleven percent of lacunar infarct patients had lower limb claudication (27, 44), a frequency not different from nonlacunar infarct patients (44). The association between lower limb claudication and the risk for lacunar infarction is not well established and should be further investigated. A comparison of the frequency of lower limb claudication in lacunar and nonlacunar stroke patients could provide insight into the frequency of generalized large vessel disease in these stroke subgroups.

Other Risk Factors

Oral contraceptives, obesity, physical inactivity, dietary potassium deficit, homocysteinuria (homo- and heterozygosity), cocaine or amphetamine abuse, hyperuricemia, sickle cell disease, and migraine are often considered as possible risk factors for stroke (32,33). These factors have not been investigated in relation to lacunar infarcts, but may warrant further study.

POSSIBLE NEW RISK FACTORS OF INTEREST FOR LACUNAR INFARCTION

The presently known risk factors account only partially for the risk of stroke in general, and the risk of lacunar infarction in particular. Additional risk factors need to be investigated (52), including heredofamilial factors, race, life-style (socioeconomic factors, personality type, etc.), diet, and environment (geographic location, season, climate, etc.) (32,52).

Only a few studies have investigated heredofamilial factors in stroke. A nearly fivefold increase in the prevalence of stroke among monozygotic compared with dizygotic twin pairs suggests that genetic factors are involved in stroke (73). Twin studies may differentiate the role of genetic and environmental influences on stroke. There are apparent racial differences in the location of vascular lesions in patients with TIA or minor stroke (74). Studies of Japanese residents of Hawaii, however, have suggested that besides race, diet, life-style, and environmental factors influence the risk of stroke (75–78). Specific effects of these factors on the risk of lacunar infarction are unknown.

IMPLICATION OF RISK FACTOR STUDIES FOR THE MANAGEMENT OF PATIENTS WITH LACUNAR INFARCTION

The established risk factors for lacunar infarction (age, sex, hypertension, diabetes mellitus, ischemic heart disease, transient ischemic attack, and cigarette smoking) are not specific for lacunar infarction because the incidence of these factors does not differ from that in nonlacunar infarcts. What determines whether mainly small (in lacunar infarcts) or mainly large (in nonlacunar infarcts) vessels will become affected in the presence of the same atherogenic circumstances remains unknown. This means that following a lacunar infarct, it is very important to treat the vascular risk factors, particularly hypertension. The effect of aspirin on secondary prevention of stroke has not been systematically studied in patients with lacunar infarcts, TIA, or stroke. It is likely, however, that aspirin has a similar preventive effect to that in nonlacunar stroke because lacunar strokes made up a proportion of the patients in the secondary prevention studies. On the other hand, it cannot be excluded that the preventive effect of aspirin on small vessel thrombosis differs from that in presumed artery-to-artery embolism from the carotid. Lacunar stroke patients with a potential cardiac or carotid embolic source pose a distinct problem. Such potential embolic causes are uncommon, and they may merely reflect more advanced generalized atherosclerosis. Very small emboli, however, may travel wherever the blood goes, and cardiogenic embolism cannot be excluded as a cause of a lacunar infarct in an individual patient.

As with the aspirin studies, lacunar infarct patients were not systematically excluded from the carotid surgery studies. This implies that carotid endarterectomy may reduce the risk of future stroke in a patient with a lacunar infarct and an ipsilateral (>70%) carotid stenosis. Subgroup analysis in both NASCET and ECST should be pursued to investigate whether lacunar TIA and stroke patients benefit from endarterectomy (79,80). More extended follow-up studies or data pooling of present series might reveal the relative contribution of a carotid stenosis or cardioembolic source to the risk of recurrent stroke in patients with lacunar stroke. With the present state of knowledge it appears that carotid endarterectomy in patients with lacunar stroke and a high-grade carotid stenosis will do more good than harm. There is a subgroup of small deep infarcts that are situated in the vascular borderzone between the basal and cortical MCA vessels, which we found to be significantly associated with a high-grade carotid stenosis and which may be caused by hypotension. It is possible that endarterectomy may be specifically indicated in these cases.

It is unknown whether anticoagulation reduces the risk of recurrent stroke in lacunar infarct patients with nonrheumatic atrial fibrillation (NRAF) on the basis of the recent primary prevention studies (81). When a patient with lacunar infarction with NRAF is identified, anticoagulation should be considered. The definitive answer to this question awaits the outcome of the European Atrial Fibrillation Trial in 1993. If a cardiac abnormality with a generally recognized emboligenic potential (recent anterior myocardial infarction, especially with mural thrombus or an akinetic wall segment, rheumatic heart disease, mitral stenosis, cardiomyopathy, left ventricular aneurysm, valve prosthesis) is detected in a patient with a lacunar infarct we would anticoagulate such a patient. Although clinical trials on the value of anticoagulation in these settings are virtually lacking, this treatment is generally indicated even in the absence of lacunar stroke. It must be stressed that lacunar infarct patients need to be considered separately in stroke treatment and prevention trials, and in studies on stroke pathophysiology in order to allow rational treatment and prevention of lacunar infarction.

REFERENCES

1. Mohr JP, Caplan LR, Melski JW, et al. Cooperative Stroke Registry: a prospective registry. *Neurology* 1978;28:754–762.
2. Gross CR, Kase CS, Mohr JP, Cunningham SC, Baker WE. Stroke in South Alabama: incidence and diagnostic features—a population based study. *Stroke* 1984;15:249–255.
3. Kunitz SC, Gross CR, Heyman A, et al. The pilot stroke data bank: definition, design and data. *Stroke* 1984;15:740–746.
4. Bamford J, Sandercock P, Jones L, Warlow Ch. The natural history of lacunar infarction: the Oxfordshire Community Stroke Project. *Stroke* 1987;18:545–551.
5. Bogousslavsky J, van Melle G, Regli F. The Lausanne Stroke Registry: analysis of 1000 consecutive patients with first stroke. *Stroke* 1988;19:1083–1092.
6. Ricci S, Celani MG, Guercini G, et al. First-year results of a community-based study of stroke incidence in Umbria, Italy. *Stroke* 1989;20:853–857.
7. Fisher CM. Lacunar strokes and infarcts: a review. *Neurology* 1982;32:871–876.
8. Mohr JP. Lacunes. *Neurol Clin* 1983;1:201–221.
9. Miller VT. Lacunar stroke. A reassessment. *Arch Neurol* 1983;40:129–134.

10. Kappelle LJ, Van Gijn J. Lacunar infarcts. *Clin Neurol Neurosurg* 1986;88:3–17.
11. Malmgren R, Warlow C, Bamford J, Sandercock P. Geographical and secular trends in stroke incidence. *Lancet* 1987;2:1196–1200.
12. Gross CR, Kase CS, Mohr JP, Cunningham SC, Baker WE. Stroke in South Alabama: incidence and diagnostic features. A population based study. *Stroke* 1984;15:249–255.
13. Chamorro A, Sacco RL, Mohr JP, et al. Clinical-computed tomographic correlations of lacunar infarction in the Stroke Data Bank. *Stroke* 1991;22:175–181.
14. Kay R, Woo J, Kreel L, Wong HY, Teoh R, Nicholls MG. Stroke subtypes among Chinese living in Hong Kong: the Shatin Stroke Registry. *Neurology* 1992;42:985–987.
15. Bonita R, Beaglehole R, North J. Event, incidence and case fatality rates of cerebrovascular disease in Auckland, NZ. *Am J Epidemiol* 1984;120:236–243.
16. Boiten J, Lodder J. Lacunar infarcts. Pathogenesis and validity of the clinical syndromes. *Stroke* 1991;22:1374–1378.
17. Myashita K, Naritomi H, Sawada T, et al. Identification of recent lacunar lesions in cases of multiple small infarctions by magnetic resonance imaging. *Stroke* 1988;19:834–839.
18. Hommel M, Besson G, LeBas JF, et al. Prospective study of lacunar infarction using magnetic resonance imaging. *Stroke* 1990;21:546–554.
19. Bamford JM, Warlow CP. Evolution and testing of the lacunar hypothesis. *Stroke* 1988;19:1074–1082.
20. Anzalone N, Landi G. Non-ischemic causes of lacunar syndromes; prevalence and clinical findings. *J Neurol Neurosurg Psychiatry* 1989;52:1188–1190.
21. Boiten J, Lodder J. Isolated monoparesis is usually caused by superficial infarction. *Cerebrovasc Dis* 1991;1:337–340.
22. Van Merwijk G, Lodder J, Bamford J, Kester ADM. How often is nonvalvular atrial fibrillation the cause of brain infarction? *J Neurol* 1990;237:205–207.
23. Bamford J, Dennis M, Sandercock P, Burn J, Warlow C. The frequency, causes and timing of death within 30 days of a first stroke: the Oxfordshire Community Stroke Project. *J Neurol Neurosurg Psychiatry* 1990;53:824–829.
24. Bamford J, Sandercock P, Dennis M, Burn J, Warlow C. Classification and natural history of clinically identifiable subtypes of cerebral infarction. *Lancet* 1991;337:1521–1526.
25. Sacco SE, Whisnant JP, Broderick JP, Philips SJ, O'Fallon WM. Epidemiological characteristics of lacunar infarcts in a population. *Stroke* 1991;22:1236–1241.
26. Hier DB, Foulkes MA, Swiontoniowski M, et al. Stroke recurrence within 2 years after ischemic infarction. *Stroke* 1991;22:155–161.
27. Norrving B, Staaf G. Pure motor stroke from presumed lacunar infarct. *Cerebrovasc Dis* 1991;1:203–209.
28. Jamrozik K, Anderson CS, Stewart-Wynne EG. What is the true incidence of each subtype of stroke?: the Perth Community Stroke Study. *Cerebrovasc Dis* 1992:2–227.
29. Landi G, Cella E, Boccardi E, Mussico M. Lacunar versus non-lacunar infarcts: pathogenetic and prognostic differences. *J Neurol Neurosurg Psychiatry* 1992;55:441–445.
30. Boiten J, Lodder J. Prognosis for survival, handicap and recurrent stroke in lacunar and superficial infarction. *Cerebrovasc Dis* 1993 (in press).
31. Brainin M, Foulkes MA, Pauly E, Seiser A, Dastmaltschi J, Steiner M. The role of hypertension and diabetes for the survival of lacunar stroke patients. *Cerebrovasc Dis* 1992:2:202.
32. Dyken ML. Stroke risk factors. In: Norris JW, Hachinski VC, eds. *Prevention of stroke*. New York: Springer-Verlag; 1991:83–101.
33. Dyken ML, Wolf PA, Barnett HSM, et al. Risk factors in stroke. A statement for physicians by the subcommittee on risk factors and stroke of the Stroke Council. *Stroke* 1984;15:1105–1111.
34. Gandolfo C, Caponnetto C, Del Sette M, Santoloci D, Loeb C. Risk factors in lacunar syndromes: a case-control study. *Acta Neurol Scand* 1988;77:22–26.
35. Norrving B, Cronqvist S. Clinical and radiologic features of lacunar versus nonlacunar minor stroke. *Stroke* 1989;20:59–64.
36. Ghika J, Bogousslavsky J, Regli F. Infarcts in the territory of the deep perforators from the carotid system. *Neurology* 1989;39:507–512.
37. Arboix A, Marti-Vilalta JL, Garcia JH. Clinical study of 227 patients with lacunar infarcts. *Stroke* 1990;21:842–847.
38. Donnan GA, Tress BM, Bladin PF. A prospective study of lacunar infarction using computerized tomography. *Neurology* 1982;32:49–56.
39. Foulkes MA, Wolf PA, Price TR, Mohr JP, Hier DB. The stroke data bank: design, methods, and baseline characteristics. *Stroke* 1988;19:547–554.
40. Fisher CM. Lacunes: small, deep cerebral infarcts. *Neurology* 1965;15:774–784.
41. Fisher CM. Lacunar infarcts. A review. *Cerebrovasc Dis* 1991;1:311–320.
42. Tuszynski MH, Petito CK, Levy DE. Risk factors and clinical manifestations of pathologically verified lacunar infarctions. *Stroke* 1989;20:990–999.
43. Dozono K, Ishii N, Nishihara Y, Horic A. An autopsy study of the incidence of lacunes in relation to age, hypertension, and arteriosclerosis. *Stroke* 1991;22:993–996.
44. Lodder J, Bamford JM, Sandercock PAG, Jones LN, Warlow CP. Are hypertension or cardiac embolism likely causes of lacunar infarction? *Stroke* 1990;21:375–381.
45. Boiten J. Lacunar stroke. *A prospective clinical and radiological study* [Doctoral Thesis]. Maastricht, The Netherlands: University of Limburg, 1991.
46. Fisher CM. The arterial lesions underlying lacunes. *Acta Neuropathol (Berlin)* 1969;12:1–15.
47. Fisher CM. Capsular infarcts. The underlying vascular lesions. *Arch Neurol* 1979;36:65–73.
48. Kannel WB, Wolf PA, Verter J, McNamara PM.

Epidemiologic assessment of the role of blood pressure in stroke: the Framingham study. *JAMA* 1970;214:301–310.

49. MacMahon S, Peto R, Cutler J, et al. Blood pressure, stroke, and coronary heart disease. *Lancet* 1990;335:765–774.
50. Weisberg LA. Diagnostic classification of stroke, especially lacunes. *Stroke* 1988;19:1071–1073.
51. Pullicino P. Small deep infarcts in diabetes. *Neurology* 1990;40:249.
52. Norris JW, Hachinski VC. Stroke prevention: past, present, and future. In: Norris JW, Hachinski VC, eds. *Prevention of stroke*. New York: Springer-Verlag; 1991:1–15.
53. Loeb C, Gandolfo C, Mancardi GL, Primavera A, Tassinari T. The lacunar syndromes: a review with personal contribution. In: Lechner H, Meyer JS, Ott E, eds. *Cerebrovascular disease: research and clinical management*. Vol 1. Amsterdam: Elsevier; 1986:107–156.
54. Hankey GJ, Warlow CP. Lacunar transient ischemic attacks: a clinically useful concept? *Lancet* 1991;337:335–338.
55. Kappelle LJ, Van Latum JC, Koudstaal PJ, Van Gijn J. Transient ischemic attacks and small-vessel disease. *Lancet* 1991;337:339–341.
56. Shinton R, Beevers G. Meta-analysis of relation between cigarette smoking and stroke. *Br Med J* 1989;298:789–794.
57. Wolf PA, D'Agostino RB, Kannel WB, Bonita R, Belanger AJ. Cigarette smoking as a risk factor for stroke. The Framingham study. *JAMA* 1988;259:1025–1029.
58. Wolf PA, Kannel WB, Verter J. Current status of risk factors for stroke. *Neurol Clin* 1983;1:317–343.
59. Tegeler CH, Shi F, Morgan T. Carotid stenosis in lacunar stroke. *Stroke* 1991;22:1124–1128.
60. Faris AA, Poser CM, Wilmore DW, Agnew CH. Radiologic visualization of neck vessels in healthy men. *Neurology* 1963;13:386–391.
61. Harrison MJG, Marshall J. Angiographic appearance of carotid bifurcation in patients with completed stroke, transient ischaemic attacks, and cerebral tumour. *Br Med J* 1976;1:205–207.
62. Hennerici M, Aulick A, Sandmann W, Freund HJ. Incidence of asymptomatic extracranial arterial disease. *Stroke* 1981;12:750–758.
63. Laloux P, Brucher JM. Lacunar infarctions due to cholesterol emboli. *Stroke* 1991; 22:1440–1444.
64. Cacciatore A, Russo LS. Lacunar infarction as an embolic complication of cardiac and arch angiography. *Stroke* 1991;22:1603–1605.
65. Kannel WB. Epidemiology of cerebrovascular disease. In: Ross Russell RW, ed. *Cerebral arterial disease*. Edinburgh: Churchill Livingstone; 1976:1–23.
66. Adams RJ, Carroll RM, Nichols FT, et al. Plasma lipoproteins in cortical versus lacunar infarction. *Stroke* 1989;20:448–452.
67. Gorelick PB. The status of alcohol as a risk factor for stroke. *Stroke* 1989;20:1607–1610.
68. Camargo CA. Moderate alcohol consumption and stroke. The epidemiologic evidence. *Stroke* 1989;20:1611–1626.
69. Wilhelmsen L, Svardsudd K, Korsan-Bengtsen K, Larsson B, Welin L, Tibblin G. Fibrinogen as a risk factor for stroke and myocardial infarction. *N Engl J Med* 1984;311:501–505.
70. Kannel WB, Wolf PA, Castelli WP, D'Agostino RB. Fibrinogen and risk of cardiovascular disease. The Framingham study. *JAMA* 1987;258:1183–1186.
71. Kannel WB, Gordon T, Wolf PA, McNamara PM. Hemoglobin and the of cerebral infarction: the Framingham study. *Stroke* 1972;3:409–420.
72. LaRue L, Altes M, Lai SM, et al. Acute stroke, hematocrit, and blood pressure. *Stroke* 1987;18:565–569.
73. Brass LM, Isaacsohn JL, Merikangas KR, Robinette CD. A study of twins and stroke. *Stroke* 1992;23:221–223.
74. Inzitari D, Hachinski VC, Taylor DW, Barnett JM. Racial differences in the anterior circulation in cerebrovascular disease. How much can be explained by risk factors? *Arch Neurol* 1990;47:1080–1084.
75. Kagan A, Popper J, Rhoads GG, et al. Epidemiologic studies of coronary heart disease and stroke in Japanese men living in Japan, Hawaii, and California: prevalence of stroke. In: Scheinberg P, ed. *Cerebrovascular diseases*. New York: Raven Press; 1976:267–277.
76. Kagan A, Popper JS, Rhoads GG, Yano K. Dietary and other risk factors for stroke in Hawaiian Japanese men. *Stroke* 1985;16:390–396.
77. Mitsuyama Y, Thompsow LR, Hayashi T, et al. Autopsy study of cerebrovascular disease in Japanese men who lived in Hiroshima, Japan, and Honolulu, Hawaii. *Stroke* 1979;10:389–395.
78. Takeya Y, Popper JS, Shimizu Y, Kato H, Rhoads GG, Kagon A. Epidemiologic studies of coronary heart disease and stroke in Japanese men living in Japan, Hawaii and California: incidence of stroke in Japan and Hawaii. *Stroke* 1984;15:15–23.
79. North American Symptomatic Carotid Endarterectomy Trial Collaborators. Beneficial effect of carotid endarterectomy in symptomatic patients with high-grade stenosis. *N Engl J Med* 1991;325:445–453.
80. European Carotid Surgery Trialist's Collaborative Group. MRC European Carotid Surgery Trial: interim results for symptomatic patients with severe (70–99%) or with mild (0–29%) carotid stenosis. *Lancet* 1991;337:1235–1243.
81. Sherman DG. Stroke prevention trials in atrial fibrillation. *Cerebrovasc Dis* 1992;2:14–17.
82. Pullicino P, Nelson RF, Kendall BE, Marshall J. Small deep infarcts diagnosed on computed tomography. *Neurology* 1980;30:1090–1096.
83. Kappelle LJ, Koudstaal PJ, Van Gijn J, Ramos LMP, Keunen JEE. Carotid angiography in patients with lacunar infarction. A prospective study. *Stroke* 1988;19:1093–1096.
84. Olsen TS, Skriver EB, Herning M. Cause of cerebral infarction in the carotid territory. Its relation to the size and the location of the infarct and to the underlying vascular lesion. *Stroke* 1985;16:459–466.

Index

Page numbers in *italics* refer to illustrations; page numbers in **boldface** refer to diagrams of arterial territories; page numbers followed by (t) refer to tables.

A

Abdomen, sensory loss, in pontine infarct, 147
Abscess, brain, pure motor hemiparesis and, 190
Acalculia, 153
Acquired immunodeficiency syndrome (AIDS), small deep infarct and, 133
Adiadokokinesia, in ataxic hemiparesis, 145
Affect, disorders of, caudate nucleus infarct and, 165
Age, lacunar infarct risk and, 217
Akinesia, psychic, pure, lenticular nucleus necrosis and, 166
Alcohol consumption, lacunar infarct risk and, 223
Alzheimer, A., 2
Alzheimer's disease, 204–205
  cerebral amyloid angiopathy and, 108
Amphetamines, vasculitis and, 111
Amyloid angiopathy, 205
  familial, 110
  putamen infarct and, 152
  small vessel lesions and, 107, 109–110, *109*
Amyloidosis, hereditary, cerebral hemorrhage with, 110
Aneurysm, miliary (Charcot-Bouchard), 103, 105
Angiitis, granulomatous, small deep infarct and, 132
Angionecrosis, 103
Angiopathy, amyloid, 205
  familial, 110
  putamen infarct and, 152
  small vessel lesions and, 107, 109–110, *109*
Anisocoria, in ataxic hemiparesis, 145
Ansa lenticularis, **47, 53**
Ansa peduncularis, **46, 52**
Anterior opercular syndrome, 182
Anticardiolipin antibody, 110
Anticardiolipin syndrome, 110
Anticoagulation, in lacunar infarct, 225
Antihypertensive drugs, lacunar state and, 182
Antiphospholipid antibody syndrome, small deep infarct and, 131
Apathy, caudate nucleus infarct and, 165
Aphasia
  internal capsule infarct and, 165
  lacunar syndromes with, 153
  lenticular nucleus infarct and, 166
  thalamic infarct and, 168
Apraxia, 153
Arndt, R., 1
Arteriolosclerosis
  dilated perivascular spaces and, 129
  hyaline
    diabetes and, 107
    hypertension and, *106*
  white matter ischemia and, 203
Arterionecrosis, hyaline, 103
Arteriosclerosis, 93
Arteritis
  fibrinoid, 103
  small deep infarct and, 132
Artery (arteries)
  auditory, internal, 34
  basilar
    anatomy of, *12, 27, 31*, 32–33, *33*
    occlusion of, embolism and, 133
    stenosis of, small deep infarct and, 131
  carotid
    internal
      anatomy of, *12*, 14
      artery-to-artery embolism from, lacunar infarct risk and, 221, 223(t)
      occlusion of
        low-flow infarcts and, 79–81, *79, 80*
        small deep infarct and, 134–135
      territory of, **44, 48, 53**
      turbulent flow in, lacunar infarct and, 129
  cerebellar
    inferior
      anterior
        anatomy of, *27, 33*, 33–34
        territory of, **59, 60, 63, 64, 69, 70**
      posterior
        anatomy of, *27, 35*, 36
        territory of, **58, 59, 60, 63, 64, 65, 66**
    superior
      anatomy of, *27, 31*, 30–31
      territory of, **58, 59, 60, 62, 63, 64, 70**
  cerebral
    anterior
      anatomy of, *11, 12*
      territory of, **43, 44, 46, 47, 51, 52**
    middle
      anatomy of, *12*, 14–17, *15, 16, 18, 20, 27*
      infarct of, hypoperfusion and, 134
      occlusion of
        borderzone infarct and, 81, *81*, 134, 135
        small deep infarct and, 134, 135
      stenosis of, small deep infarct and, 131
      territory of, **44, 45, 46, 47, 48, 49, 50, 51, 52, 53, 54, 55, 56, 57**
    posterior, anatomy of, *12*, 21–24, *20, 27, 31*
  choroidal
    anterior
      anatomy of, *12*, **19-21**, *20*, **27, 31**

229

Artery (arteries) (*contd.*)
    infarct of, 20, 163, 165
    territory of, **44, 45, 46, 47, 48, 53, 54, 55, 56, 57, 61**
  posterolateral
    anatomy of, *20, 27,* 26–27, *28*
    territory of, **44, 45, 46, 47, 48, 49, 54, 55, 56, 57, 61**
  posteromedial
    anatomy of, *20, 27,* 28–29, *31*
    infarct of, 29
    peduncular branches of, anatomy of, 29
    tegmental branches of, anatomy of, 30
    territory of, **43, 46, 47, 48, 53, 54, 55, 56, 57, 70**
  coiling of, 107, *108*
  collicular
    accessory, anatomy of, 30, *31*
    anatomy of, *27,* 30, *31*
    territory of, **43, 44, 46, 55, 56, 61, 70**
  communicating
    anterior
      anatomy of, 12
      territory of, **43, 46, 47, 52**
    posterior
      anatomy of, *12, 20, 27, 31*
      territory of, **43, 46, 53, 54**
  Heubner's
    anatomy of, *12, 13,* 13–14
    infarct of, hypoperfusion and, 134
    territory of, **43, 44, 45, 46, 47, 50, 51**
  hippocampal, anatomy of, 29
  hypophyseal, anatomy of, *12*
  hypothalamic, anatomy of, 21
  lenticulostriate
    anterior, anatomy of, 11–14, *12*
    infarct of, 163
    intermediate, anatomy of, *12,* 17
    intracerebral segments of, anatomy of, 18–19, *18,* 19(t)
    lateral
      anatomy of, *12,* 17–18, *18, 27*
      infarct of, hypoperfusion and, 134
    medial, anatomy of, *12,* 17, *18, 27*
  medullary
    anatomy of, 35–37
    arteriolosclerosis of, lacunar infarct and, 128
    infarct of, hypoperfusion and, 134
  mesencephalic, paramedian
    anatomy of, 22–25
    infarct of, 23, 24, 168, 169
      dementia and, 184
    inferior, anatomy of, 23, *22, 23, 24*
    superior, anatomy of, 24–25, *22, 23, 24, 31*
    territory of, **46, 61**
  occlusion of, 94
    lacunar infarct and, 125–129, 126(t)
  olivary, anatomy of, 35
  peduncular, anatomy of, 29, *31*
  pedunculo-subthalamic, anatomy of, 21
  pial, anatomy of, 98, *102*
  pontine
    anatomy of, 32–33, *33*
    anterolateral, 32
    inferolateral
      anatomy of, 33, *33*
      territory of, **64**
    superolateral, anatomy of, 32, *33*
  spinal, anterior, anatomy of, *34*
  splenial, anatomy of, 29
  superficial, amyloid angiopathy in, 109, *109*
  thalamic, paramedian
    anatomy of, *12,* 22–23, 25–26, *22, 23, 24, 25, 26*
    infarct of, 26, 168, 169
      dementia and, 184
    territory of, **43, 44, 46, 47, 48, 54, 55, 56**
  thalamogeniculate
    anatomy of, *20, 27,* 26
    territory of, **44, 45, 46, 47, 48, 54, 55, 56, 57**
  thalamotuberal
    anatomy of, *12, 20,* 21, *27*
    infarct of, 167–168
    territory of, **43, 44, 45, 46, 47, 48, 53, 54**
  tortuosity of, 107, *108*
  unfolding of, 107
    dilated perivascular spaces and, 129–130, *130*
  vertebral, anatomy of, *12,* 35, 36
Aspirin, in lacunar infarct, 224–225
Asterixis
  internal capsule infarct and, 165
  lacunar syndromes with, 152
  lenticular nucleus infarct and, 167
  thalamic infarct and, 168
Ataxia
  cerebellar
    contralateral, nuclear oculomotor syndrome and, 150, *150*
    definition of, 144–145
  homolateral, and crural paresis, 145
Ataxic hemiparesis, 144–146, *146*
  cerebellar diaschisis and, 184
  corona radiata infarct and, 162
  hypesthetic, 146
    internal capsule infarct and, 164
    thalamic infarct and, 167
  internal capsule infarct and, 164
  internuclear ophthalmoplegia and, 149
  intracerebral hemorrhage and, 188–189, *188*
  lacunar infarct volume in, 76
  nonvascular cause of, 190
  pontine infarct and, 170
  thalamic infarct and, 167
  variants of, 146
Ataxic tetraparesis, 146
Atheroma, lacunar infarct and, 125, 126(t), 127
Atherosclerosis, 94
  of small arteries, 103
Atrial fibrillation, small deep infarct and, 133
Atrophy, granular, *104,* 98
Autoimmune disorders, small vessel lesions and, 110–111

B

Ballism
  lacunar syndromes with, 151
  lenticular nucleus infarct and, 167
  midbrain infarct and, 169

Behavior, disorders of
    caudate nucleus infarct and, 165–166
    lenticular nucleus infarct and, 166–167
    thalamic infarct and, 168
Benedikt's syndrome, 150, 170
Binswanger's disease, 193–208
    computed tomography of, 195
    edema and, 204
    hematocrit in, 135, 204
    hypertension and, 103, 194, 203
    hypoperfusion and, 134, 204
    linear subinsular MR hyperintensities and, 82
    magnetic resonance of, 195
    multiple lacunar infarcts in, 182–183
    pathogenesis of, 98, 203–204
        hypoperfusion in, 134
        hypotension and, 134
    pathology of, 115, *116–117*
Bizzozzero, G., 1
Blindness, monocular, vasospasm and, 128
Blood-brain barrier, alteration of, dilated perivascular spaces and, 129
Body
    geniculate
        collicular artery supply to, 30
        posteromedial choroidal artery supply to, 28
        thalamogeniculate artery supply to, 26
    lateral, **46, 56, 57, 59, 69, 70**
        anterior choroidal artery supply to, 19
        coronal MR scan through, **56**
    medial, **44, 46, 56, 69**
        sagittal MR scan through, **44**
    mamillary, **54**
        hypothalamic artery supply to, 21
Bonnamour, S., 5
Brachial monoparesis, pontine infarct and, 144
Brachial monoplegia
    internal capsule infarct and, 163
    supratentorial infarct and, 144
Brachiocrural motor deficit
    internal capsule infarct and, 143, 163
    medullary infarct and, 143
Brachiofacial motor deficit, internal capsule infarct and, 163
Brainstem
    accessory collicular artery supply to, 30, *31*
    anterior inferior cerebellar artery supply to, 33–34
    arterial supply to, anatomy of, 29–37, *31*, *33*, *35*
    basilar artery supply to, 32–33
    collicular artery supply to, 30, *31*
    infarct of
        clinical features of, 168–171
        magnetic resonance of, 77
    lateral pontine artery supply to, 32–33
    medullary artery supply to, 35–36
    posterior inferior cerebellar artery supply to, 36
    superior cerebellar artery supply to, 30–32
    vertebral artery supply to, 35–36

C
Campbell, A. W., 2
Caplan, L. R., 8

Caps, of white matter hyperintensities, 87, 87(t)
Capsular claudication, 142
Capsular genu syndrome, internal capsule infarct and, 165
Capsular warning syndrome, 135, 142
Capsule
    external, **50, 51, 52**
    internal, **49**
        anterior choroidal artery supply to, 20
        anterior limb of, **47, 48, 50, 51, 52**
            hemorrhage of, 187
            infarct of
                brachiocrural motor deficit and, 143
                crural monoplegia and, 145
                hypoperfusion and, 134
                sensorimotor stroke and, 148
                vocal cord palsy and, 144
        genu of, **44, 48, 53, 59, 60**
            coronal MR scan through, **53**
            hemorrhage of, 144
            infarct of, dysarthria—clumsy hand syndrome and, 146
            MR scan through, **45, 48**
        infarct of
            aphasia and, 164
            ataxic hemiparesis and, 164
            capsular genu syndrome and, 164
            clinical features of, 162–165
            cognitive defects and, 164
            dysarthria and, 164
            dysarthria—clumsy hand syndrome and, 164
            hemiballism and, 164
            homonymous sectoranopia and, 164
            magnetic resonance of, 77
            pure motor hemiplegia and, 143
            pure motor stroke and, 163–164
            pure sensory stroke and, 164
            sensorimotor stroke and, 164
        internal carotid artery supply to, 14
        lateral lenticulostriate artery supply to, 17
        medial lenticulostriate artery supply to, 17
        posterior limb of, **47, 48, 54, 55, 56, 68, 69**
            hematoma of, 189
            hemorrhage of, 187
            infarct of
                homolateral ataxia and, 145
                sensorimotor stroke and, 148
        recurrent artery of Heubner supply to, 14
        thalamogeniculate artery supply to, 26
        thalamotuberal artery supply to, 21
Cardiac valves, prosthetic, infarct and, 133
Castaigne, J., 5
Catola, G., 5
Centrum semiovale
    low-flow infarct of, 79–81, 134
Cerebello-spasmodic paraplegia, 190
Cerebral blood flow
    anatomy of, 94, 98–100, *98*, *99*, *100*, *101*
    in Binswanger-like white matter low attenuation, 197–198
    in multi-infarct dementia, 198
    in multiple subcortical infarct state, 184
    small deep infarct and, 135
    white matter hyperintensities and, 202

Cerebral cortex, recurrent artery of Heubner
    supply to, 13
Cerebral porosis, 2, *2*
Challa, V. R., 8
Charcot-Bouchard aneurysm, 103, 107
Chavany, J. A., 6
Cheiro-oral syndrome, 147, 148, 167, 189, *189*, 190
Cholesteatoma, cheiro-oral sensory loss and, 190
Chorea
    lacunar syndromes with, 151
    lenticular nucleus infarct and, 167
    thalamic infarct and, 168
Cigarette smoking, lacunar infarct risk and, 220–221
Clarke, L., 2
Claude's syndrome, 150, *150*, 170
Claudication, lower limb, lacunar infarct risk and, 224
Claustrum, **49, 50, 51, 52, 53, 54**
Coagulopathy, small deep infarct and, 131–132
Cocaine
    small deep infarct and, 136
    vasculitis and, 111
Cogan's syndrome, small deep infarct and, 132
Cognition. *See also* Dementia
    disorders of
        caudate nucleus infarct and, 165
        internal capsule infarct and, 165
Coiling, arterial, 107, *108*
Cole, F. M., 7
Colliculus
    collicular artery supply to, 30
    inferior, superior cerebellar artery supply to, 32
        posteromedial choroidal artery supply to, 28
    superior, **43, 46, 57, 58, 70**
        thalamogeniculate artery supply to, 26
Commissure, anterior, **43, 44, 47, 52, 53, 58, 59**
    anterior communicating artery supply to, 12
    medial lenticulostriate artery supply to, 17
    recurrent artery of Heubner supply to, 14
Computed tomography. *See also* White matter low attenuation
    in Binswanger's disease, 195–198, *197*
    borderzone infarct on, 81, *81*
    contrast-enhanced, small deep infarct on, 77
    giant perivascular space on, 87
    linear subinsular infarct on, 81–82
    pathologically proven lacunar infarct on, 73, 75
    presumed lacunar infarct on, 75
Contraceptives, oral, small deep infarct and, 136
Corectopia, midbrain infarct and, 170
Corona radiata, **49, 54, 55, 68**
    infarct of
        ataxic hemiparesis and, 162
        clinical features of, 161–162
        dysarthria—clumsy hand syndrome and, 146, 162
        pure motor stroke and, 162
        pure sensory stroke and, 162
        sensorimotor stroke and, 148, 162
    lateral lenticulostriate artery supply to, 17
    lymphoma of, ataxic hemiparesis and, 190
Coronary heart disease, lacunar infarct risk and, 219

Corpus callosum
    anterior communicating artery supply to, 12
    splenial artery supply to, 29
Cortex
    frontal, recurrent artery of Heubner supply to, 13
    piriform, anterior choroidal artery supply to, 19
Cribriform cavity, 8
Crural monoparesis, 144
Crural monoplegia, internal capsule infarct and, 163
Cruveilhier, J., 1
Cryptococcus, small deep infarct and, 133
Curry, B., 9
Cysticercosis
    ataxic hemiparesis and, 190
    pure motor hemiparesis and, 190

D
De Reuck, J., 7
Dechambre, A., 1
Dementia
    in Binswanger's disease, 120, 193–194
        cerebral blood flow in, 198
        features of, 194
    lacunar, 182–184
    multi-infarct, white matter low attenuation in, 205–207
    vascular, 205–207
    white matter hyperintensities in, 199, *199*
    white matter low attenuation and, 196–197
Demyelination
    ataxic hemiparesis and, 190
    dilated perivascular spaces and, 130–131
    in multi-infarct dementia, 206
    postmortem magnetic resonance of, 84, *85*
    pure motor hemiparesis and, 190
Derouesné, C., 8
Devaux, A., 4
Diabetes
    lacunar infarct risk and, 218–219, 219(t)
    small deep infarcts and, 93, 107
Diencephalon, MR scan through, **46**
Disinhibition, caudate nucleus infarct and, 165
Down gaze palsy, midbrain infarct and, 151, 169
Drugs, abuse of, vasculitis and, 111
Dupré, E., 4
Durand-Fardel, M., 1
Dysarthria
    corona radiata infarct and, 162
    internal capsule infarct and, 164
    lacunar syndromes with, 153
    in pseudobulbar palsy, 182
Dysarthria—clumsy hand syndrome, 146
    corona radiata infarct and, 162
    intracerebral hemorrhage and, 188–189, *188*
    pontine infarct and, 170
Dyskinesia, oral, 151
    lacunar syndromes with, 151
    thalamic infarct and, 168
Dysmetria, in ataxic hemiparesis, 145
Dystonia
    lacunar syndromes with, 151
    lenticular nucleus infarct and, 167
    thalamic infarct and, 168
Dystrophic lacunar sclerosis, 5

INDEX

E

Ectasia, small artery, postmortem magnetic resonance of, 84
Edema
 Binswanger's disease and, 204
 peri-infarct, 76–77
Electroencephalography, white matter low attentuation and, 197
Embolism
 artery-to-artery
  lacunar infarct and, 127
  lacunar infarct risk and, 221, 223(t)
  small deep infarct and, 133–134
 cardiogenic
  lacunar infarct and, 126(t), 127
  small deep infarct and, 133
 lacunar infarct risk and, 221, 222(t)
 lacunar infarcts and, magnetic resonance of, 82–83, *82*
Encephalopathy
 arteriosclerotic, subcortical. *See* Binswanger's disease
 hypertensive, 207–208
 thalamic infarct and, 168
Endarterectomy, carotid, in lacunar infarct, 225
Endarteritis obliterans, small deep infarct and, 132
Epilepsy, in Binswanger-like white matter low attenuation, 197
Erythrocytosis, lacunar infarct risk and, 223
État criblé, 1, 2, 3. *See also* Perivascular space, dilated in Binswanger's disease, 194
État lacunaire, 181–182
État pré-criblé, 5
Eye, movement disorders of, lacunar syndromes with, 149–151, *150*

F

Facial palsy
 internal capsule infarct and, 163
 lacunar infarct and, 144
 supranuclear, pontine infarct and, 170
Faciobrachial paresis
 bilateral, 144
 internal capsule infarct and, 164
Factor V deficiency, small deep infarct and, 132
Falx cerebri, meningioma of, ataxic hemiparesis and, 190
Fasciculus
 lenticular, **44**, **59**
 longitudinal, medial, **46**, **56**, **57**, **62**, **63**, **64**, **65**, **69**, **70**
  basilar artery supply to, 33
  infarct of, 150
  superior paramedian mesencephalic artery supply to, 24
 thalamic, **47**, **54**
Fasciculus cuneatus, **67**
Fasciculus gracilis, **67**
Ferrand, J., 4–5, *5*
Fibrillation, atrial, small deep infarct and, 133
Fibrinogen
 blood, lacunar infarct risk and, 223
 plasma, white matter hyperintensities and, 202

Fibrinoid necrosis, 103
 diabetes and, 107
Fibrohyalinosis, in Alzheimer's disease, 204
Fields of Forel, **43**, **54**, **58**
 anterior choroidal artery supply to, 20
 pedunculo-subthalamic artery supply to, 21
Fisher, C. M., 6–7, *6*, 8, 9
 serial section studies of, 111, 125–128, 126(t)
Fogging effect, on computed tomography, 77
Foix, C., 5, 6
Foix-Chavany syndrome, 182
Formes apparentés, in Binswanger's disease, 194
Fornix, **43**, **58**
 columns of, **46**, **47**, **52**
  anterior communicating artery supply to, 12
  coronal MR scan through, **52**
Foville's syndrome, 149

G

Gait, in Binswanger-like white matter low attenuation, 197
Genetic factors, in lacunar infarct risk, 224
Glioblastoma, cheiro-oral sensory loss and, 190
Glioma
 ataxic hemiparesis and, 190
 pure motor hemiparesis and, 190
Gliosis, fibrillary, 94, 96–97
Globus pallidus, **44**, **45**, **46**, **47**, **51**, **52**, **53**, **54**, **55**, **59**, **60**, **68**
 anterior choroidal artery supply to, 20
 infarct of, clinical features of, 166–167
 internal carotid artery supply to, 14
 lateral lenticulostriate artery supply to, 18
 medial lenticulostriate artery supply to, 17
Granulomatous angiitis, small vessel lesions and, 110
Grasset, J., 5
Gray matter, periaqueductal, **46**, **57**, **70**
 posteromedial choroidal artery supply to, 28
 superior paramedian mesencephalic artery supply to, 24
Gyrus
 parahippocampal, **54**
  hippocampal artery supply to, 29
 paraolfactory, anterior communicating artery supply to, 12
 paraterminal, **50**
  recurrent artery of Heubner supply to, 13
 subcallosal, recurrent artery of Heubner supply to, 13

H

Habenula, **47**
Hallucination, visual, lenticular nucleus infarct and, 167
Hallucinosis
 lacunar syndromes with, 153
 peduncular, midbrain infarct and, 169
Heart disease, coronary, lacunar infarct risk and, 219
Hematocrit
 lacunar infarct risk and, 223
 in Binswanger's disease, 135, 204
 in presumed lacunar infarct, 135

Hematoma
  ataxic hemiparesis and, 188–189
  cavity of, 114
  dysarthria—clumsy hand syndrome and, 188–189
  pure motor hemiparesis and, 190
  pure sensory stroke and, 189, *189*
  sensorimotor stroke and, 189, *189*
  in Weber's syndrome, 149
Hemialgic syndrome, 147
Hemiballism, 151
  internal capsule infarct and, 164
  lacunar syndromes with, 151
Hemifacial spasm, pontine infarct and, 170, 171
Hemiparesis. *See* Ataxic hemiparesis; Pure motor hemiparesis
Hemiplegia. *See also* Pure motor hemiplegia
  abducens nerve palsy and, 149
  contralateral oculomotor nerve palsy and, 149
  lenticular nucleus infarct and, 166
Hemolytic-uremic syndrome, small deep infarct and, 131–132
Hemorrhage, intracerebral, 187–190, *188*, 188(t), *189*
  ataxic hemiparesis and, 188–189, *188*
  cerebral amyloid angiopathy and, 109–110
  computed tomography of, 75
  diabetes and, 107
  dysarthria—clumsy hand syndrome and, 188–189, *188*
  magnetic resonance of, 76
  miliary aneurysm and, 103
  pure motor stroke and, 187–188
  pure sensory stroke and, 189, *189*
  sensorimotor stroke and, 189, *189*
Hereditary cerebral hemorrhage with amyloidosis, 110
Herpes zoster, trigeminal, small deep infarct and, 132
Herring, A. P., 2
Heubner's arteritis, small deep infarct and, 132
Hippocampal formation, **56**, **68**, **69**
Hippocampus
  anterior choroidal artery supply to, 19
  posterolateral choroidal artery supply to, 27
Homonymous sectoranopia, 165
Horizontal gaze palsy, pure motor hemiplegia and, 149
Horizontal one-and-a-half syndrome, 150
  pure motor hemiplegia and, 149
Horner's syndrome, 150
  lacunar syndromes with, 151
  thalamic infarct and, 168
Hughes, W., 6, 7
Hyaline fatty change, 103
Hydrocephalus, normal pressure, 207
Hyperlipidemia, lacunar infarct risk and, 221, 223
Hypertension
  Binswanger's disease and, 100, 194, 203
  cocaine-induced, 136
  lacunar infarct risk and, 217–218, 217(t)
  lacunar state and, 182, 183
  lipohyalinosis and, 125
  small vessel lesions and, 100, 102–103, *106*, *108*
  white matter lesions and, 203

Hypertensive encephalopathy, 207–208
Hypesthesia, in ataxic hemiparesis, 145
Hypoperfusion, 115, 120
  amyloid angiopathy and, 205
  Binswanger's disease and, 204
  lacunar infarct and, 127–128
  small deep infarct and, 134–135
Hypophysis, hypothalamic artery supply to, 21
Hypotension, Binswanger's disease and, 134
Hypothalamus, **43**, **46**, **52**, **53**, **54**, **58**
  anterior communicating artery supply to, 12
  internal carotid artery supply to, 14
  recurrent artery of Heubner supply to, 13
Hypotonia, in ataxic hemiparesis, 145
Hypoxia/ischemia, tissue changes with, 94, *95*, *96–97*, *98*

I
Infarct(s)
  borderzone
    internal, 81, *81*
    middle cerebral artery occlusion and, 135
  deep, small. *See* Small deep infarct(s)
  definition of, 94, *95*
  hemorrhagic, magnetic resonance of, 76
  incomplete, 94, 120
  lacunar. *See* Lacunar infarct(s)
  low-flow
    hypoperfusion and, 134
    imaging of, 79–81, *79*, *80*
    sites of, *80*
  subinsular, linear, 81–82, *82*
  terminal zone, 79
    imaging of, 79, 81
  watershed, 79
    hypotension and, 134
Inflammation, meningeal, small deep infarct and, 132
Infundibulum, **52**
  hypothalamic artery supply to, 21
  internal carotid artery supply to, 14
Internuclear ophthalmoplegia, 150
  ataxic hemiparesis and, 149

J
Jacobsohn, L., 2

L
Lacunar infarct(s)
  computed tomography of, 73, 75
  dementia and, 182–184
  embolism and, 82–83, *82*
  hemorrhagic, magnetic resonance of, 76
  magnetic resonance of, 74, 75
    postmortem, 75
  multiple, 182–183
  natural history of, 214–216, 215(t)
  pathogenesis of, 111, 125–129, 126(t)
    artery-to-artery embolism in, 127
    cardiogenic embolism in, 127
    carotid turbulent flow in, 129
    embolic occlusion in, 127
    hemodynamic compromise in, 127–128
    occlusive disease in, 125–127
    perforating artery hypoperfusion in, 128–129

vasospasm in, 128–129
white matter infarcts and, 128
presumed
acute, magnetic resonance of, 77
computed tomography of, 75
definition of, 73
hematocrit in, 135
magnetic resonance of, 76
risk factor(s) for, 216–217, 216(t)
age as, 217
alcohol consumption as, 223
carotid stenosis as, 221, 223(t)
cigarette smoking as, 220–221
diabetes mellitus and, 218–219, 219(t)
emboligenic cardiac disease as, 221, 222(t)
erythrocytosis as, 223–224
fibrinogen as, 223
hyperlipidemia as, 221, 223
hypertension as, 217–218, 217(t)
ischemic heart disease and, 219
lower limb claudication as, 224
patient management and, 224–225
sex as, 217
transient ischemic attacks and, 220, 220(t)
of temporo-occipital white matter, 75
Lacunar transient ischemic attacks, 135–136
Lacune(s), 73. *See also* Lacunar infarct(s)
classification of, 8
definition of, 73, 112, 115
by Ferrand, 4–5
by Pierre Marie, 2–3
vs. small deep infarcts, 73, 111–115, *112–113*
Lacune miliaire, 5
Lamina terminalis, anterior communicating artery supply to, 12
Landry's syndrome, 149
pontine infarct and, 170
Lejonne, P., 5
Lemniscus
lateral, **43, 61, 62, 63**
anterior inferior cerebellar artery supply to, 34
pontine artery supply to, 33
superior cerebellar artery supply to, 31
medial, **43, 44, 46, 56, 57, 58, 59, 61, 62, 63, 64, 65, 66, 69, 70**
coronal MR scan through, **70**
posteromedial choroidal artery supply to, 28
superior cerebellar artery supply to, 31
Leri, A., 5
Leukoaraiosis, 94, *118–119*, 120
Leukoencephalopathy
experimental, 120
familial disorder with, 205
Lhermitte, J., 5
Lipohyalinosis, 7, 102–103
hypertension and, 125
Locked-in syndrome
midbrain infarct and, 170
vs. bilateral pure motor hemiplegia, 144
Locus ceruleus, **43, 58, 61**
superior cerebellar artery supply to, 31
Lupus anticoagulant, small deep infarct and, 131
Lyme disease, small deep infarct and, 132–133

M

Magnetic resonance scan. *See also* White matter hyperintensities
acute presumed lacunar infarct on, 77
axial
through caudal midbrain, **61**
through caudal pons, **64**
through diencephalon, **46**
through internal capsule genu, **48**
through lateral ventricles, **49**
through medulla, **66, 67**
through midpons, **63**
through midthalamus, **47**
through olivary nucleus, **65**
through rostral pons, **62**
contrast-enhanced, small deep infarct on, 77–78, *78*
coronal
through anterior thalamus, **54**
through caudate nucleus, **50**
through cerebellar peduncle, **69**
through cerebral peduncles, **68**
through columns of fornix, **52**
through geniculate bodies, **56**
through internal capsule genu, **53**
through medial lemniscus, **70**
through pulvinar, **57**
through red nucleus, **55**
through septal area, **51**
embolism on, 82–83, *82*
linear subinsular infarct on, 82, *82*
low-flow infarcts on, 79–81, *79, 80*
pathologically proven lacunar infarct on, *74*, 75
postmortem, 83–84
lesion size on, 83–84
noncystic small deep infarcts on, 84
pathologically proven lacunar infarcts on, 75
perivascular demyelination on, 84, *85*
perivascular spaces on, 84–87, *86*
small artery ectasia on, 84
validity of, 83
white matter hyperintensities on, 84, 87–89, 87(t), 88(t)
presumed lacunar infarct on, 76
sagittal
near midline, **43, 58**
through dentate nucleus, **60**
through internal capsule genu, **45**
through lateral pons, **59**
through medial geniculate body, **44**
small deep infarct on, 77
Mancardi, G. L., 8
Marche à petits pas, 181
Marfan's syndrome, small deep infarct and, 134
Marie, Pierre, 2–3, *3*, 5
Marshall, J., 7
Medulla, **57, 70**
anterolateral territory of, arterial supply to, 35
anteromedial territory of, arterial supply to, 34–35
arterial supply to, 34–37
axial MR scan through, **66, 67**
infarct of
clinical features of, 171
sensorimotor stroke and, 148

Medulla (*contd.*)
    lateral territory of, arterial supply to, 35–36
        infarct of, 36
    posterior inferior cerebellar artery supply to, 36–37
    posterior territory of, arterial supply to, 36–37
        infarct of, 37
Meningitis, lacunar infarct and, 127
Microaneurysm, 103, 106
Microatheroma, lacunar infarct and, 125, 126(t), 127
Microcirculation, anatomy of, 94, 98–100, *98*, *99*, *100*, *101*
Midbrain
    accessory collicular artery supply to, 30, *31*
    anterolateral territory of
        arterial supply to, 29, 30
        posteromedial choroidal artery supply to, 28
    anteromedial territory of
        arterial supply to, 23–25, *23*, *25*, *31*
        inferior paramedian mesencephalic artery supply to, 23
        paramedian thalamic artery supply to, *22–25*, 25–26, *27*, *31*
        superior paramedian mesencephalic artery supply to, 24–25
    caudal, MR scan through, **61**
    collicular artery supply to, 30, *31*
    infarct of
        clinical features of, 168–170
        third nerve palsy and, 169–170
        upward gaze palsy and, 169
        vertical gaze palsy and, 169
    lateral territory of, arterial supply to, 30
    posterior territory of, arterial supply to, 30
    superior cerebellar artery supply to, 31–32
Midthalamus, MR scan through, **47**
Migraine, small deep infarct and, 136
Miliary (Charcot-Bouchard) aneurysm, 103, 107
Mohr, J.P., 8
Monoparesis
    brachial, pontine infarct and, 144
    crural, 144
Monoplegia
    brachial
        internal capsule infarct and, 163
        isolated, supratentorial infarct and, 144
    crural, internal capsule infarct and, 163
Moore, M. T., 6
Movement, disorders of, 151–153
    caudate nucleus infarct and, 166
    lacunar syndromes with, 151–153
    lenticular nucleus infarct and, 167
    midbrain infarct and, 169
    pontine infarct and, 171
    thalamic infarct and, 168
Mutism, midbrain infarct and, 170

N

Necrosis, 111–112, 114–115
    fibrinoid, 103
        diabetes and, 107
    production of, 98, 100, *103*
Neglect syndrome, thalamic infarct and, 168

Nerve(s)
    abducens, **64**
    facial, **58**, **64**
        genu of, **43**
    hypoglossal, **65**
    oculomotor, paramedian mesencephalic artery supply to, 24
    sixth, palsy of, pontine infarct and, 170
    third
        intra-axial lesions of, 149
        nuclear syndrome of, lacunar syndromes with, 150
        palsy of, midbrain infarct and, 169–170
    trigeminal, **44**
        posteromedial choroidal artery supply to, 28
        superior cerebellar artery supply to, 31–32
    vagus, **65**
    vestibulocochlear, **64**
Nerve roots, trigeminal, **63**
Neurocysticercosis, small deep infarct and, 132
Neuropsychological disorders
    caudate nucleus infarct and, 165–166
    lenticular nucleus infarct and, 166–167
    thalamic infarct and, 167–168
Nicolesco, I., 5
Normal pressure hydrocephalus, 207
Nuclear oculomotor syndrome, contralateral cerebellar ataxia and, 150, *150*
Nucleus (nuclei)
    abducens, **43**, **58**
        anterior inferior cerebellar artery supply to, 34
        basilar artery supply to, 32
    of abducens nerve, **64**
    accumbens septi, **50**, **51**
    amygdaloid, **53**, **54**, **61**
        anterior choroidal artery supply to, 19
    of Broca, **43**, **58**
    caudate, **44**, **45**, **46**, **47**, **48**, **49**, **50**, **51**, **52**, **53**, **55**, **56**, **57**, **59**, **60**, **68**, **69**, **70**
        coronal MR scan through, **50**
        hemorrhage of, 188
        infarct of, clinical features of, 165–166
        infarct of
            dementia and, 183
            sensorimotor stroke and, 148
        lateral lenticulostriate artery supply to, 18
        recurrent artery of Heubner supply to, 14
    cochlear, **64**
    cuneate, **43**, **58**, **65**, **66**
    of Darkschewitsch, **46**, **56**, **69**
    dentate, **44**, **45**, **59**, **60**, **63**
        sagittal MR scan through, **60**
    emboliform, **63**
    facial, **43**, **58**
        anterior inferior cerebellar artery supply to, 34
    of facial nerve, **64**
    fastigial, **63**
    globose, **43**, **58**, **63**
    hypoglossal, **65**, **66**
    of inferior colliculus, **43**
    interstitial, of Cajal, **46**, **56**, **69**
        superior paramedian mesencephalic artery supply to, 24

lenticular
  hemorrhage of, 188
  infarct of, 166–167
    sensorimotor stroke and, 148
mesencephalic, of trigeminal nerve
  posteromedial choroidal artery supply to, 28
  superior cerebellar artery supply to, 31–32
motor, trigeminal, **63**
oculomotor, **56, 69**
  collicular artery supply to, 30
olfactory, **51**
olivary
  axial MR scan through, 65
  superior, anterior inferior cerebellar artery supply to, 34
pontine, **63**
  pontine artery supply to, 33
  reticular, basilar artery supply to, 32
of posterior commisure, superior paramedian mesencephalic artery supply to, 24
pretectal, posteromedial choroidal artery supply to, 28
pulvinar, **70**
  thalamogeniculate artery supply to, 27
red, **43, 46, 55, 58, 68**
  anterior choroidal artery supply to, 20
  coronal MR scan through, 55
  MLF, superior paramedian mesencephalic artery supply to, 24
septal, **51**
  coronal MR scan through, 51
solitary, **66**
subthalamic, **44, 46, 54, 55, 59, 68**
  anterior choroidal artery supply to, 20
tegmental, dorsal, superior paramedian mesencephalic artery supply to, 24
thalamic
  anterodorsal (anterior), posteromedial choroidal artery supply to, 29
  anteroprincipal (anterior), **43, 48, 53, 54, 58**
    posteromedial choroidal artery supply to, 29
  central (centromedian), **44, 47, 56, 59, 69**
    thalamogeniculate artery supply to, 26
  dorso-oral, thalamotuberal artery supply to, 21
  dorsocaudal (lateral posterior), **44, 45, 48, 55, 57, 59, 60, 68, 69, 70**
    thalamogeniculate artery supply to, 26
  fascicular, **47**
  lateropolar (ventral lateral), **43, 44, 47, 58, 59**
    thalamotuberal artery supply to, 21
  medial (dorsomedial), **43, 47, 48, 54, 55, 56, 58, 68, 69**
    thalamotuberal artery supply to, 21
  median, posteromedial choroidal artery supply to, 29
  parafascicular, **54, 55, 68**
    thalamogeniculate artery supply to, 26
  pulvinar, **57**
  reticular, **53**
    thalamogeniculate artery supply to, 26
    thalamotuberal artery supply to, 21
  superficial, dorsal, (lateral dorsal), **44, 55, 56, 59, 68, 69**

ventro-oral, thalamotuberal artery supply to, 21
ventrocaudal (ventral posterolateral), **44, 45, 47, 55, 56, 59, 60, 68, 69**
  thalamogeniculate artery supply to, 26
ventrolateral (ventral lateral), **58**
trigeminal, **63, 64, 65, 66**
  anterior inferior cerebellar artery supply to, 34
  pontine artery supply to, 33
of trigeminal nerve, 59
vagal, **65**
of vagus nerve, **66**
vestibular, **64**
  anterior inferior cerebellar artery supply to, 34
Nucleus accumbens, **46**
Nucleus ambiguus, **65**
Nucleus basalis of Meynert, **45, 60**
Nucleus gracilis, **65, 66**
Nucleus prepositus hypoglossi, **64**
Nucleus solitarius, **64, 65**
Nystagmus, in ataxic hemiparesis, 145

O

Obersteiner, H., 1
Ocular overshoot, lacunar syndromes with, 151
Ocular tilt reaction, midbrain infarct and, 170
Oculomotor nerve palsy
  contralateral, pure hemiplegia and, 149
  lacunar syndromes with, 149
Olive, inferior, **43, 58**
One-and-a-half syndrome
  horizontal, 150
  pure motor hemiparesis and, 170
  vertical, 151
Ophthalmoplegia, internuclear, 150
  ataxic hemiparesis and, 149
  unilateral, pontine infarct and, 170, 171
Optic chiasm
  anterior communicating artery supply to, 12
  internal carotid artery supply to, 14
Oral contraceptives, small deep infarct and, 136

P

Painful ataxic hemiparesis, 146
Palsy
  abducens nerve, pure hemiplegia and, 149
  down gaze, midbrain infarct and, 169
  facial
    internal capsule infarct and, 163
    ipsilateral, lacunar syndromes with, 151
    lacunar infarct and, 144
    supranuclear, pontine infarct and, 170
  horizontal gaze, pure motor hemiplegia and, 149
  oculomotor, lacunar syndromes with, 149
  pseudobulbar, 181–182
    cortico-subcortical form of, 182
    pontine form of, 182
    striate form of, 182
  sixth nerve
    lacunar syndromes with, 151
    pontine infarct and, 170

Palsy (*contd.*)
  third nerve, midbrain infarct and, 169–170
  upward gaze, midbrain infarct and, 169
  vertical gaze
    lacunar syndromes with, 151
    midbrain infarct and, 169
    thalamic infarct and, 168
  vocal cord, 144
    internal capsule infarct and, 163
Paresis, faciobrachial, internal capsule infarct and, 164
Parkinsonism
  disappearance of
    internal capsule infarct and, 164
    thalamic infarct and, 168
  lacunar syndromes with, 152
  lenticular nucleus infarct and, 167
Peduncle
  cerebellar
    coronal MR scan through, **69**
    inferior, **44**, **63**, **64**, **65**
    middle, **45**, **60**, **62**, **63**
      anterior inferior cerebellar artery supply to, 34
    superior, **43**, **44**, **56**, **57**, **58**, **59**, **61**, **62**, **63**, **69**, **70**
    superior cerebellar artery supply to, 31
  cerebral, **44**, **45**, **46**, **54**, **55**, **59**, **60**, **61**, **68**, **69**
    anterior choroidal artery supply to, 19
    basilar artery supply to, 32
    collicular artery supply to, 30
    coronal MR scan through, **68**
    hemorrhage of, 188
    pedunculo-subthalamic artery supply to, 21
    posteromedial choroidal artery supply to, 28
    pure motor hemiplegia and, 143
    thalamogeniculate artery supply to, 26
    inferior paramedian mesencephalic artery supply to, 23
  thalamic, inferior, **46**, **47**, **52**, **53**
Percheron, artery of, 29
Periarteritis nodosa
  parkinsonian syndrome and, 152
  small deep infarct and, 132
Perivascular space, 1
  dilated, *74*
    in Binswanger's disease, 194
    magnetic resonance of, 84–87, *85*, *86*
    pathogenesis of, 129–131, *130*
      arterial unfolding in, 129–130, *130*
      blood-brain barrier in, 129
      demyelination in, 130–131
      inflammation in, 130
      lytic agent in, 130
    postmortem magnetic resonance of, 85–87, *86*
    vs. small deep infarct, 114
  normal, postmortem magnetic resonance of, 84–85
Pes hippocampi, **54**
Petit foyers pisiformes, 1
Pick, A., 1, 5
Plasma cell dyscrasia, small deep infarct and, 132
Plasma viscosity
  in Binswanger-like white matter low attenuation, 197
  in Binswanger's disease, 204

Plasmatic vascular destruction, 103
Plexus, choroid, posterolateral choroidal artery supply to, 27
Poirier, J., 8
Polyarteritis nodosa, small vessel lesions and, 110
Polycythemia, small deep infarct and, 132
Pons, **55**, **56**, **68**, **69**
  anterior inferior cerebellar artery supply to, 33–34
  anterolateral territory of, arterial supply to, 32, *33*
  anteromedial territory of, arterial supply to, 32, *33*
  arterial supply to, 32–34, *33*
  caudal, axial MR scan through, **64**
  hemorrhage of, 188
  infarct of
    ataxic hemiparesis and, 170
    clinical features of, 170–171
    dysarthria—clumsy hand syndrome and, 170
    magnetic resonance of, 76
    pure motor stroke and, 170
    pure sensory stroke and, 170
    sensorimotor stroke and, 148, 170
  lateral
    arterial supply to, 32–34
    sagittal MR scan through, **59**
    mid-, axial MR scan through, **63**
  posterior territory of, arterial supply of, 34
  pure motor hemiplegia and, 143, *143*
  rostral, axial MR scan through, **62**
  superior cerebellar artery supply to, 34
Porosis, cerebral, 2, *2*
Positron emission tomography
  in pure motor hemiparesis, 77
  white matter hyperintensities on, 202
Posture, abnormalities of, lenticular nucleus infarct and, 167
Preoptic area, **46**
Prineas, J., 7
Probst, M., 2
Proust, A., 1
Pseudobulbar palsy, 181
  cortico-subcortical form of, 182
  pontine form of, 182
  striate form of, 182
  types of, 182
Ptosis, 150
  lacunar syndromes with, 151
  midbrain infarct and, 170
Pulvinar, **47**, **48**, **59**, **60**
  coronal MR scan through, **57**
Pupil, eccentric, midbrain infarct and, 170
Pure motor hemiparesis, 141–144
  atheromatous stenosis in, 126(t), 128
  bilateral, internal capsule infarct and, 163
  incidence of, 141
  lacunar infarct volume in, 76
  nonvascular cause of, 190
  one-and-a-half syndrome and, 170
  onset of, 142
  partial, 143–144
  pontine infarct and, 170
Pure motor hemiplegia, 9, 141–144, *143*
  bilateral, vs. locked-in syndrome, 144

capsulolenticular infarct and, 142–143
cerebral blood flow in, 184
clinical outcome of, 142
diagnosis of, 142
horizontal gaze palsy and, 149
horizontal one-and-a-half syndrome and, 149
Pure motor quadriparesis, medullary infarct and, 171
Pure motor quadriplegia, 144
  medullary infarct and, 144
Pure motor stroke, 143–144
  bilateral, 144
  corona radiata infarct and, 162
  internal capsule infarct and, 163–164
  intracerebral hemorrhage and, 187–188
  medullary infarct and, 171
  midbrain infarct and, 168
  partial, 143–144
  pontine infarct and, 170
  thalamic infarct and, 167
Pure paresthetic stroke, 147
Pure sensory deficit, nonvascular cause of, 190
Pure sensory stroke, 147, *148*
  corona radiata infarct and, 162
  internal capsule infarct and, 164
  intracerebral hemorrhage and, 189, *189*
  lacunar infarct volume in, 76
  pontine infarct and, 170
  thalamic infarct and, 167
Putamen, **44, 45, 46, 47, 48, 50, 51, 52, 53, 54, 55, 56, 59, 60, 68, 69**
  hemorrhage of, 188, *188*
  infarct of
    clinical features of, 166–167
    low-flow, 79–81
    postmortem magnetic resonance of, 75(t)
  lateral lenticulostriate artery supply to, 18
  medial lenticulostriate artery supply to, 17
  recurrent artery of Heubner supply to, 14

Q

Quadriparesis, motor, pure, medullary infarct and, 171

R

Rims, of white matter hyperintensities, 87, 87(t)
Ripping, L. H., 1
Rueling, R., 2

S

Sectoranopia, homonymous, 165
  internal capsule infarct and, 165
Segmental arterial disorganization, 7, 102. *See also* Lipohyalinosis
Sensorimotor stroke, 147–148
  classification of, 148
  corona radiata infarct and, 162
  internal capsule infarct and, 164
  intracerebral hemorrhage and, 189, *189*
  lacunar infarct volume in, 76
  nonvascular cause of, 190
  pontine infarct and, 170
  thalamic infarct and, 167
Septum pellucidum, anterior communicating artery supply to, 12

Sex, lacunar infarct risk and, 217
Sheath, perivascular, inflammation of, 130
Sickle cell trait, white matter infarcts and, 128
Sixth nerve palsy
  lacunar syndromes with, 151
  pontine infarct and, 170, 171
Skew deviation, 150
  lacunar syndromes with, 151
Small artery ectasia, postmortem magnetic resonance of, 84
Small deep infarct(s)
  acute, magnetic resonance of, 77
  in Binswanger-like white matter low attenuation, 197, *197*
  computed tomography of, 75
    enhanced, 77
    volume change and, 76–77
  curative effects of, 152–153
  definition of, 73
  diabetes and, 107
  hypertension and, 100, 103, 105, 107, *106, 108*
  magnetic resonance of, 76
    enhanced, 77–78, *78*
    volume change and, 76–77
  measurement of, 88–89
    methods of, 89
  noncystic, postmortem magnetic resonance of, 84
  pathogenesis of, 131–136
    arteritis in, 132
    artery-to-artery embolism in, 133–134
    atrial fibrillation in, 133
    cardiogenic embolism in, 133
    coagulopathies in, 131–132
    cocaine abuse in, 136
    hypoperfusion in, 134–135
    imaging characteristics and, 78–83, *79, 80, 81, 82*
    infection in, 132–133
    lacunar transient ischemic attacks in, 135–136
    large artery disease in, 131
    migraine in, 136
    oral contraceptives in, 136
  volume changes in, 76–77
    imaging characteristics of, 76–77
  vs. lacunes, 73, 111, 114, 115, *112–113*
Somatosensory evoked responses, in pure motor stroke, 142
Spasm, hemifacial, pontine infarct and, 170, 171
Spinothalamic tract, posteromedial choroidal artery supply to, 28
Stenosis, atheromatous, 94
  lacunar infarct and, 125–126, 127–128, 136
Stria medullaris, **53**
Striatum, anterior, recurrent artery of Heubner supply to, 14
Stroke. *See* Pure motor stroke; Pure sensory stroke; Sensorimotor stroke
Stuttering, internal capsule infarct and, 165
Subcallosal area, **51**
Subcortical arteriosclerotic encephalopathy. *See* Binswanger's disease
Substantia innominata, **45, 53, 60**

Substantia nigra, **43, 44, 46, 54, 55, 56, 58, 59, 61, 68, 69**
    anterior choroidal artery supply to, 19
    inferior paramedian mesencephalic artery supply to, 23
    posteromedial choroidal artery supply to, 28
Supranuclear bulbar palsy, 181–182
Supranuclear facial palsy, pontine infarct and, 170
Syndrome
    anticardiolipin, 111
    antiphospholipid antibody, small deep infarct and, 131
    Benedikt's, 150, 170
    capsular genu, internal capsule infarct and, 165
    cheiro-oral, 147, 148, 167, 189, *189*, 190
    Claude's, 150, *150*, 170
        contralateral cerebellar ataxia and, 150, *150*
    Cogan's, small deep infarct and, 132
    dysarthria—clumsy hand, 146
        corona radiata infarct and, 162
        intracerebral hemorrhage and, 188–189, *188*
        pontine infarct and, 170
    Foix-Chavany, 182
    hemialgic, 147
    hemolytic-uremic, small deep infarct and, 131–132
    horizontal one-and-a-half, pure motor hemiplegia and, 149
    Horner's, 150
        thalamic infarct and, 168
    Landry's, pontine infarct and, 170
    locked-in
        midbrain infarct and, 170
        vs. bilateral pure motor hemiplegia, 144
    Marfan's, small deep infarct and, 134
    neglect, thalamic infarct and, 168
    nuclear, of third nerve, lacunar syndromes with, 150
    one-and-a-half
        horizontal, 150
        vertical, 151
    opercular, anterior, 182
    pseudobulbar palsy, 181
    top of the basilar, 153
    Weber's, 149, 170
Syphilis
    pure motor hemiparesis and, 190
    small deep infarct and, 132
Systemic lupus erythematosus, 205–207
    small deep infarct and, 131
    small vessel lesions and, 110–111

T
Tegmentum
    midbrain, anterior choroidal artery supply to, 19
    pontine
        basilar artery supply to, 32
        pontine artery supply to, 33
Temporal lobe
    anterior choroidal artery supply to, 19
    posterolateral choroidal artery supply to, 26
Tetraparesis, ataxic, 146
Tetraplegia, midbrain infarct and, 170
Thalamotomy, stereotactic, cheiro-oral sensory loss and, 190
Thalamus
    anterior
        coronal MR scan through, **54**
        internal carotid artery supply to, 14
    anterior choroidal artery supply to, 20
    hemorrhage of, 188, 189
    hypothalamic artery supply to, 21
    infarct of, 75
        aphasia and, 168
        ataxic hemiparesis and, 167
        behavioral change and, 168
        clinical features of, 167–168
        dementia and, 183–184
        language function and, 153
        magnetic resonance of, 76, 77–78, *78*
        movement disorders and, 168
        neuropsychological features of, 167–168
        pure sensory stroke and, 167
        sensorimotor stroke and, 167
    paramedian thalamic artery supply to, 25–26, *22, 24, 26*
    pedunculo-subthalamic artery supply to, 21
    posterior communicating artery supply to, 21, *22*
    posterolateral choroidal artery supply to, 27, *28*
    posteromedial choroidal artery supply to, 28, 29, *28*
    thalamotuberal artery supply to, 21, 22
Third nerve
    intra-axial lesions of, 149
    nuclear syndrome of, lacunar syndromes with, 150
    palsy of, 150
        midbrain infarct and, 169–170
Thrombocythemia, small deep infarct and, 132
Tongue, deviation of, in ataxic hemiparesis, 145
Tonsil, cerebellar, **66**
Top of the basilar syndrome, 153
Tortuosity, arterial, 107, *108*
Tract
    corticospinal, **67**
        basilar artery supply to, 32
        pontine artery supply to, 33
    mamillothalamic, **43, 46, 47, 54, 58**
        thalamotuberal artery supply to, 21
    optic, **43, 53, 54, 55, 58, 68**
        anterior choroidal artery supply to, 19
        hypothalamic artery supply to, 21
        internal carotid artery supply to, 14
    prerubral. *See* Fields of Forel
    pyramidal, **62, 63, 64, 65, 66, 67**
    spinocerebellar, **63, 64, 66, 67**
    spinothalamic, **65, 67**
        superior cerebellar artery supply to, 31
    tegmental, central, **43, 46, 56, 57, 58, 61, 62, 63, 64, 69, 70**
        anterior inferior cerebellar artery supply to, 34
        superior cerebellar artery supply to, 32
    trigeminal, spinal, **44, 59, 64, 65, 66, 67**
    trigeminothalamic, **65**

Transient ischemic attack
  lacunar, 135–136
  lacunar infarct risk and, 220, 220(t)
  prodromal, 142, 147
Tremor
  essential, cure of, internal capsule infarct and, 165
  thalamic infarct and, 168
Trigone
  olfactory, recurrent artery of Heubner supply to, 13, 14
Tuberculoma, ataxic hemiparesis and, 190
Tuberculosis, small deep infarct and, 133
Tuberothalamic artery syndrome, unilateral, 153

U

Uncus, 61
  anterior choroidal artery supply to, 19
  hippocampal artery supply to, 29
  internal carotid artery supply to, 14
Unfolding, arterial, 7, 107
  dilated perivascular spaces and, 129–130, *130*
Upward gaze palsy, midbrain infarct and, 169
Urinary incontinence, in Binswanger-like white matter low attenuation, 197

V

Vaginalite destructive, 3, 4, 5
  dilated perivascular spaces and, 130
Vander Eecken, H., 7
Varicella, childhood, small deep infarct and, 133
Vasculitis
  drug abuse and, 111
  small deep infarct and, 132, 133
  small vessel lesions and, 110
Vasospasm
  cerebral ischemia and, 128–129
  monocular blindness and, 128
Vassale, G., 2
Ventricles, lateral, axial MR scan through, **49**
Ventriculomegaly, white matter hyperintensities and, 199, 202, 207
Ventrolateral formation, **43, 44, 48, 54, 58, 59**
Vertical gaze palsy
  lacunar syndromes with, 151
  midbrain infarct and, 169
  thalamic infarct and, 168
Vertical one-and-a-half syndrome, 151
Virchow-Robin space. *See* Perivascular space
Viscosity, plasma
  in Binswanger-like white matter low attenuation, 197
  in Binswanger's disease, 204
Vocal cord palsy, 144
  internal capsule infarct and, 163
Vogt, C., 5, 130
Vogt, O., 5, 130

W

Weber's syndrome, 170
White matter
  demyelination of, 193–194. *See also* Binswanger's disease
  infarct of, 128
    hypoperfusion and, 134
    postmortem magnetic resonance of, 75, 84
White matter hyperintensities
  Binswanger-like, 195–198, *197*
    clinical findings in, 196–197
    incidence of, 196
    investigations of, 197–198, *197*
  caps of, 87, 87(t)
  cerebral blood flow and, 202
  confluent, 88, 88(t)
  differential diagnosis of, 87–89, 87(t), 88(t)
  focal, 86, *86*, 87–88, 88(t)
  heterogeneity of, on magnetic resonance, 198
  incidence of, on magnetic resonance, 198
  infarcts and, 84
  magnetic resonance of, 84–89, *85, 86, 87*, 87(t), 88(t), 198–202, *199*
  pathological correlations with, *199, 200*, 201–202, 202–203
  pathology of
    computed tomography and, 202–203
    magnetic resonance and, *199, 200*, 201–202, 202–203
  perivascular demyelination and, 84–85, *85*
  perivascular space dilation and, 85–87, *86*
  postmortem magnetic resonance of, 84
  rims of, 87, 87(t)
  small artery ectasia and, 84
White matter low attenuation
  Binswanger-like, 195–198, *197*
    in Alzheimer's disease, 204–205
    in amyloid angiopathy, 205
    clinical findings in, 196–197
    in hypertensive encephalopathy, 207–208
    incidence of, 196
    investigations in, 197–198, *197*
    in leukoencephalopathy, 205
    in normal pressure hydrocephalus, 207
    in vascular dementia, 205–207
  giant perivascular space and, 87
  pathological correlation of, 202–203
  stroke risk and, 197

Y

Yates, P., 7

Z

Zona incerta, **43, 44, 54, 55, 58, 59, 68**
  anterior choroidal artery supply to, 20
  pedunculo-subthalamic artery supply to, 21
  thalamogeniculate artery supply to, 26